MW00846035

Atlas of Chinese Tongue Diagnosis

SECOND EDITION

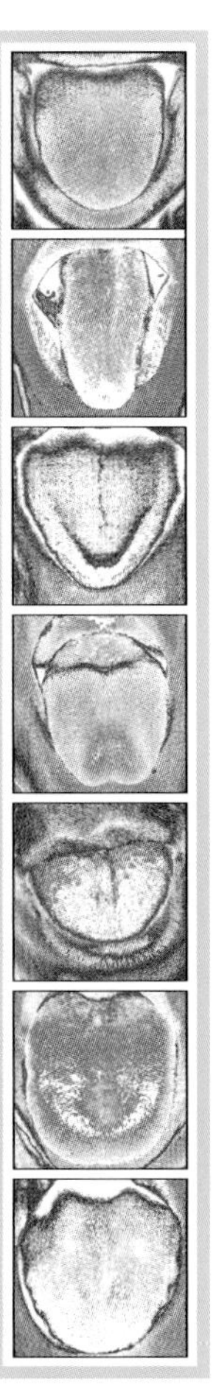

Atlas of Chinese Tongue Diagnosis

Second Edition

Barbara Kirschbaum

Foreword by
Dominique Hertzer

Eastland Press
SEATTLE

Portions of this work were originally published in German
by Verlag für Ganzheitliche Medizin Dr. Erich Wühr GmbH as
Atlas und Lehrbuch der Chinesischen Zungendiagnostik (1998) and
Atlas und Lehrbuch der Chinesischen Zungendiagnostik, Band 2 (2002), and
in English by Eastland Press as *Atlas of Chinese Tongue Diagnosis*, Vol. 1 (2000)
and *Atlas of Chinese Tongue Diagnosis*, Vol. 2 (2003).

Eastland Press, Inc.
P.O. Box 99749
Seattle, WA 98139, USA
www.eastlandpress.com

Library of Congress Control Number: 2010930524
ISBN: 978-0-939616-71-8
Printed in Korea

4 6 8 10 9 7 5 3

English translation by Barbara Kirschbaum

Book design by Gary Niemeier

TABLE OF CONTENTS

CHAPTER 2 Pale Tongue Signs

CHAPTER 3 Tongue Signs Associated with Kidney Disharmonies

CHAPTER 4 Tongue Signs Associated with Stomach Disharmonies

CHAPTER 5 Tongue Signs Associated with Lung Disharmonies

CHAPTER 6 Tongue Signs Associated with Heart Disharmonies

A C K N O W L E D G E M E N T S

WHEN, IN THE 1980s, the excellent book *Tongue Diagnosis in Chinese Medicine* by Giovanni Maciocia appeared, it awakened my interest in this art. For the structured conveyance of his knowledge, I wish to thank him. Thanks also to my first teacher, J. D. van Buren, who taught me the art of observation; Ted Kaptchuk, who introduced me to Chinese herbalism; and Dr. Huang Yun-Rui, of the Chengdu University of Traditional Chinese Medicine, who taught me the practice of Chinese medicine.

To those collegues and friends who gave me the courage and support to write this book, my hearty thanks. A very special thanks to Jeni Barnet for her help with the English edition, and her continuing friendship. Thanks to Dr. Dominique Hertzer for her constructive support, which was also expressed in her excellent Foreword. I am indebted to my students and patients, as this tongue book could not have been realized without them.

Finally, a very special thanks to Walter Geiger. Not only did he permit me to use tongue photographs of some of his patients, but he also contributed with his helpful observations and criticisms to the completion of this book.

Any mistakes in the book are entirely my own.

FOREWORD

ACCORDING TO CHINESE sources the first time 舌 *(shé)*, the Chinese character for tongue, appeared was as an inscription on oracle bones. Even in this ancient context it revealed a great deal about the importance of the tongue.

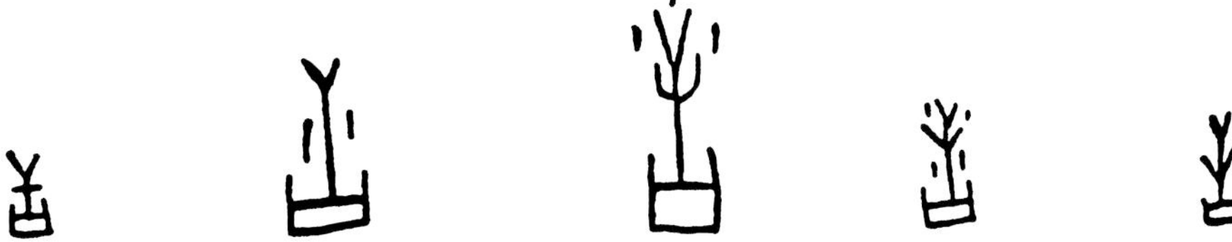

The original representation shows a bell with a wooden clapper, which appears to be moving to and fro. The body of the bell, which is placed upside-down, forms the upper part of the picture, while the lower part of the picture shows a clapper, which sticks out like a protruding tongue.[1]

It is interesting to note that the original symbol for tongue, inscribed on the bones, matches the style of writing of two other characters; thus, several words with different meanings are united in the characters. Unlike modern Chinese, which utilizes many different independent characters, ancient Chinese used only one character which, out of necessity, needed to express many things.

The development of the Chinese language and its writing can be clearly marked. For instance the word *shé* is also used to mean *gào,* 'to communicate with,' while *yán,* the Chinese word meaning 'to talk' or 'to speak words,' also means 'a bell with a wooden clapper.' This meaning emanates from the oldest of traditions when the eldest of the clan wanted to communicate with his people. Because he first had to ring a bell to gather them together, the 'ringing of the bell' was a sign of forthcoming 'communication.' This connection can be found in the oldest Chinese dictionary, the *Shuo wen jie zi*:

> *Shé* [the tongue] is that with which one talks in the mouth as well as differentiating taste.[2]

As the essential function of the tongue is spoken communication, the character *shé* was already used in many classical texts to mean 'to talk' and 'to communicate.'

In one of the chapters from the *Lun yu,* Confucius in conversation with his pupils discussed the following question:

> "How is the superior man able to observe and maintain forms and rituals when he occupies himself, because of his being, with essential things?"
>
> Ji-Cheng said: "The superior man is concerned with the essence, why is it necessary for him to bother with the forms?"
>
> Zi-Gong replied: "Your understanding of the superior man is truly regretful. A four-in-hand cannot catch up with [the speed of your] tongue."[3]

Zi-Gong, a favorite pupil of Confucius, regretted the thoughtless words uttered by Ji-Cheng, where the character 舌 *(shé)* was obviously used to mean 'verbal expression.'

The application of the character *shé* along with further associations are found in the *Yi jing*, namely in the commentaries on the trigrams where the symbolic meaning of the eight trigrams is discussed.[4]

Here the tongue is assigned to the trigram *duì,* where a yin line is positioned above two yang lines. While this represents 'a lake,' it is also an essential characteristic of 'the merry' or 'the joyous.' The commentary notes:

> The joyous is the lake, it is the youngest daughter, it is the magician, it is the mouth and the tongue. It is the undoing and the destruction. With regard to the earth it means hardness and saltiness. With regard to his seraglio, it is the second woman, not the first. It is the sheep.[5]

Here the 'tongue' appears in the context of speaking and communicating. For example, it is a distinctive mark of the magician to give her words and abilities a special meaning and power. If we look more closely at the fundamental quality of the trigram *duì* in relation to the 'the joyous,' we find, in the context of Chinese medicine, a unison of qualities which represents the essential qualities of the Heart. The 'talking tongue' is the off-shoot of the Heart, and the Heart's body opening is the mouth. While its vocal manifestation is laughter, its emotional expression is joy.

So in every sense of the word, both literally and metaphorically, the tongue has the power of expression.

On one hand the tongue, as an organ, enables us to communicate with our environment through language. It is through the tongue that thoughts and emotions are brought from the inside to the outside; it is the connecting link between our inner and outer worlds. On the other hand, in the context of Chinese medicine, the tongue is a diagnostic tool. By using tongue diagnosis, an experienced practitioner can judge the exterior flow of energy in the yin organs and the interior flow of energy in the yang organs. The tongue, therefore, connects the 'inside' and the 'outside' of a person.

The first person who is said to have applied tongue diagnosis is Bian Que,[6] one of the most renowned doctors in pre-Han China. He practiced during the Warring States period (471-221 B.C.). Before becoming a physician he worked in a boarding house in the ancient state of Cheng, which today is the province of Hebei. One of his customers was a great physician, Chang Sang-Jun, who traveled incognito, and legend has it that Bian Que became his pupil, having followed a prescription given to him by Chang.[7]

Bian Que took the medicine for 30 consecutive days, after which, it is said, he had the ability to see the 'insides' of people. Bian Que then received all of Chang's prescriptions and studied all of his books. Using this knowledge he traveled around from state to state practicing successfully as a doctor in many different areas of medicine, from gynecology to pediatrics to illnesses of the ear, nose, and throat. Bian Que didn't limit himself to tongue diagnosis; it was said that he was very proficient in the use of herbs and acupuncture, and was highly knowledgeable in pulse diagnosis. His fame, however, was not solely attributable to his enormous abilities as a doctor. Against a background of competing arguments concerning the history of ideas led by different philosophical schools such as Daoism, Confucianism, Mohism and Naturalism, Bian Que's work and abilities represented a changing view of society, namely, from a religious to a rational conception of the world.

Bian Que fought for a medicine whose success was not based on shamanistic techniques, as had been the case in the Shang (1766–1122 B.C.) and early Zhou (1122–221 B.C.) eras. In the so-called 'demon medicine' of that time, where the causes of illness were attributed to evil demons,[8,9] treatment was aimed at expelling demonic spirits. Success or failure was, as a rule, inexplicable.

At the time of the Warring States, new philosophical ideas and the move toward rational thinking was reflected in a changing theoretical understanding as well as in the practical application of medicine. It was at this time that Bian Que introduced an objective and comprehensive method of diagnosis using the tongue and the pulse. If properly studied, anyone, not just a few shamans, could observe and describe the quality of an illness by using these methods. Bian Que demonstrated that through tongue and pulse diagnosis it was possible to gain insight into the present condition of a patient, as well as review their past and predict future developments.

Thus, the observation of the tongue—its shape, color, and consistency—became one of the most important aspects of Chinese medicine. By observing the patient closely, and utilizing the senses of sight, sound, smell, and touch, one could reach a comprehensive description of the whole person.

The first differentiated and concrete statements concerning the significance of the tongue coating and its body are found in the *Nei jing:* "When the evil qi penetrates the lesser yang channel of the hand, this will cause a blockage in the neck, the tongue curls upward, the mouth is dry, and the Heart is restless."

This is a commonly cited passage about tongue diagnosis, as it reflects not only the connection of the Triple Burner channel to the tongue, but also a pathology that appears in connection with pathogenic heat.

The next passage describes the long and soft tongue: "If the tongue is long and protrudes, and is without strength, and if the patient is frightful, choose the lesser yin channel of the foot."

Here the long tongue is also defined as soft, and when it is retracted it gives the appearance of being without strength. This is a description of Kidney yin deficiency, and the illness would be treated via the Kidney channel.

The effects of pathogenic heat on the five yin organs are discussed in Ch. 32 of the *Su wen*.

Discussing the effects of heat on the Lung, the tongue coating is described as follows:

> "If the patient has fallen sick from heat in the Lung, he will have chills at first. The smallest hairs are raised and he will dislike wind and cold. The tongue coating is yellow and the body is hot." [10]
>
> "The Lung channel begins in the middle burner, has a connection to the Large Intestine, and encircles the Stomach as well as the mouth. When heat is present in the Lungs, it penetrates to the Stomach and from there ascends; the tongue coating will be yellow and the body will be hot." [11]

Even if these historical passages do not give a clearly systematized and specific description of tongue diagnosis, we still find in the *Nei jing* important statements about the essential elements of tongue diagnosis, that is, the shape and coating of the tongue.

In the framework of the general development of diagnosis and treatment strategies, we find in many classical works of Chinese medicine, over a thousand year period, more and more specific observations in relation to tongue diagnosis.

The first text to deal exclusively with tongue diagnosis dates from 1341 during the Yuan (Mongol) dynasty. This was published by Du Qing-Bo. His work, entitled *Ao shi shang han jin jing lu*, is based upon a textbook of tongue diagnosis from an otherwise unknown man named Ao. This book contains 12 color illustrations with descriptions of the tongue body and coating. Du Qing-Bo added another 24 illustrations and assigned to the different tongues their corresponding patterns and pulses.[12]

Unfortunately, the illustrations did not survive, but the tradition of pictorial illustration of the tongue coatings and shapes continued. In a work entitled *Kou chi lei yao*, illustrations of different tongues were not only assigned corresponding patterns, but a corresponding prescription as well. The following drawings are samples drawn from this work:[13]

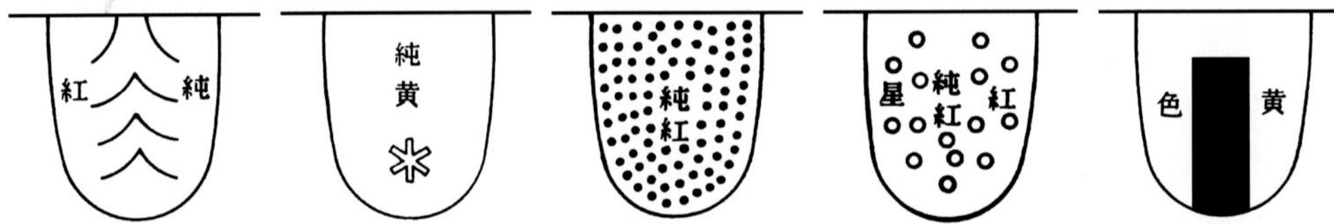

These illustrations, with their descriptions, clearly show the development of Chinese medicine in its quest toward more refined and specific diagnostic techniques, with corresponding treatment strategies, and its application of existing knowledge to examine and integrate new findings. Against this background it was only a matter of time before the Chinese absorbed Western medicine into their culture to work alongside Chinese medicine. Western medicine has been adopted in China in part because of a common belief that it is superior to Chinese medicine but also because it is thought to enrich Chinese medicine, rather than competing with it. In Chinese medicine, as in many other areas of Chinese thinking, the question is never 'either/or' but 'as well.'

Barbara Kirschbaum stands firmly in this tradition with her *Atlas of Chinese Tongue Diagnosis*. According to official sources, many diseases like skin complaints, chronic fatigue syndrome, and AIDS are more common in the West than in China, and as such have not been described, in detail, in the Chinese literature. Here, Barbara Kirschbaum integrates, within the parameters of Chinese medical diagnosis, her own insights, and provides examples of many new, or typically Western, illnesses. This is done without losing the essential characteristics of Chinese medicine: precise observation and clear diagnosis. Beginning with the diagnosis of individual organs, tongue signs with their corresponding patterns are clearly explained, and documentation of their pathogenesis, from mild to severe cases, are set forth in detailed case histories.

This *Atlas* is both a reference book and a useful study guide for diagnosis, both for the beginner as well as the advanced practitioner. It will be of invaluable help in daily clinical practice.

The quality of the tongue photographs, together with their precise descriptions, are unique in the Western literature on Chinese medicine, and, from own my research, in the native Chinese literature as well. I hope this book will set a new standard for Chinese medical publications and contribute to the wider circulation and recognition that it truly deserves.

—Dominique Hertzer, M.D.

Endnotes

1 Compare the representation and meaning of *shé* on the oracle bones inscription with Xu Z, ed. *Jia gu wen ci dian.* Chengdu: Sichuan Provincial Publishing House, 1990:208.

2 *Zhong zheng xin yin yi cong he da ci dian.* Taipei: Zhongzheng shuju, 1990:1436

3 *Lun yu, "Yan yuan"* 12/.8 in *Xin yi si shu du ben.* Taipei: Sanmin shuju, 1985: 161.

4 For the symbolic meaning of the trigrams, see Hertzer D. "Das alte und neue Yijing. Die Wandlunges des Buches der Wandlungen." *Diederichs Gelbe Reihe* 126, S. 137-143, München, 1996.

5 *Zhou yi yin de: Concordance to Yijing.* Taipei: Harvard Yenching Institute Sinological Index Series, 1966:52.

6 Li J-W, et. al. *Zhong yi da ci dian.* Beijing: Peoples Medical Publishing House, 1995:1178.

7 Chuang Y. *Historical Review of the Development of Chinese Acupuncture.* Taipei, 1978:47-49.

8 Unschuld P. *Medizin in China.* Munich: Eine Ideengeschichte, beck, 1980:28-48.

9 Guo A-C, ed. *Huang di nei jing su wen xiao zhu.* Beijing: Peoples Medical Publishing House, 1995:769.

10 Ibid., 428

11 Ibid.

12 Ding F-B. *Zhong guo li dai yi yao shu mu.* Taipei: Nan tian shu ju, 1979:378.

13 Chen M-L, et al. *Gu jin tu shu ji cheng yi bu quan lu.* Beijing: Peoples Medical Publishing House, 1995; 5(2):80-85.

INTRODUCTION (SECOND EDITION)

1.1 The Importance of Tongue Diagnosis in Clinical Practice

This new edition of *Atlas of Chinese Tongue Diagnosis* combines, and to some extent reconfigures, the content of the two volumes in the original edition of this work into one new volume. The many photographs in the first volume of different tongue shapes, colors, and coatings that are commonly seen in the clinic have been combined with a number of case histories from the second volume. The sequence of the tongue photographs within a chapter shows the increasing degree of imbalance among the body's energies. The book seeks to enhance awareness of the importance of tongue diagnosis in assessing the energetic condition of the patient.

In each chapter, detailed case histories are presented in order to facilitate the step from theory to practice. By analyzing several different case histories related to a particular organ system, the diagnostic procedures and treatment strategies become clearer. The cases serve to illustrate the integration of the tongue signs, symptoms, and other clinical findings in the process of diagnosis and defining an appropriate treatment.

I have added a few photographs that are particularly good examples of a specific tongue color or tongue sign. At the same time, some of the case histories in the original edition have been removed to enhance the readability of the book and thus make it more useful as a reference book for tongues. During the last ten years I have personally arrived at the conclusion that the overall appearance of the tongue, especially the tongue body shape and color, are of greater significance than a single crack or a distinctive marking on the tongue. This understanding is reflected in this new edition.

The analysis of the case histories in this volume, and especially the evaluation of certain signs and symptoms, reflects thirty years of clinical practice. In many respects, my approach to treatment, especially the application of Chinese herbal medicine, changed and became clearer as a result of the training I received at various hospitals in Tianjin, Chengdu, and Kunming. I encountered many physicians who took pride in their years of experience, reputation, and individual styles of treatment. Physicians, especially those with decades of experience, impressed on me the need to read and study the classics and to learn classical prescriptions by heart in order to really understand their functions and workings. A few Western practitioners of Chinese medicine also influenced my style of practice in certain areas, for example, Steve Clavey in gynecology and Mazin Al-Khafaji in dermatology. Finally, besides the work with my patients, it was the feedback as well as the problems my students encountered in clinical practice that forced me to become clearer in my own work.

The case histories here reflect these various influences. Based on my experience, I believe in the importance of a discussion that clearly narrates the steps used to formulate treatment strategies and that allows practitioners to share their findings. I have found that this process increases and improves the awareness of the participants by helping them synthesize all the signs and symptoms while incorporating the 'nature' of the patient in the formulation.

Practicing Chinese medicine for three decades has inevitably changed my understanding of illness and how I treat it. My experience has been shaped by many successes as well as failures. I have observed that even after a course of treatment, a patient may be free of pain but still feel unwell; there remains an inner tension, a sense of restlessness, or an inner emptiness. In stark contrast, symptoms associated with a chronic illness may linger, but the patient suddenly feels that he, or she, can endure the ensuing problems and even feel better. I have come to the conclusion that the underlying constitution of a patient, their vitality, and the harmony of their spirit, must not be ignored; all of these factors contribute to the healing process and help shape the treatment. With regard to tongue diagnosis in particular, I am convinced that the color and shape of the tongue body are of greater importance than a single crack, a slight swelling, etc.

1.2 Tongue Diagnosis and the Patient's Constitution

In cases of chronic disease, tongue diagnosis helps enormously in discerning the underlying constitution[1] of the patient in relation to the condition of the blood, qi, yin, and yang. The constitutional strength of a patient will contribute to the progression of a disease and may allow a prognosis for the healing process. Having specialized in the treatment of cancer, I have found, for example, that the effect of chemotherapeutic drugs on the body's energies and therefore on the tongue color and coating are drastic, yet at the same time most instructive for the practitioner of Chinese medicine. The majority of those drugs have a hot nature that injures the blood and yin. In contrast to the normal progression of illness and its subsequent reflection on the tongue, here the changes occur within days or weeks. Because most patients with the same cancer, say an estrogen positive tumor, receive basically the same chemical agents, it is the constitution of the particular woman that determines how she will cope with the treatment. Here, the tongue color and coating prior to chemotherapy may give an indication about the tolerance of this treatment and be very helpful in providing the patient with specific advice based upon her constitution. In my experience, the pulse qualities also change based upon a particular treatment, but they seem not to differ much from person to person.

A strong constitution does not automatically guarantee a long life. Its quality does, however, influence a person's ability to cope with physical or mental illness and with other threatening situations. The constitution encompasses an individual's charisma and physique as well as more medical qualities, such as susceptibility to illness and infectious disease and the course taken by these maladies, including the healing process.

The *Divine Pivot* devotes several chapters to the subject of the human constitution. A passage in Chapter 6 states that the build of the body, the strength of the muscles, the elasticity of the skin, and the quality of the pulse make up the constitution of an individual.[2] In Chapter 72, five different types of people are analyzed with respect to their character, individual attributes, and constitution. For example, a person in whom the yin and yang are balanced is presented as quietly self-confident,[3] and a person in whom the power of yin is dominant may exhibit a relaxed and reflective manner. Those who have this type of constitution often prefer calm activities, like reading, as opposed to physical activities, and their tongue bodies will be pale and swollen.[4] Those in whom the power of yang is dominant often have an urge to move physically. A dominance of yang, with a tongue body that is often reddish or unusually long,[5] can lead to headaches or inner restlessness. If someone with this constitution suffers from blazing Heart fire, denoted by a deep red tip of the tongue, he may present with inner restlessness and irritability. On the other hand, if the individual has a yin constitution and a red tongue tip, while the body of the tongue is pale and swollen, then the injury from Heart fire will not be as severe. Thus it is possible to deduce a person's disposition by referring to the tongue body color and shape, and this evidence can then be used to evaluate the course or outcome of an illness and to provide prophylactic action to strengthen a particular constitution or conserve the balance of energies. For this reason, the constitution is frequently mentioned in the case histories.

1.3 Tongue Signs as Aspects of an Energetic Whole

One purpose of this book is to dispel dogmatic thinking about the interpretation of tongue signs, an approach that is inappropriate in Chinese medicine. For example, a red tongue does not automatically indicate Kidney yin deficiency, nor does a rootless coating always imply Stomach or Kidney yin deficiency, any more than hot feet always denote Kidney yin deficiency. It should therefore be apparent that, in Chinese medicine, one sign or symptom is not enough to establish a diagnosis or treatment strategy. The relationship among the vitality, nature, and emotional background of the patient, as well as the various signs and symptoms, must all be considered as a whole. The tongue signs are but one element of the diagnosis in that they often reflect the contours of the energetic structure of the body.

Most of the case histories in this book, especially those involving chronic and/or serious illnesses, clearly demonstrate that many different patterns can appear simultaneously. These patterns influence the pathology in varying degrees. Clinical practice shows that a 'pure' pattern rarely exists. For example, it is unusual for a patient to suffer from a pattern of Spleen qi deficiency alone. Rather, it is more likely that they will also have, for example, Heart blood deficiency and an accumulation of heat toxin, both of which may play an important role in the patient's illness. Evaluating diverse disease mechanisms often poses a challenge for the practitioner, and it is here that tongue diagnosis becomes an important aid in reaching a more precise diagnosis. Thus an additional purpose of presenting the case histories is to show the various facets of the overall pathomechanism and to demonstrate the different layers of the disease process.

It is noteworthy that during an acute illness, the localization, color, and consistency of the tongue coating is more significant than the color and shape of the tongue body. These findings are especially important when an externally-contracted pathogenic factor is responsible for the illness, an issue that is discussed at greater length in Ch. 9.

Each case history includes a diagram that identifies the proposed patterns of disharmony that have contributed to the energetic imbalance, that is, the overall pathomechanism. The diagrams show the individual patterns of disharmony—with the dominant pattern or patterns clearly demarcated in bold type—and their interrelationships. This is followed by an analysis of the primary disease-inducing mechanisms, which explores their relationship to the findings on the tongue.

Several case histories are included here where a patient's progress could not be followed after the initial treatment, or where the patient declined to continue treatment. There are also examples of patients whose complaints have not been treated successfully, which, of course, is part of everyday life in the clinic, but I have chosen to include these histories because of remarkable tongue signs or unusual pathomechanisms.

In the treatment strategy section of the case histories, Chinese herbal prescriptions and combinations of acupuncture points are mentioned in order to show the actual steps that were taken to deal with the pathomechanism. Because they are not included for instructional purposes in the practice of Chinese pharmacology or acupuncture, they are not explained in much detail.

1.4 The Limitations of Tongue Diagnosis

It must be emphasized that tongue diagnosis represents just one of the diagnostic techniques in Chinese medicine. Occasionally, findings based on tongue diagnosis have less meaning than other signs. This is also true of pathologies originating from an accumulation of phlegm, the presence of which is sometimes difficult to detect by tongue diagnosis. In this case, pulse diagnosis is often more accurate. Occasionally, the tongue bears signs of injury to the yin or fluids from a previous illness, but these signs do not play an important role in the new or acute illness.

In addition, tongue diagnosis cannot be used to identify the specific location of damp-heat in the lower burner. The posterior third of the tongue reflects the energetic state of the lower burner, which includes the Kidneys, Bladder, and Small and Large Intestines. A yellow, thick coating on the posterior third of the tongue reflects damp-heat in one or more of these organs. The coating denotes the strength and quality of the existing damp-heat. However, its precise location can only be determined from the symptoms. Pulse diagnosis, in this case, is much more accurate since the individual pulse positions will reflect the state of each of the above-mentioned organs.

Nor is the gravity of an illness always discernible on the tongue. The frequently asked question about why seriously ill people can have a 'good' tongue or seemingly healthy people can have a 'bad' tongue cannot always be answered satisfactorily. In the elderly, a very red tongue body is not unusual. Here the tongue body color does not always signal a serious pathology, but instead reflects the physiological decline of yin in old age. In addition, blue, distended sublingual veins, or bluish spots on the tongue body, are common in those over the age of seventy. They are less meaningful than they would be if presented in a younger person, since the elderly have a tendency to develop blood stasis due to the physiological weakening of qi and blood that comes with age.

In this context it is worth mentioning the relationship between blood stasis and cancer. Many practitioners equate distended sublingual veins or blue spots on the tongue body with a tendency to form knots or cancerous lumps. This is not so! By themselves, these signs merely signal that the circulation of qi and blood in the body has slowed down. Again, a pattern of blood stasis can only be properly diagnosed based on *all* the signs and symptoms.

It is important to note that Chinese medicine is extremely accurate when diagnosing patterns of disease and constitution but is inferior to Western medicine in diagnosing cellular processes. This would suggest that practitioners of Chinese medicine are unable to diagnose illnesses defined by biomedicine using tongue and pulse diagnosis. But surely, over time and with plenty of experience, it should be possible to make an educated guess at the corresponding diagnosis.

Empirical experience, years of clinical practice, and intuition are equally important in the formulation of a diagnosis. Applying the four diagnostic techniques of Chinese medicine sharpens the perception when treating energetic disturbances. In my own practice, I have found that tongue analysis alongside other diagnostic techniques accurately reflects not only the pathomechanism of an illness, but also the underlying constitution of the patient. Besides the pulse, tongue diagnosis is, in my view, one of the most important diagnostic techniques in Chinese medicine.

1.5 How to Read This Book

This book is written for the benefit of practitioners of Chinese medicine. Each chapter stands as a self-contained unit, with an extensive discussion of the theory needed to understand the material presented in the case histories. At the beginning the reader will find typical signs of disharmony for a particular *zāng* or *fŭ* organ. The cases at the end of each chapter include a list of signs, symptoms, and background to the disease; the history of the patient; an analysis of the case; and the treatment strategy used to treat the patient.

Items of special interest are highlighted in italics or bold letters.

As noted above, a diagram accompanies many of the case histories which illustrates the pathomechanism in the case. The heavier lines and arrows represent the primary disease factor or pattern. The regular lines represent supporting patterns, or those which develop from the primary pattern, and the broken lines represent patterns which are indirectly related or caused by the other patterns. The underlying causes of the disorder are often highlighted in bold.

- Ch. 1 discusses the fundamentals of Chinese tongue diagnosis: the topography of the tongue and how to do an inspection, as well as the basic elements of tongue body color, shape, and coating.
- Ch. 2 focuses on Spleen qi deficiency, which is denoted by pale and swollen

tongues, leading to blood deficiency, or where Spleen qi deficiency is accompanied by deficiency of Kidney essence, source qi, and/or Kidney yang.

- Ch. 3 focuses on patterns of Kidney yin and/or Kidney essence deficiency that occur either alone or as part of a combined pattern.
- Ch. 4 focuses on disharmonies of the Stomach where yin deficiency plays a major role in the pathomechanism, or where there is blockage of the middle burner as a result of an attack by acute external cold. For the former, additional factors include other patterns of deficiency or patterns of excess such as heat in the Stomach, phlegm-heat in the Stomach, accumulated food, or Liver qi stagnation.
- Ch. 5 focuses on disease patterns of the Lungs. The sequence of the photographs is structured to show the development from a pattern of Lung qi deficiency to one of Lung yin deficiency, not the severity of the condition.
- Ch. 6 focuses on pathologies of the Heart that contain predominantly patterns of deficiency or patterns of excess. There is an additional focus on tongue signs that reflect pathologies of the Heart that are characterized by either a constitutional disharmony or an acquired disease pattern.
- Ch. 7 focuses on various manifestations of Liver pathologies such as qi stagnation, ascending Liver yang, Liver fire, or Liver blood deficiency.
- Ch. 8 focuses on blood stasis. There is also a discussion about the diagnostic use of sublingual veins. The relevance of distended veins to 'masses' in the body and to chest pain is also discussed.
- Ch. 9 focuses on the tongue signs associated with heat or damp-heat.
- Ch. 10 focuses on different aspects of tongue coatings, incluing wet and slippery, greasy, dry and white or yellow, and black or gray.
- Ch. 11 considers a range of special tongue signs, among them cracked, tofu-like, patchy, black and hairy.
- Ch. 12 looks at how the tongue changes over the course of treatment with acupuncture and herbal medicine.
- The index to this book will be most helpful in one's search for particular tongue signs or combinations of signs, disease patterns or pathomechanisms, specific symptoms, and biomedically-defined disorders.

Endnotes

1 The term 'constitution' in this book refers to the quality of an individual's qi, blood, yin, yang, Kidney essence, and source qi. It does not refer to a constitution based on the five elements.

2 Anonymous. *Huang di nei jing ling shu yi shi* [Translation and Explanation of the Yellow Emperor's Inner Classic: Divine Pivot], edited by Nanjing College of Traditional Chinese Medicine, Traditional Chinese Medicine Department. Shanghai: Shanghai Science and Technology Press, 1997: 6:62.

3 Ibid., 72:435.

4 An imbalance in favor of yin can reduce the activity of yang and impair the circulation of qi and blood to the tongue. This is discussed in Ch. 2.

5 An excess of yang can move the blood and fluids too much, resulting in the discoloration and change in the shape of the tongue body.

CHAPTER 1

The Foundations of Tongue Diagnosis

1.1 Relationship of the Tongue to the Interior of the Body

1.1.1 Channel Connections to the Tongue

The external aspect of a person can be perceived through their vitality, exuberance, body posture, and quality of the hair and skin, all of which reflect on the individual's internal energetic condition. The external aspects, along with the different tissues in the body, are supplied by qi, blood, and body fluids that are produced, transformed, and transported by the organs. This is especially true for the tongue. However, unlike the skin and hair, the tongue lies somewhere between the 'interior' and the 'exterior' and has an immediate connection to the interior. Because of this direct relationship to the interior, the tongue is extremely well suited for the diagnosis of various energies and the circulation in the body.

The texture of the tongue shows the quality of the individual's energy production and inherited constitution. The color and shape of the tongue body reflect the quality of the circulation of qi, blood, yin, yang, fluids, and essence. The tongue coating mirrors the condition of the body fluids, the functioning of the organs, and the strength and depth of pathogenic factors present in the body.

The tongue has an especially close relationship with the Stomach and Spleen. Liquids and solids are received by the Stomach where they are transformed and transported by the power of the Spleen qi. The Stomach is regarded as the source of fluids and its ability to produce fluids is directly reflected in the tongue's moisture. The quality of the nutritive qi and blood depends on the strength of Spleen qi to extract the essence from ingested foods, which contributes to the healthy pale-red color of the tongue body.

In its function as a sensory organ, the tongue is an 'offshoot' of the Heart, which means that the Heart qi communicates with the tongue. The Heart governs taste and speech. In addition, Heart qi controls blood circulation and supplies the tongue with blood, thus giving the tongue body its pale-red color. A direct connection from the Heart to the tongue is made through the collateral vessels of the Heart, which reach the root of the tongue.

All the other organs directly or indirectly supply the tongue via the channels. An internal branch of the Spleen channel ascends to the tongue and spreads out beneath it. The Kidney channel ascends to the tongue and ends at its root. The Liver channel and the secondary channels of the Bladder, Stomach, and Triple Burner also reach the tongue. Only the Lung, Large Intestine, Small Intestine, and Gallbladder channels have no direct connection to the tongue; but they do have indirect contact, either through their coupled partner organs or through deep internal channel connections. As a result of all these connections, the tongue can be used as a source of information about the status of qi, blood, and fluids throughout the body.

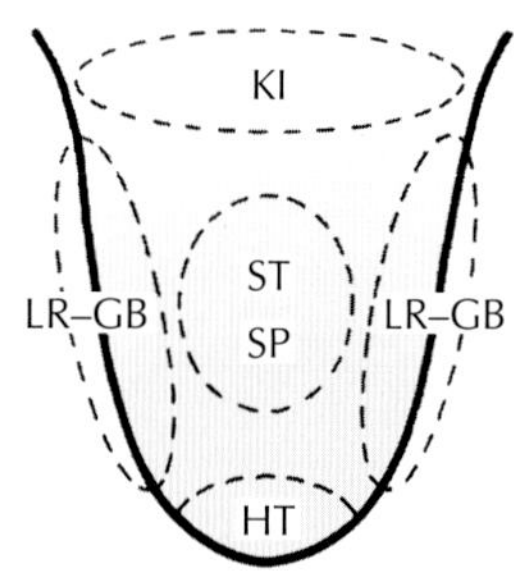

Fig. 2

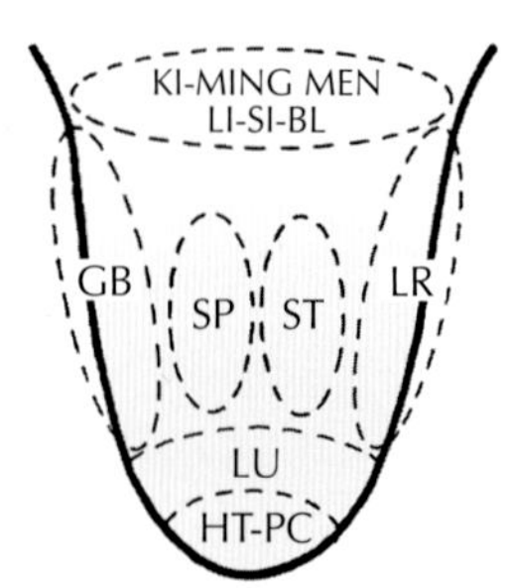

Fig. 3

1.1.2 Topography of the Tongue

To assess an individual's general energetic condition, the entire structure of the tongue is inspected. For a more detailed diagnosis, the tongue is divided into three zones or areas (Fig. 1):

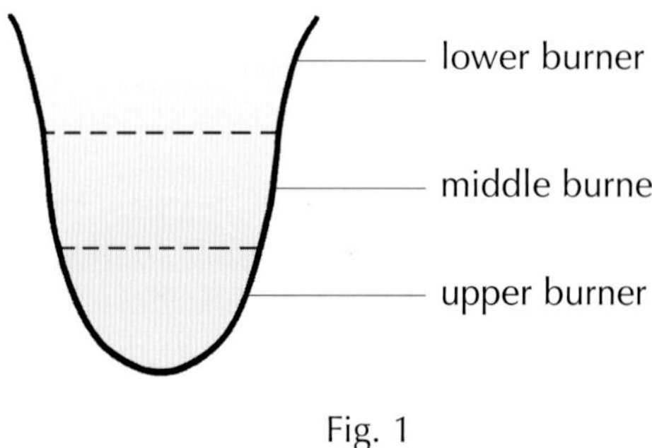

Fig. 1

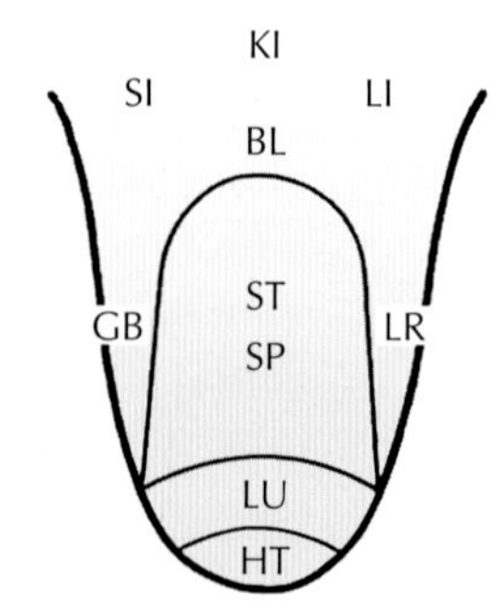

Fig. 4

1. The first (anterior) third of the tongue reflects the condition of the upper burner, which encompasses the Heart, Pericardium, and Lung.
2. The second (middle) third reflects the condition of the middle burner, which encompasses the Spleen, Stomach, Liver, and Gallbladder.
3. The third (posterior) third reflects the condition of the lower burner, which encompasses the Kidney, Bladder, Small Intestine, Large Intestine, and *mìng mén* (gate of vitality).

In contrast to the pulse positions, which have been the subject of much discussion in the history of Chinese medicine, the topography of the tongue is less controversial. The most common topographic representations, which deviate only a little from each other, are shown in Figs. 2 through 4.[1]

The blueprint for the tongue pictures in this book is shown in Fig. 5.

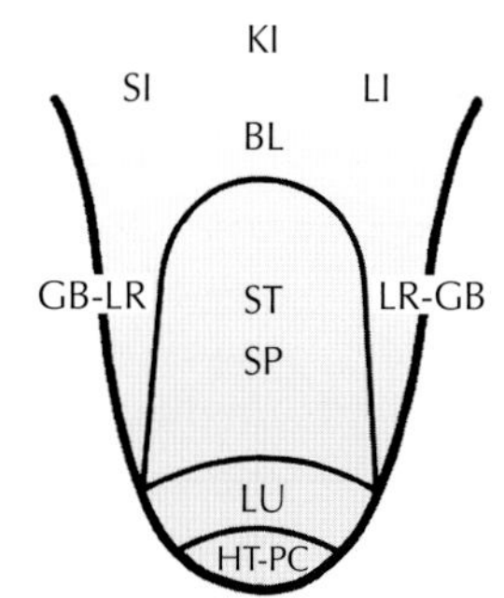

Fig. 5

1.2 General Information Regarding Inspection of the Tongue

1.2.1 Three-Step Procedure

In the daily practice of Chinese medicine it is often difficult to synthesize a complete picture of the patient's condition, even though all the information has been retrieved from the history, face, pulse, and tongue. Practitioners often ask which is the more important of the two, tongue or pulse diagnosis, and what is the best way to evaluate the signs, symptoms, and findings. This subject will be discussed more thoroughly in Section 1.2.7.

Tongue diagnosis represents only one aspect of the diagnostic process in Chinese medicine. It is, therefore, extremely important to view each diagnostic finding in the context of the overall picture. When undertaking tongue diagnosis, a clear understanding of the entire person and pathology is required to evaluate either general or specific tongue signs. The process thus involves three steps:

1. First, one should form a general impression. In tongue diagnosis, this means observing the tongue's vitality.
2. Second, collect and identify the individual signs concerning the tongue's color, shape, and coating. In order to assess these signs, a topographic map of the tongue should be used.
3. Third, reevaluate the general impression in light of the individual signs. Through this synthesis, a diagnosis can then be formulated.

1.2.2 Conditions for an Accurate Tongue Diagnosis

An accurate interpretation of the tongue color and shape is only possible when the patient presents the tongue in a relaxed manner. If a patient is very nervous or frightened, the tongue may be only partially extended, and then only in a tense fashion. Wait for the patient to relax and try again. However, even when the tongue is presented in a tensed manner, it can be used as a diagnostic sign of the quality of the patient's energy flow. I find that this is especially true with the appearance of curled-up tongue edges, which are only formed when the tongue has a certain amount of muscle tension. This often represents a condition of Liver qi constraint that is rarely visible in a relaxed tongue.

It is recommended that the color of the tongue body be observed and noted immediately, as it changes with activity of the tongue. It can, for example, change to a deeper red when it is extended for a long time. For this reason, the tongue should not be extended for longer than about 20 seconds, and with as little effort as possible.

When inspecting the tongue, lighting is very important. The most objective results are achieved with daylight. Fluorescent light falsifies the color and the tongue body may appear to be lighter than it really is. If artificial light must be used, halogen light is preferred, as it is closest to daylight. To avoid confusion, always try to maintain the same position and location.

If one part of the tongue body (usually the center) is noticeably red or discolored, ascertain when the patient last ate. Some foods discolor the tongue body, especially coffee, black tea, and spices like curry or cayenne pepper. Alcoholic beverages may lead to a reddening of the tongue body. Sucking sweets or licorice, as well as the coating of some tablets, discolors the center of the tongue or leads to the disappearance of the coating in the center. In general, it is best to check whether the patient is taking medication, as some medicinal substances discolor the tongue body.

Special attention should be given to the thickness of the tongue coating. Inspection starts at the tip and ends at the root of the tongue. In the case of a noticeably yellow, brown, or black coating, check when the patient last ate. Cigarettes or cigars, for example, have a drying effect upon the coating and give the tongue a yellow discoloration. Hot spices, like curry or mustard, have the same effect. Tea or coffee may cause the coating to develop a brownish color, while fatty foods often give it an oily consistency. The frequent drinking of fluids, or the intake of large amounts of fluids, may lead to an increase in tongue moisture; conversely, a small intake of fluids reduces moisture.

Occasionally the tongue surface will look rough, often with a thin coating. This can occur when patients haven taken to brushing their tongue on a daily basis. For the sake of an accurate tongue diagnosis, ask your patients to refrain from this habit.

1.2.3 Tongue Body Color

The color of the tongue body provides information about the state and quality of the blood, yin, and fluids, as well as the yang and qi. Spleen qi deficiency may lead to a pale tongue body since the qi, in this case, is too weak to transport the blood to the tongue. In the case of serious qi and yang deficiency, blood is not being moved adequately, which can lead to blood stasis; this manifests as a pale-blue tongue. In the case of blood deficiency, the tongue body will appear noticeably pale, while a reddening of the tongue body is seen with yin deficiency.

Disorders of heat and cold also show themselves in the color of the tongue body. When externally-contracted heat, for example, enters the blood, the tongue body may turn dark or crimson red. If cold blocks qi and yang in the interior, the tongue body becomes noticeably pale. As a generalization, the tongue body color tends to reflect the state of qi, yang, blood, and yin. In acute diseases, its color can also provide information about the quality and depth of penetration of a pathogenic factor. Thus a continuing high fever lasting over a few days may change the color of the tongue body to a dark red. In the case of a chronic disease, the tongue body can reflect long-term pathological disharmony as well as constitutional weakness.

1.2.4 Relationship between Tongue Body Color and Shape

The color and shape of the tongue body are very closely linked to one another and should not be considered in isolation. Together they reflect the strength of normal qi (*zheng qi*).

In general, tongue body color shows, with the exception of acute illnesses, the underlying pattern of disharmony in a person's constitution. A very pale, swollen tongue body may indicate Kidney yang deficiency, a dark-red body without coating Kidney yin deficiency. If there is a strong contrast in color from a healthy pale-red tongue body, this commonly reveals the onset of a more serious illness, usually involving the internal organs. In addition, where there are contradictory symptoms—for example, a patient with all the signs of Kidney yin deficiency but experiencing an intense internal feeling of cold ('false cold, true heat'), or of an underlying Kidney yang deficiency but experiencing hot flushes—the tongue body color is a reliable indicator.

As a rule, the normal tongue shape changes only when pathology persists over a long period of time. A pale, swollen tongue body shows that the qi in the body has been deficient for quite a while. It indicates that the qi is not only failing to bring blood to the tongue (hence the pale color) but is also failing to transform and transport the fluids (swollen tongue body). A red tongue with a normal tongue body can indicate the beginning of Kidney yin deficiency or of the penetration of heat into the blood level. A red tongue with a small, contracted body may reveal Kidney yin deficiency with a severe loss of fluids. This combination of color and shape is an indication that the yin has been exhausted over a long period of time: yin deficiency has given rise to heat, which in turn has injured the fluids, eventually leading to the contracted appearance of the tongue body.

Thus the combination of tongue body color and shape provides precise information about the condition of the qi, blood, yin, yang, and fluids. In the case of chronic illness, it is especially important to use the results of this diagnostic procedure to assess the severity of the illness.

In relation to the eight principles, the tongue body color and shape reflect the state of yin and yang as well as the presence of heat and cold. Yin deficiency produces heat, which is represented by a red tongue body, and, in severe cases, by a contracted body as well. By contrast, the internal cold that develops with yang deficiency is reflected in a very pale, swollen tongue body. Again, the tongue body color and shape are important indicators when assessing chronic illness.

Cracks, depressions, and localized swellings on the tongue body reflect energetic disharmonies in specific organs. For example, if the anterior third of the tongue is noticeably swollen, this implies retention of phlegm in the Lungs. If such a patient complains of a cough, it must be given immediate attention. However, if there are no Lung symptoms, it is of no special significance, and should simply be noted.

Sometimes the tongue does not reflect a pattern of disharmony. This, in my experience, is especially true of patterns involving the Liver. For example, it is inadvisable to differentiate a pathology caused by ascending Liver yang or Liver fire based entirely on the appearance of a specific tongue sign, namely, redness or red points on the side of the tongue. An accurate diagnosis is possible only by considering the pulse qualities in conjunction with the symptoms experienced by the patient, since both of the aforementioned tongue signs can denote ascending Liver yang as well as Liver fire.

This is also the case with skin disorders. Heat in the blood may cause atopic eczema, for example, but this does not always show up on the tongue. Patients who have suffered with long-term skin disorders manifested in itchy skin, sensations of heat, and redness of the skin will often present with a tongue that is pale or show no signs at all of heat in the blood. Thus, for the diagnosis and treatment of skin disorders where the most obvious signs are skin lesions, indicators on the tongue are of little, if any, importance and occasionally must be ignored.

These examples will serve to underscore that tongue diagnosis must be integrated with other Chinese diagnostic techniques. It is only one aspect, albeit a very informative and important one, of the entire diagnostic protocol in Chinese medicine.

1.2.5 Relationship between Tongue Body Shape and Tongue Coating

While the shape and color of the tongue body are inseparably linked in tongue diagnosis, the body and coating of the tongue are not quite so tightly connected and occasionally can be judged independently of each other. The tongue coating reveals the location of an illness. According to the eight principles, it shows whether the illness is situated in the exterior (*biǎo*) or interior (*lǐ*). The thickness of the tongue coating indicates its excessive or deficient nature. The color and the texture of the coating reflect whether it is hot or cold. For example, a slippery, yellow coating suggests the presence of damp-heat while a dry, yellow coating indicates the predominance of heat.

In the case of an acute illness, that is, one caused by externally-contracted cold, which is indicated by a thin, white coating, it is mainly the tongue coating that shows the strength of the pathogenic factor and how deeply it has penetrated into the interior. Just by observing the tongue coating, the quality of the pathogenic factor can be ascertained without necessarily having to consider the color of the tongue body. Besides changing the tongue coating, a strong, penetrating pathogenic factor may also alter the moisture as well as the color of the tongue. Strong heat, for example, can cause a dry, red tongue body.

In the case of mild chronic illness, the tongue coating often reflects the underlying pattern of disharmony. Often a swollen, pale tongue body is accompanied by a moist, white tongue coating while a red tongue body is accompanied by a dry, yellow coating. However, this is not always true because, in severe cases, a red tongue body may present with a white, powdery tongue coating, which indicates the presence of heat instead of cold.

When diagnosing acute disorders that are characterized by fever, flu symptoms, or acute digestive problems, the tongue coating takes precedence over the shape of the tongue body. It is especially important to note the thickness, location, and texture of the tongue coating.

1.2.6 Observation of the Sublingual Veins

It is always important to examine the sublingual veins and to note their color and thickness. The patient should be asked to touch the palate with the tip of the tongue. If the veins are clearly blue, filled, or swollen, this may indicate the presence of blood stasis in the body. It is important to repeat this procedure during various visits of the patient in order to receive correct findings.

1.2.7 Comparison of Pulse and Tongue Diagnosis

Qi moves the blood. The quality and dynamics of the movement of qi reveals itself in the pulse. The pulse mainly describes the present energetic condition of an individual. By feeling the pulse the practitioner enters into a close relationship with the patient, perceiving the quality of the patient's pulsating energy. An example from my own practice is illustrative. A 60-year-old woman, who always put the needs of others before her own, complained about intense inner tension. Her tongue was normal. The pulse was very wiry (*xián*) and thin (*xì*). From the pulse and symptoms it was clear that she had developed Liver qi constraint. In the course of treatment the woman was eventually able to begin fulfilling her own wishes rather than those of others. Slowly, the pulse became less wiry, and this was accompanied by a greater sense of joy in her life.

In this case it was the pulse, much more than the tongue, that reflected the true energetic state of the patient. The pulse, however, did not provide any indication of the length or depth of the Liver qi stagnation. For its part, the normalcy of her tongue did not reflect any disharmony, or might have suggested that it was not that deep or serious. This example illustrates that pulse diagnosis can be quite accurate when the tongue signs are inconspicuous. In this case, the pulse was given priority over the tongue.

The tongue reflects the condition of the blood, body fluids, and essence more clearly than does the pulse. There are pulse qualities, of course, like the choppy (*sè*) pulse, which indicate blood deficiency. However, the depth and severity of such deficiency is difficult to judge from the pulse alone, and can only be made by an experienced practitioner. Yet a thin, dry, or contracted tongue makes the condition easy to detect, especially if the color, shape, and texture of the tongue obviously deviate from normal. In such cases, the tongue is given priority over the pulse.

Occasionally, the pulse and tongue signs deviate from each other. If the tongue body, for example, is pale and swollen, the practitioner may expect a slow (*chí*) or submerged (*chén*) pulse. But if the pulse were fast (*shuò*) and floating (*fú*), this could be the result of nerves (arriving late for the appointment, or fear of the consultation itself), shock, coffee, or medication. The pulse can change very quickly in response to the most recent event in a patient's life, while the tongue will remain unchanged.

To summarize, the qualities of the pulse accurately reflect the present energetic condition of an individual. The qualities of the tongue, especially its body, color, and shape, allow one to predict long-term changes in the energetic state. The tongue coating is a very important indicator in cases of acute illness (see Ch. 10).

1.3 The Normal Tongue

The normal tongue reflects energetic harmony within the body. The right interplay of yin and yang, qi, blood, and fluids is reflected in the color, shape, and coating of the tongue body. As previously noted, the first step in the examination of the tongue is to gain an overall impression, especially of the vitality of the tongue. A vital tongue has a fresh-looking body that is well supplied with blood, giving it a fresh, pale-red color. When the tongue is full of vitality, it moves easily and can protrude from the mouth without difficulty. The normal tongue should also be a little moist, indicating the presence of adequate fluids.

During the second step of the examination, the following individual aspects of the tongue should be evaluated:

a) The normal tongue color is pale red.

The red coloration indicates that the qi and yang are strong enough to transport blood to the tongue. It also reflects the quality and quantity of the blood circulation in the body. The tongue has a pale tinge due to the supply of fluids that ascend from the Stomach to the tongue (see Ch. 5).

The clear part of the fluids (*jīn*) also serves the function of thinning the blood. If there is a deficiency of fluids in the body, the blood will be correspondingly less dilute. This will cause the tongue to appear redder. In a healthy person, the pale-red tongue body color arises from the appropriate mixture of blood and fluids. If a tongue is lighter than pale red, it is called pale. If it is darker than pale red, it is called reddish or red.

b) The normal tongue body shape is neither too thick nor too thin.

The tongue body should move easily and look neither too soft nor too stiff. The tongue's surface should be smooth and soft and show no cracks. The size of the tongue body usually corresponds to the constitution of the individual and therefore does not necessarily imply pathology. It could thus be said that the tongue fits the body shape of the individual. A big, strong person normally has a big tongue body, while a thin, small person has a thin, smallish tongue.

The volume of the tongue body, however, is important. It should be neither too thin nor too thick. A slight tapering toward the tip of the tongue is also normal. The tongue body shape reflects the condition of a person in relation to their long-term energetic development. It can, for example, take years before a contracted or extremely swollen tongue body develops. The formation of cracks in the tongue body may also represent a lengthy pathological process.

c) The normal tongue coating is white and thin.

A thin, white tongue coating is regarded as normal, although it can also indicate acute, externally-contracted wind-cold. If the tongue shows no coating but is moist and of a normal color, this is also normal and does not suggest pathology. A slightly thick, pale-yellow tongue coating at the root of the tongue arises from the physiological activity of Stomach qi during the process of digestion. Fermentation of the ingested liquids and solids results in 'steam,' which materializes as a form of turbid moisture on the coating of the tongue. This coating is thickest at the root of the tongue and steadily thins out toward the tip. Due to the turbidity rising up, it is normal for the tongue coating, at the root, to be of a pale-yellow color. If there is coating in the middle and anterior parts of the tongue, but none on the posterior, this is indicative of a condition characterized by deficiency (see Section 3.6). This so-called 'rootless' coating originates most commonly from deficiency of Stomach qi, Stomach yin, and Kidney yin.

d) Veins underneath the tongue are not distended.

In the case of a normal tongue, the sublingual veins are either barely visible or not visible at all. Their color should be light and not of a dark-blue or purple color. When examining the veins underneath the tongue, particular attention should be paid to the following:

- The patient should be asked to curl the tongue up lightly and gently, and rest the tip of the tongue on the palate.
- If the patient does this more than once within a short space of time, the veins can become an intense bluish color. Similarly, if the patient has been talking a lot before the examination, the veins may also appear more bluish and distended. In such cases, the practitioner must be careful in formulating a diagnosis of blood stasis based on the changed appearance of these veins (see Section 8.3).

1.3.1 Examples of Normal Tongues

Tongue 1

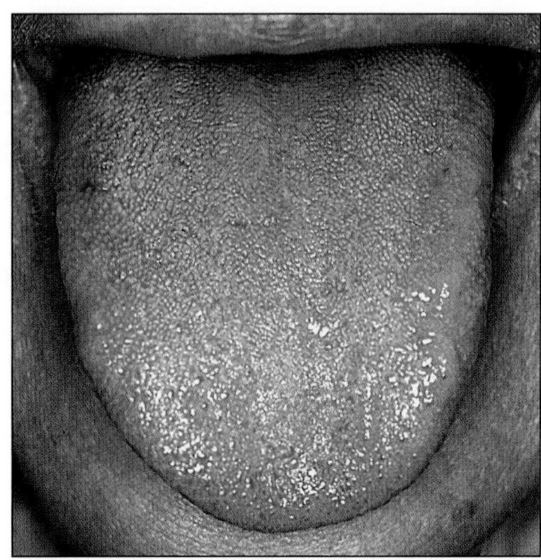

A 50-year-old woman who has never been seriously ill. Occasionally, she complains about exhaustion. The tongue body shape is normal, neither too thick nor too thin. The tongue has a fresh appearance and is moist. The tongue body color is pale red, which indicates a healthy supply of qi and blood throughout the body. The tongue coating is thin and slightly yellow at the posterior third. At the right edge of the tongue a small, bluish point is visible, which sometimes signifies blood stasis. However, as the patient has no other signs or symptoms of any kind, this particular tongue sign is not indicative of a pathological process.

Surprisingly enough, this woman returned for treatment ten years later with diagnosis of Liver cirrhosis of unknown origin.

Tongue 2

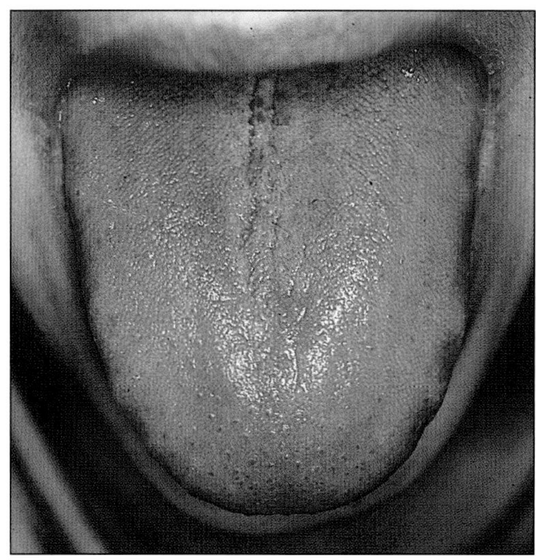

A 49-year-old woman who feels healthy. The tip of the tongue shows a few red points that reflect heat in the Heart. This occasionally manifests as difficulty in falling asleep. The tongue body, shape, and color, however, are normal. The tongue is moist and has vitality. On the posterior third of the tongue are red points that are not considered pathological. This woman has no symptoms.

Endnote

1. Compare Maciocia G. *Tongue Diagnosis in Chinese Medicine*, rev. ed. Seattle: Eastland Press, 1995:24-26.

CHAPTER 2

Pale Tongue Signs

2.1 Pale and Swollen Tongues

A pale tongue with a normal tongue shape and coating indicates only a slight deficiency of Lung and Spleen qi. In this case, the qi is not strong enough to transport the blood to the tongue, resulting in a paler coloration of the tongue body. The paleness of the tongue body is proportional to the degree of the deficiency: The paler the tongue body, the more serious the qi and yang deficiency.

A pale and swollen tongue is very common. The tongue is pale because the yang qi is too weak to transport sufficient blood to the tongue. The tongue is also swollen as a result of qi and yang deficiency, which results in inadequate fluid transformation. Since the fluids are inadequately transformed, they accumulate and transform into dampness. The degree of swelling of the tongue body is inversely related to the strength of the yang and source qi, that is, a weak yang and source qi will result in a swollen tongue body. Physical overwork, excessive exercise, and overconsumption of raw foods and dairy products can cause deficiency of Spleen qi and yang. If the pale tongue has a normal body shape, the deficiency is not as serious and can be rectified through a proper and regular diet as well as periods of rest.

Pale and swollen tongues are often accompanied by teeth marks. The deeper and more distinctive the marks, the more serious the weakness of Stomach and Spleen qi, and/or Spleen and Kidney yang.

Tongue description ---------- **Chinese diagnosis**

Tongue description	Chinese diagnosis
Slightly pale, normal shape	Slight Spleen qi and blood deficiency
Red points at the tip	Normal*
Slightly white-yellowish, greasy coating at the posterior third	Slight food stagnation

Fig. 2.1.1
Female
31 years old

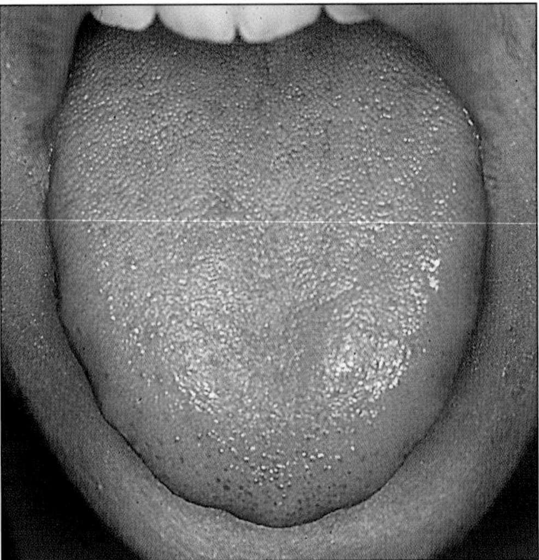

Symptoms

Fatigue
Constipation
Bouts of no appetite
Epigastric fullness

Western diagnosis

None

Background to disease

Overwork
Irregular eating habits, excessive consumption of sweets

**See Section 6.2*

Tongue description ---------- **Chinese diagnosis**

Tongue description	Chinese diagnosis
Pale, swollen, short, slightly wet	Spleen qi deficiency (accumulation of dampness and blood deficiency)

Fig. 2.1.2
Male
50 years old

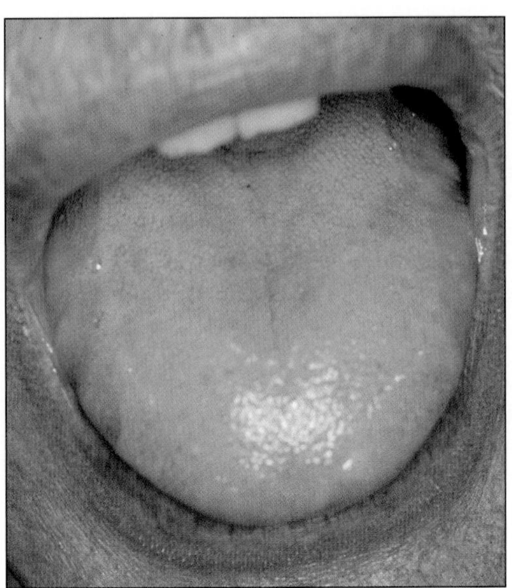

Symptoms

Loud gurgling in the abdomen
Soft stools
Excessive sputum
No appetite
Panic attacks
Difficulty in falling asleep, severe fatigue

Western diagnosis

None

Background to disease

Excessive consumption of raw foods
Excessive worrying
Lack of sleep due to work schedule t(night shift)

Tongue description

Slightly pale, swollen

White, thin, slippery coating

Yellow coating at the root

Chinese diagnosis

Spleen qi deficiency

Accumulation of dampness

Damp-heat lodges in the lower burner

Symptoms

Fatigue, especially after meals
Lack of concentration
Difficulty in falling asleep
Loose, smelly stools

Western diagnosis

None

Background to disease

Excessive consumption of dairy products
Long fasting periods in the past

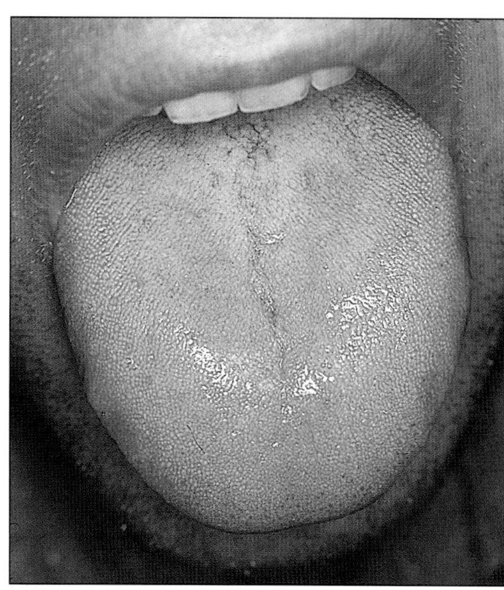

Fig. 2.1.3
Male
37 years old

Tongue description

Pale, swollen, teeth marks

Chinese diagnosis

Spleen yang deficiency (accumulation of dampness)

Symptoms

Watery stools in the morning without smell
Frequent nausea
No drive
Intense feeling of cold
Migraines, diarrhea, and vomiting preceding menstruation

Western diagnosis

None

Background to disease

Treated for a long time with tetracyclines for acne vulgaris
Frequent illnesses in childhood

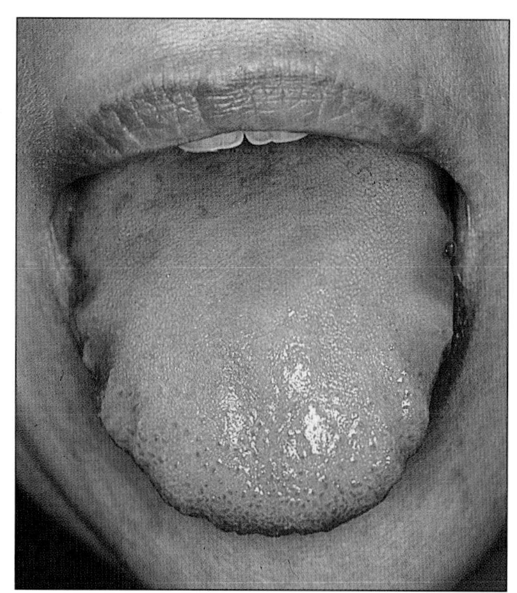

Fig. 2.1.4
Female
33 years old

Tongue description	**Chinese diagnosis**
Pale, very swollen, wide	Spleen qi and yang deficiency (accumulation of dampness)
Small, vertical cracks in the center	Stomach qi deficiency
White, thin coating	Normal

Fig. 2.1.5
Female
27 years old

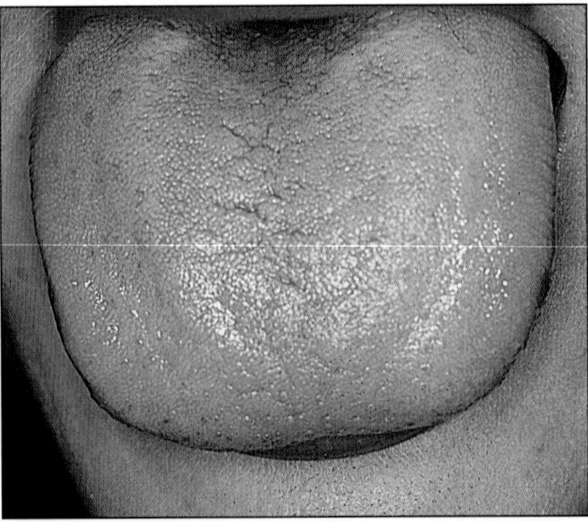

Symptoms

Exhaustion
Feeling of pressure in the center of the stomach with stress
Weight gain
Pain
Tingling and numbness in the right arm and hand

Western diagnosis

None

Background to disease

Overwork
Irregular eating habits
Excessive consumption of raw foods and cold fruit juices

Tongue description	**Chinese diagnosis**
Pale, very swollen, teeth marks	Kidney yang, Spleen yang, and Heart yang deficiency

Fig. 2.1.6
Female
67 years old

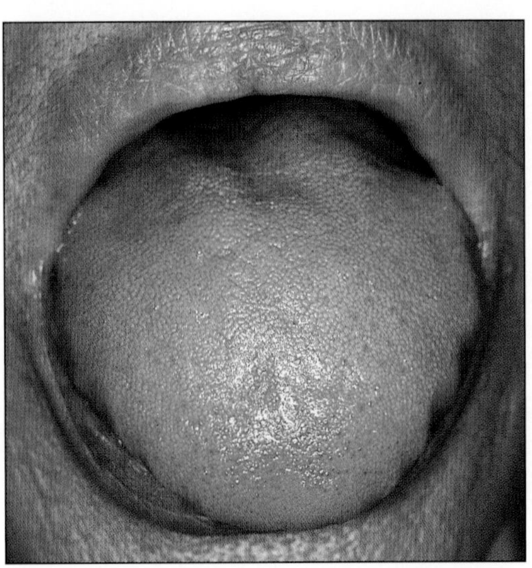

Symptoms

Extreme physical weakness
Cold feeling, cold extremities
Sensation of cold in the stomach
Stomach pain

Western diagnosis

Chronic gastritis

Background to disease

Chronic physical overwork

2.2 Pale Tongues with a Depression at Their Root

With the help of the eight principles and tongue diagnosis, acute and chronic patterns of disease can be analyzed quite accurately. Tongue diagnosis is used to gain insight into the 'energetic present' condition of the individual. There are also tongue signs that inform us about the person's 'energetic past.' These signs may include deep cracks, dents, hollows, or crevices in the tongue body, or a contracted tongue body. These and other changes to the tongue body, shape, and color, plus other specific signs, are most commonly caused by deep energetic deficiencies, for example, a chronic deficiency of Spleen and Stomach qi or Kidney yin. Generally speaking, these deficiencies will, over time, lead to a depletion or insufficient nourishment of the essence.

The essence is a very rarified and dense form of energy that is fluid in nature. It has the potential for building and nourishing the body. It supplies the energetic material for physical and mental development in childhood, and for the development and function of the reproductive system. The quality and strength of the essence is also of great importance in the production of marrow and in controlling the functions of the brain, bone marrow, and spinal cord. Finally, an increased output of essence is required to offset the shock and trauma associated with accidents.

If one follows a regular lifestyle, the essence will decrease slowly and gradually decline in old age, accompanied by such things as the loss of acute hearing or loose or falling teeth. Young or middle-aged individuals, however, may also show signs of weakening essence. The most common causes are:

- Chronic inadequate nutrition
- Chronic overwork
- Chronic lack of sleep
- Too many pregnancies and births
- Births that follow too closely together
- Excessive loss of sperm
- Extremely profuse and frequent menstrual bleeding
- Serious chronic illnesses
- Frequent colds and flu[1]
- Serious shocks
- Many operations
- Constitutional weakness, that is, inherited illness or physical and mental disabilities
- Diets that are inappropriate to the season
- Irregular eating habits, often in conjunction with overwork
- Insufficient rest after operations, infections, or other illnesses.

The essence is responsible for the conservation and quality of 'substance,' and a deficiency of essence implies loss of this substance, as reflected in brittle bones or loss of teeth.

Consider the following example: A young woman had been suffering for a long time from anorexia nervosa. Her symptoms included the cessation of periods as well as osteoporosis. The tendency to starve herself had caused the exhaustion of the postnatal essence, which in turn failed to replenish the Kidney essence. The young woman's loss of substance manifested in brittle bones.

The practitioner is first alerted to a deficiency of essence by the patient's history and corresponding symptoms, as well as through specific pulse qualities. In order to formulate an accurate diagnosis and prognosis, it is of great importance to assess the quality and strength of the essence. Alongside all the other collected data, the diagnosis of the tongue can contribute a great deal of information about the quality of the essence.[2]

Owing to its fluid nature and substantial qualities, the essence is yin in nature relative to the dynamic power of qi and yang; it thus has a strong affinity to Kidney yin. Because of this, Kidney yin deficiency can lead to deficient essence. All processes in the body that lead to a loss of fluids like severe and long-lasting diarrhea, extreme sweating, or long-lasting febrile disease, will eventually injure the yin. The loss of fluids and yin will produce dry, red tongues (Fig. 3.6.5), which can be an indication of severe deficiency of Kidney yin and of declining essence. In clinical practice these tongues are most commonly found in severely ill, elderly, or in those patients who suffer from a serious internal disease.

The interplay between Kidney yin and Kidney yang depends on the strength and quality of the essence and source qi. The essence, through the Kidney yang and the gate of vitality (*mìng mén*), supplies the material necessary for the transforming and warming actions needed to produce Kidney qi. The tongue coating is highly dependent on these actions. If the fluids are not transformed, either because of Kidney yin or Kidney yang deficiency, then the Kidney qi is unable to rise to moisten the tongue. In extreme cases, this becomes visible in a very pale, swollen tongue body that is dry. Here, Kidney yang is too weak to transform (swollen body) and transport (dry tongue) the fluids. This is rarely seen in the clinic; more commonly, a dry tongue appears as a result of deficient fluids, blood, and Stomach or Kidney yin.

However, as mentioned in Ch. 1, the lack of tongue coating is primarily associated with the function of the Stomach and Spleen qi. The fermentation of solids and liquids by the Stomach qi and the healthy, damp climate of the Stomach contribute to a turbid 'steam' that ascends and becomes the foundation of the tongue coating. If the energies of the middle burner function without any problems, there will be an evenly distributed thin coating that is closely attached to the tongue's surface. A deficiency of Stomach qi, Stomach yin, and especially Kidney yin can lead to a coating without a root. This coating is characterized by its uneven distribution, which gives it an old, peeled appearance and looks as if it could be easily scraped off (Fig. 3.6.5).

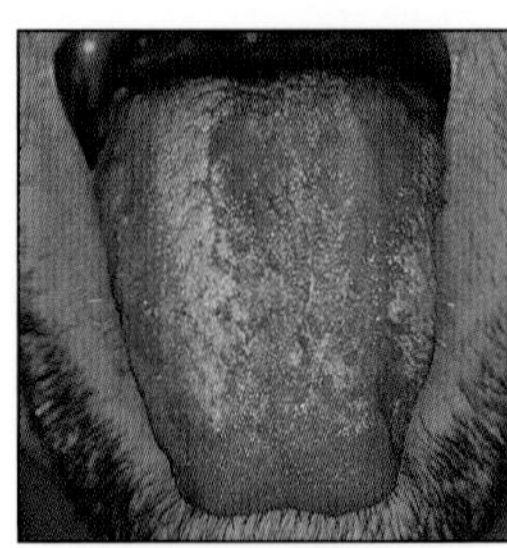

Fig. 3.6.5

The lack of a tongue coating coupled with a pale tongue body indicates a lack of Stomach qi. This combination plus the appearance of superficial cracks in the center of the tongue may signal the onset of a decline in fluids and Stomach yin.

The primary channel of the Kidney ascends along the throat and terminates at the root of the tongue. The texture and form of the tongue root can be used to assess the condition of the Kidneys. When there is weakness, the root will be seen to contract (Fig. 2.6.2). A depression at the root of the tongue shows a loss of substance or material, and denotes deficiency of Kidney essence.

In general, the tongue coating at the root reflects the condition of the Large Intestine, Small Intestine, and Bladder. The complete interpretation of the coating at the root requires knowledge of the patient's symptoms. An absence of coating at the tongue root reflects deficiency of the Kidneys, and in the case of a red root, of Kidney yin deficiency and an exhaustion of the body fluids (Fig. 3.6.4). A very red and dry root signifies that Kidney fire has arisen from deficiency of the Kidney yin.

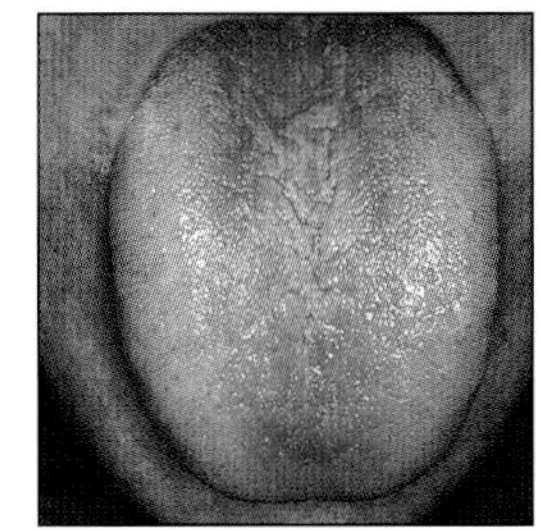
Fig. 3.6.4

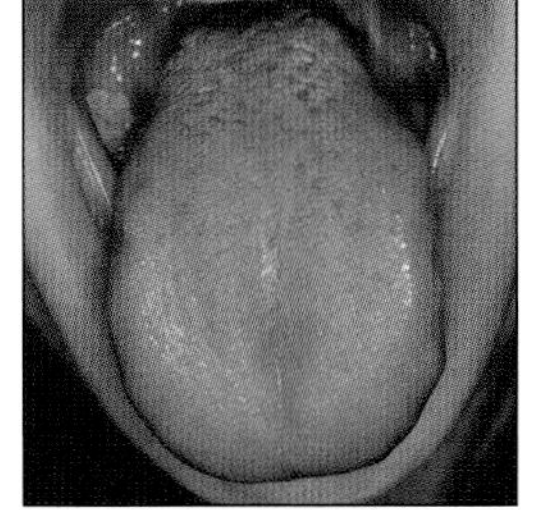
Fig. 3.7.2

The texture and form of the root of the tongue also mirrors the condition of the Kidneys. A contracted root (Fig. 3.7.2) or a depression at the root represents a deficiency of essence. These tongue shapes are the result of a loss of substance or material; as a result, the tongue lacks appropriate volume or shape. If the tongue root is of a normal color, the deficiency has not yet advanced to the stage of internal heat.

An incipient lack of essence may also be associated with pale tongues. The incipient deficiency of essence manifests as a pale tongue with a depression at its root; it is as if there were a lack of substance to fill the root of the tongue. This condition is characterized by the combination of qi deficiency symptoms (fatigue, lack of appetite, sweating upon the slightest exertion, loose stools) as well as symptoms indicating deficiency of essence. Thus, fatigue may evolve into exhaustion that is not alleviated by regular sleep, there may be a lack of concentration, failure of memory, or head hair may turn prematurely gray. In such cases, it is not enough to simply tonify the qi. The essence as well as Kidney yin and yang must also be nourished.

As the following figures illustrate, it is possible to evaluate the condition of the essence and the extent to which substance has been lost by examining the tongue body shape, and not just the tongue body color and coating. In these figures, pale tongue bodies that form as a result of essence deficiency are compared with those that result from Spleen qi or yang deficiency, or Kidney yang deficiency.

Tongue description

Slightly pale, slightly swollen
Slight depression at the root

Chinese diagnosis

Spleen and Lung qi deficiency
Slight deficiency of essence

Symptoms

Exhaustion
Insomnia
Heavy feeling in the legs
Tendency to catch colds
Coughing

Western diagnosis

Mononucleosis
Chronic fatigue syndrome following influenza

Background to disease

Chronic overwork

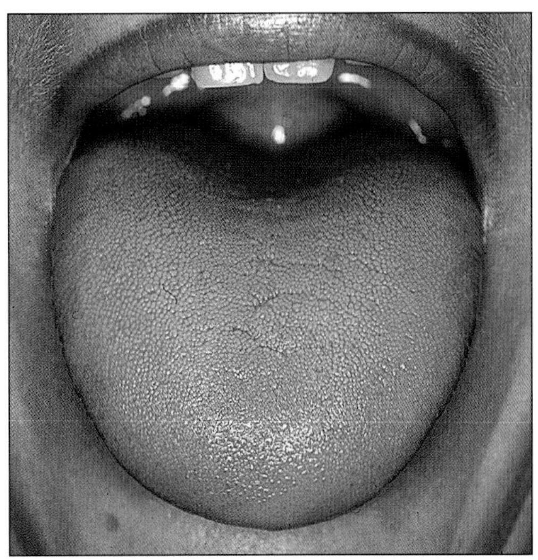

Fig. 2.2.1
Female
35 years old

Tongue description ------------------------- **Chinese diagnosis**

Tongue description	Chinese diagnosis
Slightly pale, swollen	Spleen qi deficiency (accumulation of dampness)
Slight teeth marks, moist	Early stage of Spleen yang deficiency
Depression at the root	Slight deficiency of essence

Fig. 2.2.2
Female
38 years old

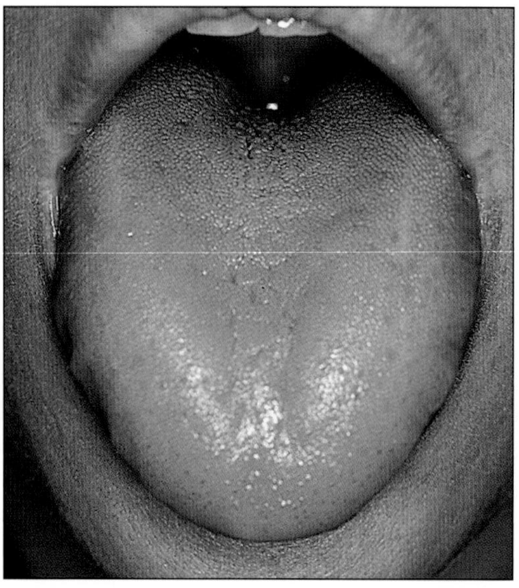

Symptoms

Exhaustion
Depression
Inability to concentrate
Feeling cold
Hair loss

Western diagnosis

Poisoning from amalgam in tooth fillings

Background to disease

Six pregnancies, four children
Overwork

Tongue description ------------------------- **Chinese diagnosis**

Tongue description	Chinese diagnosis
Very pale, swollen, slight teeth marks	Spleen yang deficiency (accumulation of dampness)
White coating in the center	Accumulation of cold-dampness in the Stomach
Depression at the root	Essence deficiency

Fig. 2.2.3
Female
39 years old

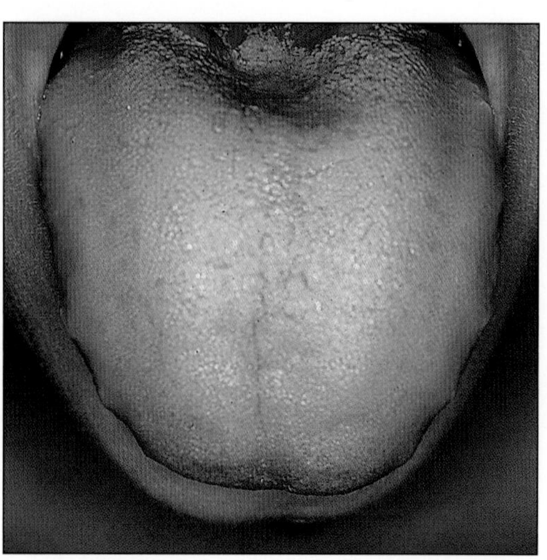

Symptoms

Exhaustion, fatigue
Inability to fall asleep
Epigastric pain with emotional stress
No appetite
Intense feeling of cold

Western diagnosis

No findings except underweight

Background to disease

Chronic overwork (works at night)
Irregular eating habits
Excessive consumption of raw foods
Infection of viral meningitis 2 years ago

2.3 Pale and Thin Tongues

A lack of blood and body fluids causes a decline in the volume of the tongue body, which is manifested in a thinning, shrinking, or contracting of the tongue body. Depending on the individual's constitution or life circumstances, Spleen qi deficiency may lead either to accumulation of dampness or a lack of blood. Both are secondary aspects of a disharmony of Spleen qi. Any long-term deficiency will lead to impairment in the transformation of food into blood. Because of this, every pale tongue reflects an element of blood deficiency. However, when blood deficiency is an important contributory factor to an illness, it is expressed in a pale and thin tongue body. At the onset of such a pathology, it will be pale and dry. This is especially true in women who suffer from profuse menstrual bleeding, breast feed for long periods of time, or follow improper dietary habits.

A thin, pale tongue is an important feature in individuals who suffer from a lack of blood. If this condition is not treated, Kidney yin deficiency may develop, as blood nourishes the yin. The development of this particular pathology is visible when the pale tongue body changes its shape or takes on an intense red or orange tinge. If the pale tongue is dry, the deficiency is not so severe, that is, the blood has lost its moistening function but the deficiency is not yet significant. Typical symptoms of blood deficiency are dry or itchy skin, hair loss, a pale tinge to the skin, numbness in the extremities, dizziness, and a tendency to insomnia and anxiety.

Tongue description	**Chinese diagnosis**
Pale, thin	Spleen qi deficiency (blood deficiency)
Curled-up edges	Liver qi constraint
Reddish center	Heat in the Stomach
Depression at the root	Essence deficiency

Symptoms

Deep exhaustion
Burning around the anus
Anal pain
Constipation
Lack of appetite
Insomnia

Western diagnosis

Inflamed hemorrhoids

Background to disease

Strong demands at work and home
Unhappy marriage
Constant frustration
Four pregnancies
Caffeine abuse

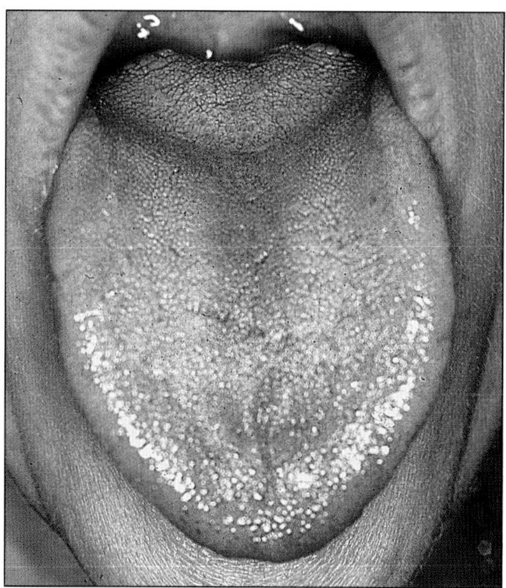

Fig. 2.3.1
Female
38 years old

Tongue description ------------------------ **Chinese diagnosis**

Tongue description	Chinese diagnosis
Pale, thin	Slight Spleen qi deficiency (blood deficiency)
Pale edges	Liver blood deficiency
Slightly dry, thin crack in the center	Slight Stomach yin deficiency

Fig. 2.3.2
Female
35 years old

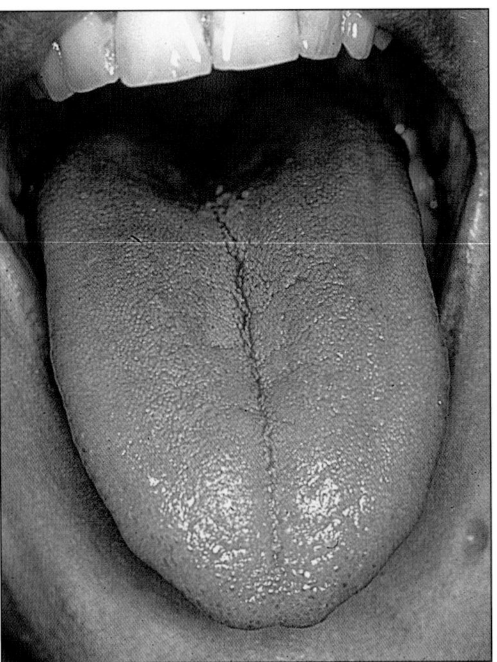

Symptoms

Exhaustion
Acute diarrhea with blood and mucus
Hair loss
Short menstrual cycle
Intense fears

Western diagnosis

Ulcerative colitis

Background to disease

Helminthes that were improperly treated in India
Emotional problems
Vegetarian diet
Fasting

2.4 Special Tongue Shapes of the Pale Tongue

2.4.1 Pale and Narrow Tongues

Pale, slightly swollen, and narrow tongue bodies may indicate deficiency of blood and improper circulation of Liver qi. In such cases, the narrow tongue will look slightly contracted (Fig. 2.4.1.1). This type of tongue arises from a deficiency of Spleen qi that lacks the strength to circulate qi and produce blood. The consequence can be an insufficient supply of qi and blood to the channels, collaterals, and muscles, leading to weakness and pain in the extremities.

In rare cases, only one side of the tongue is contracted or drawn in. This change suggests Liver qi constraint and lack of Liver blood flow since the sides of the tongue reflect the circulation of Liver and Gallbladder qi. Pain or a sense of weakness along the Liver or Gallbladder channels can be a manifestation of this pathology. This is a common tongue sign, particularly in women who suffer from various breast diseases. The contracted side of the tongue does not always correspond to the side of the affected breast.

Tongue description

Slightly pale, swollen, teeth marks
Narrow on both sides and drawn in

Chinese diagnosis

Spleen qi deficiency (Liver blood deficiency)
Liver qi constraint, possibly blood stasis

Symptoms

Pain in the left thigh and shoulder
Migraines with sensitivity to light during menstruation

Western diagnosis

Organized hematoma in the thigh

Background to disease

Overwork
Side effect of contraceptive pill

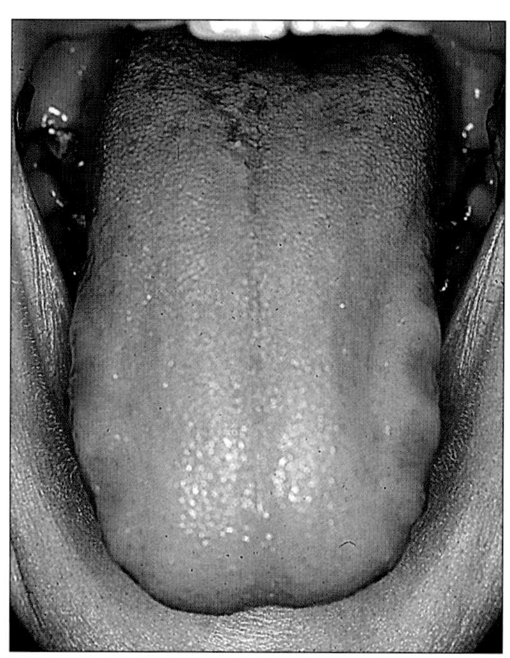

Fig. 2.4.1.1
Female
37 years old

Tongue description

Slightly pale, swollen
Drawn in on both sides

Chinese diagnosis

Spleen qi deficiency (Liver blood deficiency)
Lack of nourishment of sinews and tendons due to qi and blood deficiency

Symptoms

Pain in the right arm and shoulders
Tingling and numbness of the thumb
Muscular tension
Ringing noise in the right ear

Western diagnosis

Brachial plexus neuropathy

Background to disease

Whiplash

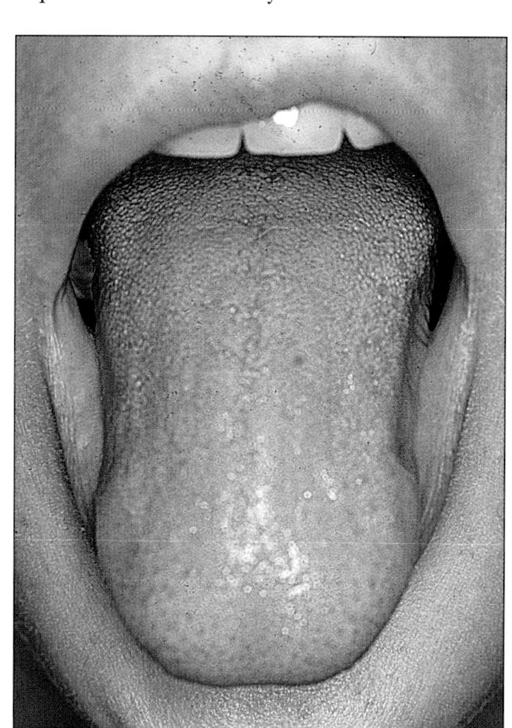

Fig. 2.4.1.2
Female
28 years old

Tongue description	**Chinese diagnosis**
Pale	Spleen qi deficiency (blood deficiency)
Strongly drawn in, especially on the left side	Liver qi constraint

Fig. 2.4.1.3
Female
38 years old

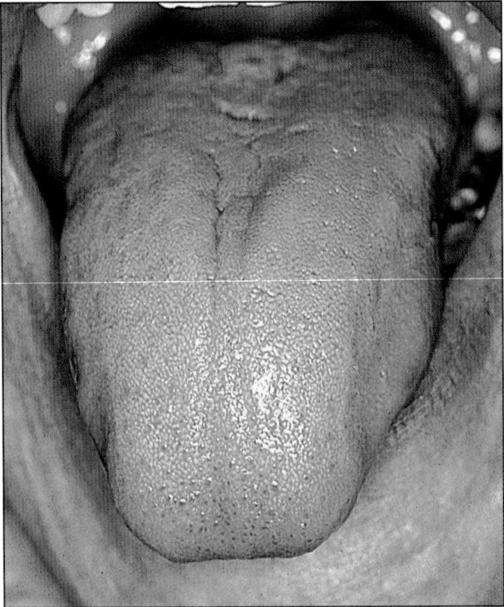

Symptoms

Weight loss
Fatigue
Swollen axillary lymph nodes
Pain under the right hypochondrium

Western diagnosis

Bilateral breast cancer*
Liver metastases

Background to disease

Suppressed anger
Overwork

**Patient died one year after this photo was taken.*

2.4.2 Uneven Sides of the Tongue, or Swollen on Half of the Tongue

The nutritive qi flows with the blood. Together they nourish the organs, muscles, tendons, and sinews and circulate and fill the channels and collaterals. Qi and blood deficiency presents not only with a pale tongue body, but also with uneven sides to the tongue (Fig. 2.4.2.1). In my experience this tongue sign represents impaired circulation of qi and blood in relation to the right or left half of the body. Again, the affected side of the tongue does not necessarily correspond to the affected side of the body.

The same interpretation obtains when only one-half of the tongue is swollen. In this case, the swelling shifts the midline of the tongue (Fig. 2.4.2.3). Symptoms associated with this type of tongue are weakness in one-half of the body, and lack of strength or stamina in one arm or leg. Occasionally, this type of tongue will be seen in atrophy disorders.

Tongue description

Pale

Uneven teeth marks on the left side

Light yellow, greasy coating

Chinese diagnosis

Spleen qi deficiency

Lack of nourishment in the channels and collaterals due to qi and blood deficiency

Acute food stagnation

Symptoms

Sharp pains in the left hip upon exertion
Lack of mobility of the hip joint
Extreme muscular tightness of the quadriceps
Acute stomachache
Loose stools

Western diagnosis

Bilateral degenerative joint disease of the hip

Background to disease

Excessive consumption of spicy foods
Lack of exercise
Mother took opiates during pregnancy

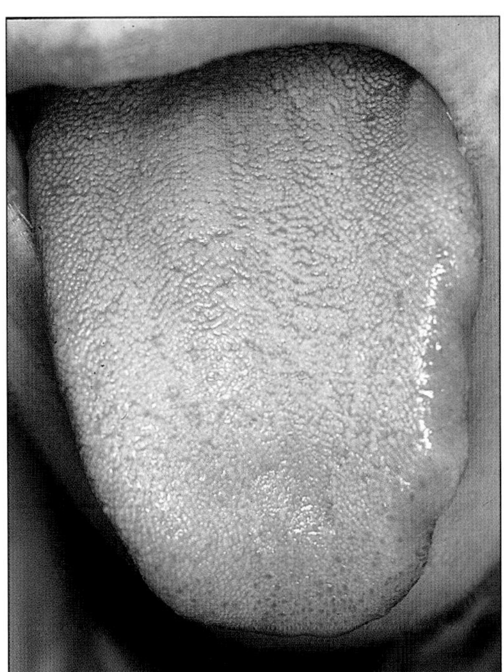

Fig. 2.4.2.1
Female
35 years old

Tongue description

Pale, slight teeth marks

Swollen center

Uneven sides to the tongue

Chinese diagnosis

Spleen yang deficiency (accumulation of dampness)

Phlegm obstructs the Stomach

Lack of nourishment in the channels and collaterals due to qi and blood deficiency

Symptoms

Tendency to catch colds
Fatigue
Blocked nasal passages or runny nose with copious white discharge
Fullness in the epigastrium
Feeling of weakness on the left side of the body
Feeling cold

Western diagnosis

None

Background to disease

Excessive physical exercise in connection with dancing competition
Irregular eating habits
Excessive consumption of dairy products and chocolate

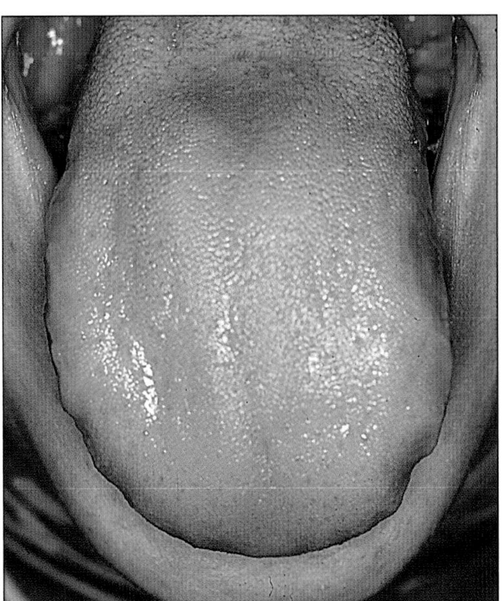

Fig. 2.4.2.2
Female
30 years old

Tongue description	**Chinese diagnosis**
Slightly pale	Spleen qi deficiency → blood deficiency
Slightly swollen edges	Spleen qi deficiency
Pale edges	Liver blood deficiency
Shifted midline	Malnourishment of the channels

Fig. 2.4.2.3
Female
64 years old

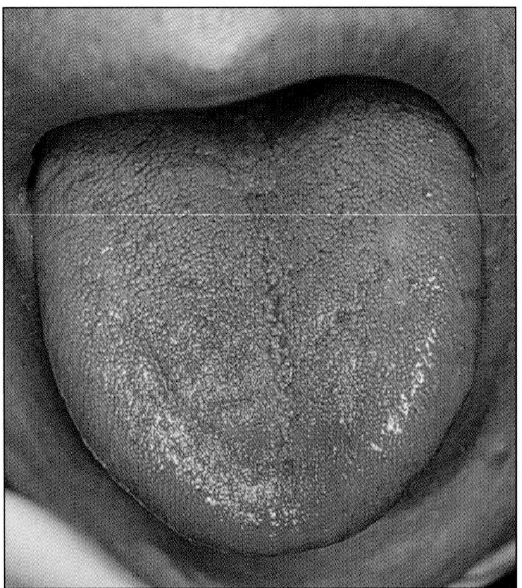

Symptoms

Muscle spasms, muscle weakness, difficulty walking
Tingling in the soles of the feet
Tiredness
Depressive moods

Western diagnosis

Psychosomatic disorder

Background to disease

Brooding and worrying

2.4.3 Swollen Tongue Sides

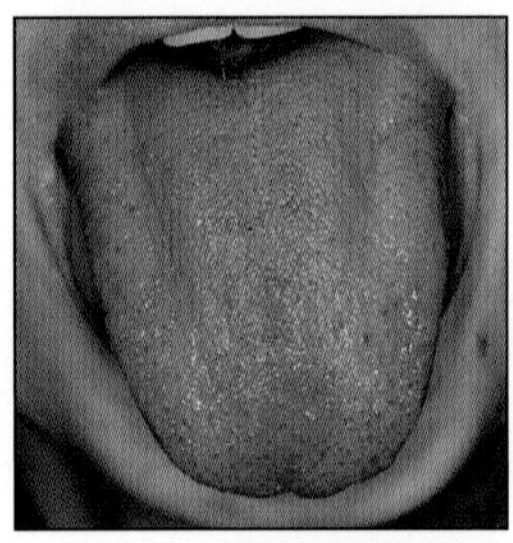

Fig. 7.1.2.1

A deficiency of Spleen qi and yang presents with a swollen tongue body as well as broad swelling on both sides of the middle third of the tongue. Note that the sides are swollen only in the middle of the tongue. This sign must not be confused with swollen sides that extend over the entire length of the tongue body (Fig. 7.1.2.1), which signifies a disharmony of the Liver.

Tongue description — **Chinese diagnosis**

Slightly pale, swollen, especially the middle part of the sides — Spleen qi deficiency (accumulation of dampness)

Slightly dry — Blood deficiency

Depression at the root — Essence deficiency

Symptoms

Migraines since 9 years of age
Migraines now preceding and following menstruation
Severe hair loss
Panic attacks since childhood

Western diagnosis

None

Background to disease

Family history of migraines
Overwork at home and on the job
Irregular eating habits

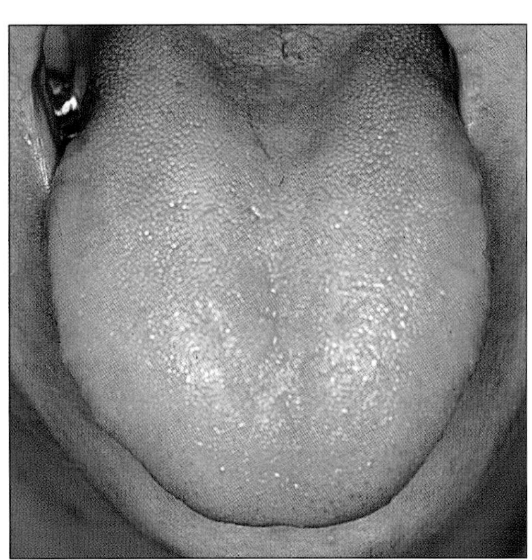

Fig. 2.4.3.1
Female
40 years old

Tongue description — **Chinese diagnosis**

Pale, slightly thin, middle part of sides swollen — Spleen qi and blood deficiency

White, thin, slippery coating — Accumulation of cold-dampness

Symptoms

Headaches
Pain at the nape of the neck
Fatigue
Weight gain

Western diagnosis

None

Background to disease

Excessive consumption of sweet foods
Excessive worrying

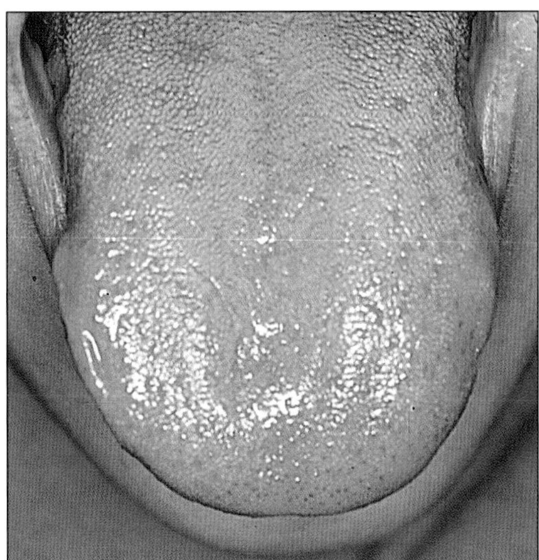

Fig. 2.4.3.2
Female
25 years old

2.5 Case Histories: Pale and Swollen tongues

The case histories serve to illustrate the application of tongue diagnosis in relation to other clinical signs and symptoms. The various functions of the Spleen are discussed and a corresponding treatment strategy is offered.

In general, a pale tongue body color, that is, one that lacks the normal reddish color, can result from either blood deficiency or qi that is too weak to transport the blood to the tongue body. A pale *and* swollen tongue body can be caused by either retention of dampness or blood deficiency associated with Spleen qi deficiency. As previously noted, Spleen qi deficiency may lead to retention of fluids that could develop into dampness. This accumulation of pathogenic yin enlarges the volume of the tongue body and gives it a swollen appearance. The greater the swelling of the tongue body, the greater the retention of dampness. However, swelling of the tongue body must always be considered in conjunction with the tongue body color. Spleen qi deficiency is only associated with retention of dampness when the tongue body is pale or pale red.

Characteristically, a pale, thin, and dry tongue body is synonymous with blood deficiency. However, a thin and dry tongue body may also originate from Kidney yin deficiency, although the tongue body color would be red and not pale.

Cases 2.5.1 and 2.5.2 are examples of the Spleen‘s important role in the production of blood, as a deficiency of Spleen qi can lead to Liver blood or Heart blood deficiency. If the Spleen function of containing the blood within the vessels[3] is weakened, bleeding (e.g., menstrual bleeding) may last longer and spotting may also occur. The Spleen helps to hold up the organs, ensuring that the inner organs remain in their proper place and that, for example, a prolapse of the uterus is avoided. Hence, sinking Spleen qi can be associated with spotting, painless hemorrhoids, or spider veins.

Fig. 2.5.1 shows a pale but only slightly swollen tongue body. In Fig. 2.5.2, the body of the tongue is also pale, but it displays a slight orange tinge, predominantly on the sides. This is an obvious sign of serious blood deficiency related to blood loss as well as to a deep-seated Spleen qi deficiency.

Tongue description	**Chinese diagnosis**
Slightly pale	Spleen qi deficiency → blood deficiency
Swollen	Retention of dampness
Whitish, thin coating	No pathology
Slightly reddish tip	Heat from deficiency in the Heart

Symptoms

Extreme, severe menstrual bleeding with clots
Pulling-down sensation in the lower abdomen
Water retention preceding menstruation
Excessive brooding, tiredness, and exhaustion

Western diagnosis

Menorrhagia, hemorrhoids

Background to disease

Excessive brooding and sadness
Unwanted abortion
Irregular eating habits

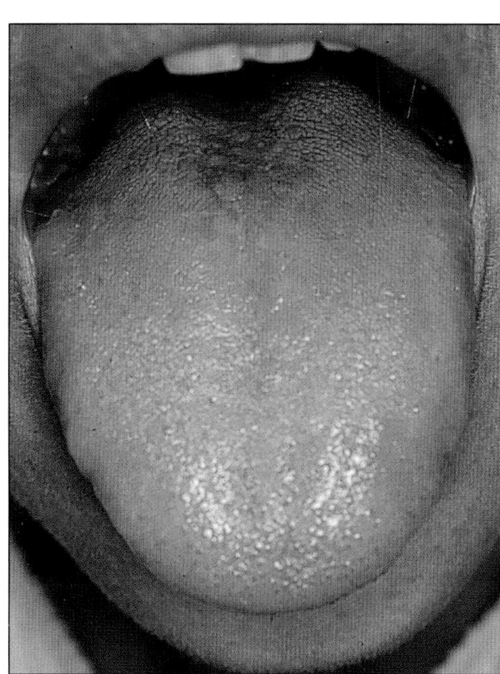

Fig. 2.5.1
Female
44 years old

CASE HISTORY Seven years ago this patient had an abortion, and since then she has suffered severe menstrual bleeding. With the onset of her period, she experienced pain in her lower abdomen, which she described as a 'pulling down' sensation spreading to the thighs. The second day of bleeding was extremely heavy and often incapacitating. The menstrual blood was red, thin, and odorless. The bleeding lasted about six days and occurred in a regular 28-day cycle. Menstruation caused her to feel tired and exhausted.

Since she began living with her new partner, her bleeding had become much worse. She had been extremely unhappy with her marriage as her husband was pathologically jealous. She felt hopeless and sad and was forever brooding about how to change her situation. Her pulse was thin and weak.

Analysis. The tongue body reflects the good constitution of the patient. The shape of the tongue body, though slightly swollen, is of a good texture and has vitality. This corresponds with the impression that the patient gives: She radiates a sense of vitality despite the severe loss of blood and resulting tiredness.

The underlying Spleen qi deficiency, shown in the pale and swollen tongue body, is partly responsible for the severe bleeding and is central to the patient's pathomechanism. The patient's constant brooding and irregular eating habits have weakened her Spleen qi. The blood, therefore, is not being contained in the vessels, which is contributing to her heavy menstruation.

The loss of blood and underlying Spleen qi deficiency cause blood deficiency, reflected in the slight paleness of the tongue body. The odorless, thin consistency of the menstrual blood underlines this deficiency. The extreme blood loss exacerbates the patient's qi deficiency and adds to her exhaustion and tiredness. The pulling-down sensation, which spread to the thighs, points toward the sinking of Spleen qi (see below for a discussion of a second pattern that

Pathomechanism

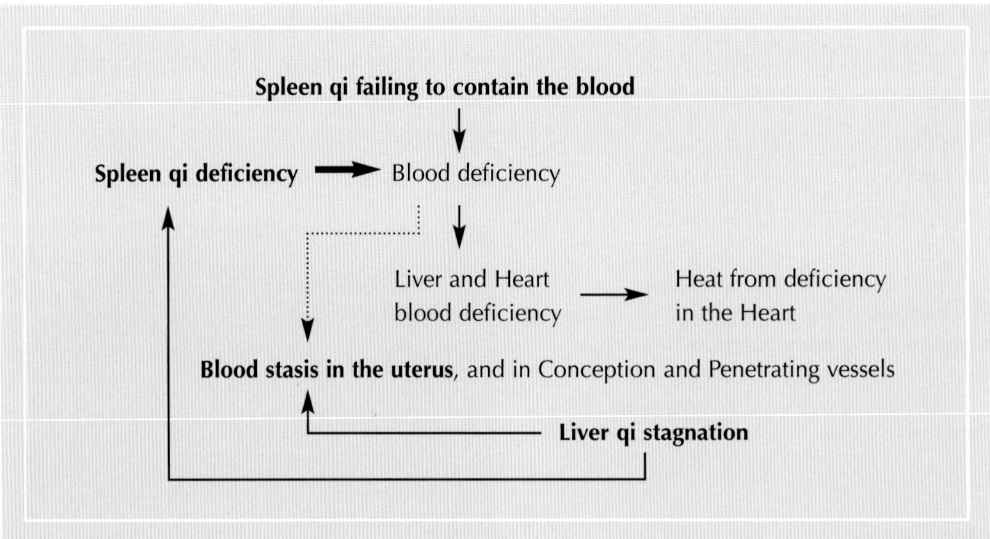

could explain the path taken). The thin pulse denotes blood deficiency, while its weakness reveals qi deficiency.

The swollen tongue body indicates retention of dampness caused by impairment of the transportive and transformative functions of the Spleen. Retention of dampness in this patient shows up as water retention shortly before the onset of menstruation.

The patient constantly feels that she cannot change her living situation. Her emotional state leads to constraint in the free flow of Liver qi that, in turn, affects the Spleen and further weakens it. The constrained Liver qi inhibits the movement of blood to the uterus, and, together with the insufficient qi, contributes to the development of blood stasis in the uterus, as evidenced by the big clots in the menstrual blood.

The patient explained that her menstrual bleeding had become much worse since her abortion. Operations involving the uterus are known to cause qi stagnation and blood stasis in the uterus or lower abdomen. In this case, the operation may well have contributed to the qi stagnation and blood stasis in the Conception and Penetrating vessels. These extraordinary vessels are vitally important to the nourishment and healthy movement of blood to the uterus. Here, the stagnation in the Penetrating vessel is more pronounced than in the Conception vessel. The path of the pain, starting in the lower abdomen and radiating downward to the inner thigh, follows an internal branch of the Penetrating vessel, which begins at ST-30 (*qì chōng*) and travels along the inner aspect of the thigh down to the foot. The intensity and localization of the pain are further evidence of stagnation in the Penetrating vessel as well as sinking of the Spleen qi.

In clinical practice, severe menstrual bleeding is often attributed to heat in the blood (Fig. 9.2.5) rather than to weakness of the Spleen qi that is unable to contain the blood. In this case, however, the qualities of the menstrual blood (thin and odorless), as well as the findings of the tongue, point to Spleen deficiency. The entire body of the tongue is pale. The tip of the tongue is slightly reddish, signalling the beginning of heat from deficiency of the Heart caused by the underlying blood deficiency.

By contrast, the pattern of heat in the blood often presents with bright red, odorous, and quite thick menstrual blood. This pattern may also include, for example, symptoms of irritability or inner restlessness. Often a reddish tongue body, red tip, or red edges can be seen in this pattern. Here, however, the tongue does not reflect the development of heat in the blood.

Instead, in this case, because of the blood deficiency, the Heart and Liver have not received sufficient nourishment. Liver blood deficiency is accountable, especially, for the patient's indecisiveness and her lack of vision concerning her 'life situation.' The combined deficiency of Heart and Liver blood has given rise to sadness and a sense of hopelessness.

Treatment strategy. Strengthen the Spleen qi, regulate the Liver qi, nourish and regulate the blood, and stop menstrual bleeding.

The patient was prescribed a modified form of Tonify the Middle and Augment the Qi Decoction (*bǔ zhōng yì qì tāng*), and Sudden Smile Powder (*shī xiào sǎn*). After four months of treatment, the menstruation was regulated and had become lighter and painless.

Tongue description	**Chinese diagnosis**
Very pale	Spleen qi deficiency → blood deficiency
Swollen	Retention of dampness
Slightly orange-colored sides	Blood deficiency
Whitish, thin, slightly rootless coating	Stomach qi deficiency

Symptoms

Mood swings, sadness, irritability
Tiredness, little appetite
Protracted menstrual spotting
Occasional nightmares

Western diagnosis

None

Background to disease

Stillbirth 12 months prior
Four children, between 17 and 28 years of age

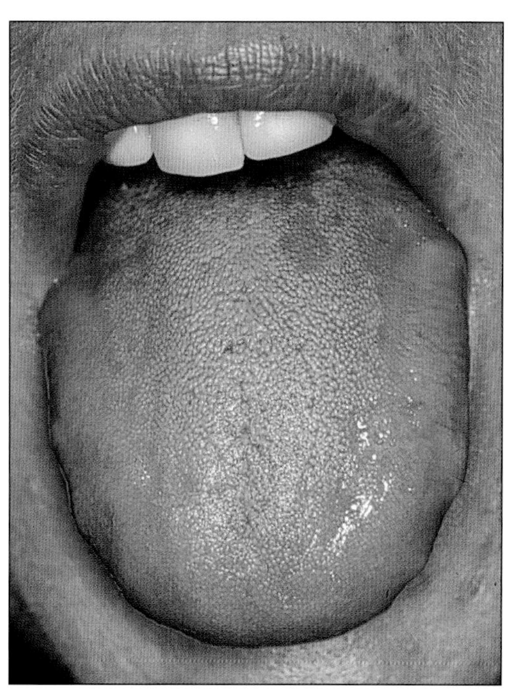

Fig. 2.5.2
Female
46 years old

CASE HISTORY Since the birth of her stillborn child 12 months before, this 46-year-old patient had been severely depressed. Her constant sadness was now turning into bouts of irritability. Since the birth she was always tired and her menstruation had changed. Before the pregnancy her cycle had been regular and her menstruation pain-free. Even though her cycle remained regular, the bleeding lasted for an extra five days and was characterized by spotting. The menstrual blood had become much thinner and lighter in color, and the bleeding lasted for a total of nine days.

Since the loss of her child, she experienced occasional nightmares, her appetite had decreased, and her facial pallor had become noticeably yellow and sallow. Her pulse was rough and slightly weak.

Analysis. Every pregnancy consumes essence, qi, and blood in order to nourish the fetus. The qi and blood decline in women after the age of 35. From the age of 42, the blood diminishes steadily, and the Penetrating vessel is not sufficiently filled.[4] Pregnancy after the age of 35 may seriously draw on the already diminished essence, and thereby weaken the qi and blood as well.

Pathomechanism

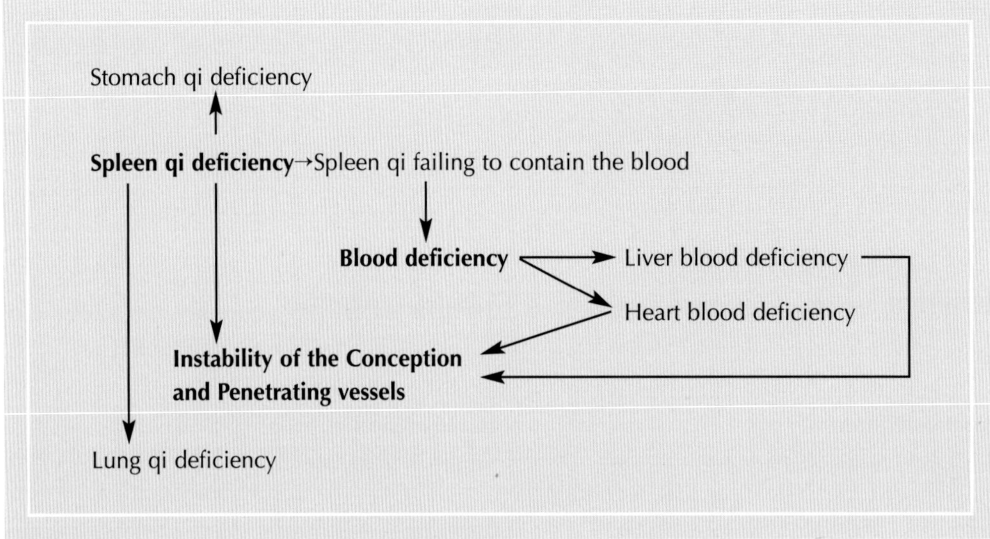

In this case, the pale and swollen tongue body reflects the lack of qi and blood. Especially noteworthy are the slightly orange sides and the intense paleness of the entire tongue body, both of which are important indications of severe blood deficiency. The deficiency of blood manifests here in the following indications:

- *Heart blood deficiency*. In human beings the Heart encompasses all the spiritual and mental faculties. Our mental powers also depend on the state of Heart blood: "Through which all things are conducted, that is the Heart."[5] If the spirit is not sufficiently nourished by Heart blood, the individual will suffer feelings of depression.
- *Liver blood deficiency*. The Liver is not storing enough blood, and this contributes to the instability of the Conception and Penetrating vessels. Because of the Liver blood deficiency, the Liver is not sufficiently pacified, adding to the development of Liver qi stagnation. This is experienced by the patient as occasional irritability.
- *Instability of the Conception and Penetrating vessels*. The instability of the two extraordinary vessels, as evidenced by the spotting, is caused by several factors: Spleen qi deficiency, Liver blood deficiency, the stillbirth of her child, and, most importantly, the patient's age.
- *Insufficient nourishment of the essence*. Over the long term, blood deficiency may result in insufficient nourishment of the essence. Blood and Kidney essence are interrelated since the essence helps with the production of blood. The Kidney essence of the patient was already weakened as a result of her previous four pregnancies.

Spleen qi deficiency, the stillbirth, and the light-colored, thin, and long-lasting menstrual bleeding are all causally related. The Spleen qi is too weak to contain the blood in the vessels, which manifests in constant spotting.

Since it takes some time for the tongue body to change its shape, a swollen tongue body reflects an accumulation of dampness. Here it is an indication that, even before her pregnancy, she suffered from Spleen qi deficiency. The presence of Spleen qi deficiency, as well as the accumulation of dampness, can also be deduced from her pale-yellow facial color.[6] The insufficient transformation of ingested food and the accumulation of dampness led to her lack of appetite. The long-standing Spleen qi deficiency also led to Stomach qi deficiency, which exacerbated the lack of appetite.

The Spleen qi deficiency, which was aggravated by the pregnancy and stillbirth, is responsible for the patient's tiredness. Long-standing and deep sorrow injures the Lung qi. Because the Spleen is weak, it has failed to sufficiently nourish its 'child', and thereby aggravated the pre-existing Lung qi deficiency. This intensifies the tiredness.

The Lungs, which are "the place of the corporeal soul (*pò*),"[7] are responsible for dream activity and hence the nightmares of the patient. *Basic Questions* observes: "With a lack of qi and retracting qi, man dreams of abstruse things; it can lead to complete confusion."[8]

The tongue coating is unremarkable, except for a small peeled-off area in the posterior third of the tongue, which indicates the onset of Stomach qi deficiency caused by the long-standing Spleen qi deficiency. However, because the remainder of the tongue body has a coating, this sign is not considered significant.

Treatment strategy. Strengthen the Spleen, Stomach, and Lung qi, nourish the blood, and stabilize the Conception and Penetrating vessels.

Stabilize the Penetrating Decoction (*gù chōng tāng*) was prescribed. This decoction worked quickly as the patient's next menstruation had no spotting and she felt much stronger. She then took Restore the Spleen Decoction (*guī pí tāng*) in the form of tablets for three months. By this time she felt much stronger and more balanced. In addition, the tongue body color appeared less pale after this course of treatment.

The tongue body portrayed in Fig. 2.5.3 is quite pale, wide, and swollen, which is mainly confined to the sides of the tongue. The tongue body reflects retention of dampness and its appearance indicates that the Spleen qi deficiency is more extensive. The Spleen function of lifting the 'clear yang' is impaired. Therefore a person may experience fatigue, epigastric fullness, or loose stools.

Tongue description

Very pale
Swollen with slight teeth marks
Small cracks in the center

Chinese diagnosis

Spleen qi deficiency → blood deficiency
Retention of dampness
Stomach qi deficiency

Symptoms

Hair loss, tiredness, dry skin
Soft, odorless stools
Strong menstrual bleeding
Anxiety

Western diagnosis

Iron deficiency anemia

Background to disease

Condition began after infection with salmonella bacteria two years prior
Overwork

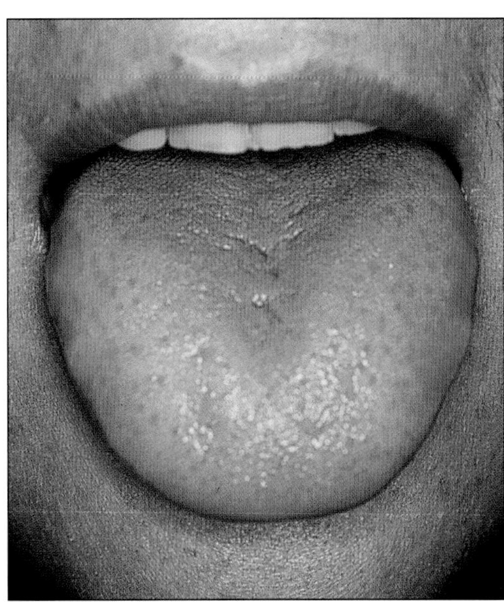

Fig. 2.5.3
Female
25 years old

CASE HISTORY This 25-year-old student held down two jobs in order to finance her studies. She felt constantly tired and stressed. Two years previously, a salmonella infection was initially treated with antibiotics, which resulted in diarrhea. Her stools were soft and odorless, and she had two bowel movements per day. Her diet was balanced, and her appetite and thirst were normal.

Her menstrual bleeding, which was red with no clots, was so heavy that it caused anemia. Over a period of time, the menstruation had exhausted her.

For months she had suffered from hair loss. Anxiety inhibited her, and her inner restlessness drained her. She felt constantly on the verge of a breakdown. Her pulse was deep and weak.

Analysis. The pale, swollen tongue body and teeth marks are characteristic of Spleen qi deficiency. This accounts for her tiredness, strong menstrual bleeding, and diarrhea.

The deficiency of Spleen qi has affected its ability to transform fluids. The resulting dampness sinks downward and causes loose stools. The ability of the Spleen to supply food qi, which is ultimately transformed into nutritive qi, is also impaired, and this manifests as tiredness.

The Spleen's function of containing the blood is also weakened here and leads to heavy bleeding. The monthly menses exacerbate the lack of qi and blood, resulting in increased tiredness after menstruation. The blood deficiency is responsible for the hair loss, and the patient's dry skin is the result of insufficient moistening by the deficient blood.

The Heart, in particular, relies on a sufficient supply of blood since blood provides the material basis for the spirit (*shén*). Thus, Heart blood deficiency manifests in mild depressive moods and insomnia, but also in anxiety accompanied by restlessness.[9] The pale tongue body, especially the pale anterior third of the tongue, reflects Heart blood deficiency. This, together with the patient's feeling of hopelessness, are indicative of Spleen qi deficiency and the ensuing Heart blood deficiency. If the Spleen qi is chronically weakened, a prolapse or sinking sensation may manifest on a physical level, while the fear of an inner breakdown may appear on the psychological level.

The body of the tongue shows no heat signs at all, but it accurately reflects the qi and blood deficiency. The prognosis is favorable as the tongue shows vitality and the patient is young.

Treatment strategy. Strengthen the Spleen qi and nourish the Heart blood.

The patient was advised to reduce her working hours and to eat a strengthening soup and warm foods on a regular basis. Further, she had five acupuncture treatments that were aimed at strengthening the Spleen qi and nourishing the Heart blood. Opening the Yin Linking (*yin wei*) vessel with the addition of KI-9 (*zhú bīn*) improved her mood considerably. Using a tonifying method, the following points were subsequently needled:

SP-4 (*gōng sūn*)	Strengthens the Spleen and calms the spirit
ST-36 (*zú sān lǐ*)	Strengthens the qi and blood

Pathomechanism

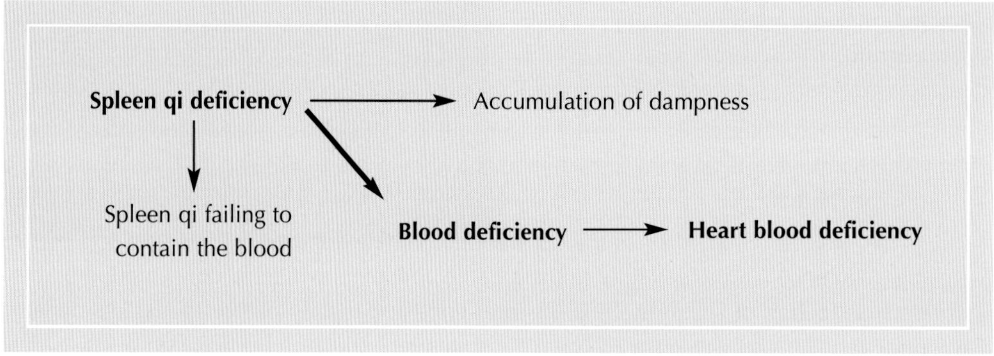

CV-4 (*guān yuán*)	Nourishes the source qi and Spleen qi and benefits the uterus
CV-6 (*qì hǎi*)	Strengthens the qi and blood

The diarrhea improved after tonifying SP-6 (*sān yīn jiāo*) and draining SP-9 (*yīn líng quán*). This pair of points is perfect for strengthening the Spleen and eliminating dampness.

Fig. 2.5.1 shows a pale but only slightly swollen tongue body. By contrast, Fig. 2.5.4 shows an extremely swollen tongue body. In the former case, the slight swelling of the tongue body suggests that the developing pathology is not dominated by internal dampness. Indeed, the tongue body shape and color deviate only slightly from a normal tongue, which suggests a good prognosis. By contrast, the tongue body of the patient in Fig. 2.5.4 is extremely pale and very swollen. This large swelling can be attributed to impairment of the function of the Spleen qi and yang, resulting in insufficient transformation of fluids in the body. The extreme swelling and pale color indicate a severe illness as well as the exhaustion of yang, which is too weak to transport the blood to the tongue. The degree of paleness and swelling of the tongue body denote a weakening of the Yang.

Tongue description	**Chinese diagnosis**
Very pale and swollen	Spleen qi and yang deficiency → retention of dampness
Yellow coating at the root	Retention of damp-heat in the Large Intestine

Symptoms

Physical weakness, muscle weakness
Tiredness, flatulence, bloating, bland taste in the mouth, belching, soft stools
Occasional feeling of pressure under the ribs
Tendency to catch colds
Depressive moods

Western diagnosis

Chronic hepatitis B

Background to disease

Viral infection through coitus
Overexertion

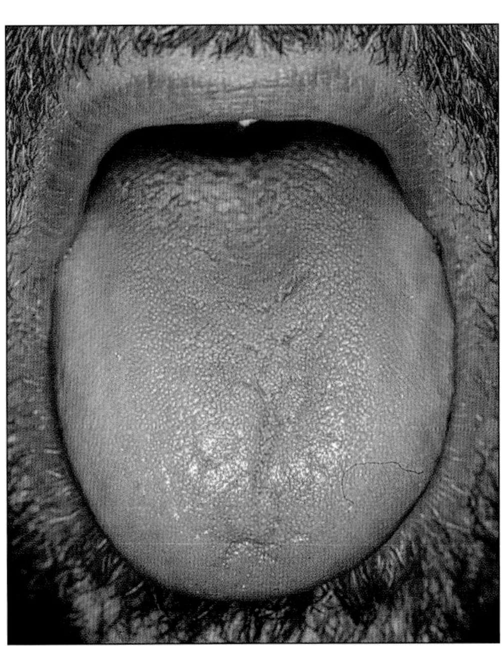

Fig. 2.5.4
Male
50 years old

CASE HISTORY This patient, a professional dancer, was infected with the hepatitis B virus 15 years previously. This resulted in an elevation of his liver enzymes, which has continued. The viral load was much increased. A liver biopsy confirmed the beginning of fibrocystic change.

The patient constantly felt sick and was depressed by his physical weakness and persistent tiredness. His numerous dancing performances added to his exhaustion. He rested as much as his job permitted.

His diet was very limited since the consumption of fatty foods and dairy products caused belching, flatulence, and a feeling of fullness in the abdomen, while the consumption of meat increased his feeling of sickness. Thus, his diet consisted mainly of raw foods. His appetite was good, and his thirst was normal. The patient was very thin, and his facial color was a little yellowish. He gave the impression of being both exhausted and depressed. His pulse was very deep, weak, and thin.

Analysis. The vital energies of the patient were substantially injured by the hepatitis B virus. Since the onset of his illness 15 years earlier, he complained of physical weakness and digestive problems. The persistent viral activity may be taken as an indication of the long-standing presence and accumulation of heat toxins in the Liver, which contributed to the development of a pattern of blood stasis in the Liver. This manifested as a cirrhotic change in the liver cells. The occasional feeling of pressure under the ribs signifies constrained flow of Liver qi resulting in a pattern of blood stasis. The tongue, however, does not reflect the characteristic signs of materialized blood stasis, namely, a bluish discoloration of the tongue body or distended sublingual veins.

The tongue does, however, provide important indications of the pathomechanism and the differential diagnosis in this case. In clinical practice, patients infected with the hepatitis B or C virus mainly present with signs of damp-heat, which often obstruct the flow of Liver qi. In these cases, the tongue has a thick and yellow tongue coating.[10] Due to the chronic nature of the illness, the majority of these cases show injury to the yin, blood, and essence, which is often reflected in a red tongue body color. If the color is red and there are signs of blood stasis, the prognosis is often unfavorable. These tongue signs, in conjunction with the diagnosis of chronic hepatitis, often suggest that the yin and liver tissue have been damaged.

The tongue body of this patient, however, is very pale and extremely swollen, and only shows a coating in the posterior third. The existing Spleen qi and yang deficiency, which is severe and is responsible for the lack of strength in the patient, is clearly indicated in the pale and swollen tongue body. These tongue signs clearly illustrate that the developing heat is not very strong, which is confirmed by other symptoms. This implies that the progressive destruction of yin and tissue in this patient is slow, which suggests a more favorable prognosis (see below).

The swollen tongue body shape also indicates that a pattern of excess dampness has arisen as a result of the Spleen qi and yang deficiency. A diet of mainly raw foods has injured the

Pathomechanism

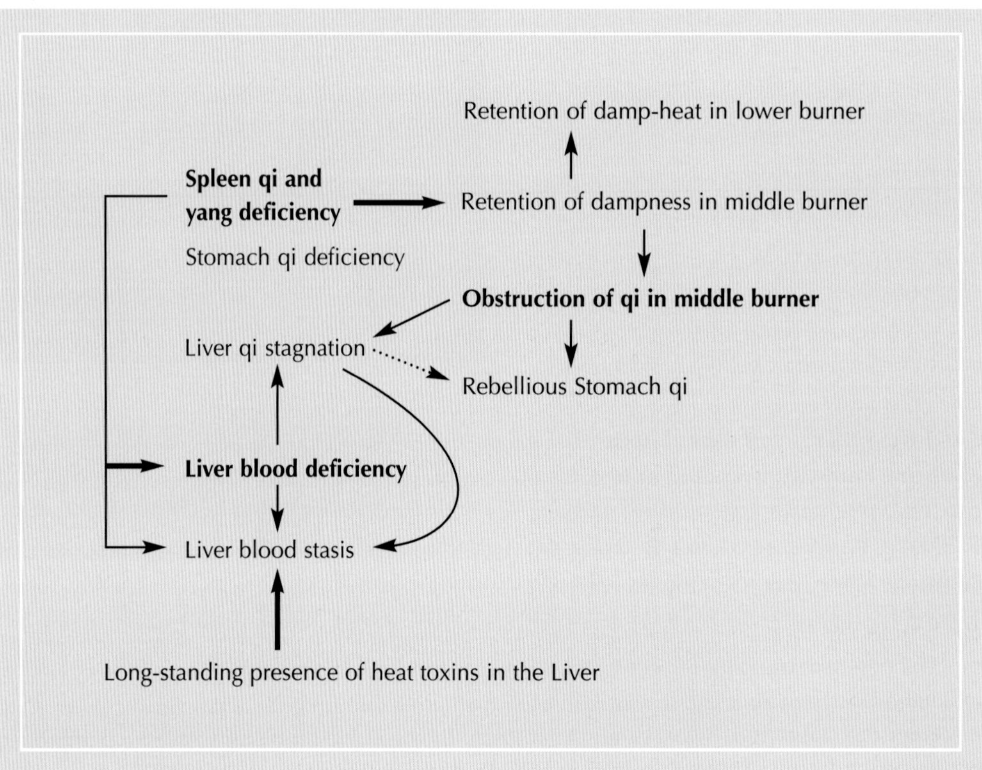

Spleen yang, resulting in an accumulation of fluids in the middle burner that is then changed into dampness. The soft stools are caused by sinking dampness, which, by its very nature, is heavy.

The dampness has also caused fullness in the middle burner, which obstructs the proper flow of Stomach qi, triggering the frequent belching. The distended abdomen, however, is not only a sign of this blockage, but also that of constrained Liver qi. This constraint is caused by the accumulation of dampness and the obstruction of the qi mechanism in the middle burner. When the patient eats foods that are difficult to digest like meat or fat the onset of belching and/or flatulence is immediate. This pathology is a clear example of both obstruction of the qi mechanism in the middle burner, due to dampness, and the serious impairment of the transportive and transformative functions of the Spleen qi and yang. Because of this impairment in the production and transportation of nutritive qi, the patient feels exhausted. The impaired flow of Spleen qi manifests in the pale, sallow facial color and bland taste in the mouth, which *Basic Questions* interprets as a sign of constrained qi in the abdomen caused by Spleen qi deficiency.[11] All the digestive disturbances are a result of this obstruction, which also impairs the lifting and ascending function of the Spleen, as well as the flow of Liver qi.

Generally, the patient's stools are loose and odorless; only after eating rich food does he notice a strong smell. Rich foods are difficult to digest and therefore stay longer in the digestive tract, particularly in the intestines, which may add to the development of damp-heat. In this case, the retention of damp-heat in the Large Intestine is minor, as reflected in the thin tongue coating. The occasionally smelly stools are the only sign indicative of this pattern.

Chronic Spleen qi deficiency often leads to a pattern of Liver blood deficiency, shown here in the extreme paleness of the tongue body. The Liver controls the sinews and tendons. Where there is Liver blood deficiency, the sinews and tendons will not be sufficiently nourished. If this occurs alongside an underlying Spleen qi deficiency, the patient will experience muscular weakness. Since the Spleen is responsible for circulation of the nutritive qi to the extremities,[12] the muscles and sinews will atrophy in cases of Spleen qi and yang deficiency. As *Basic Questions* puts it, "The Spleen rules the muscles and the flesh."[13] The weak, deep, and thin pulse confirms the lack of qi and blood.

As previously noted, the pattern of Liver blood stasis in this patient, reflected in the onset of cirrhotic change in the liver cells, has several causative factors:

- severe Spleen qi deficiency
- Liver blood deficiency
- Liver qi stagnation
- chronic retention of heat toxin

The pattern of blood stasis portends a dangerous development in the course of the illness. However, this has not yet materialized as symptoms in the patient. His complaints are essentially caused by the severe Spleen qi and yang deficiency, reflected in the tongue body. The degree of its paleness and swelling is very important in establishing the differential diagnosis.

Heat toxin is always present in chronic hepatitis B and can often trigger a feeling of malaise and exhaustion. If heat toxin remains in the body for too long, it consumes the qi and yin. Here, the normal (*zhēng*) qi is especially affected. The strength of this protective qi is impaired by both the chronic nature of the illness, which weakens the Kidneys, and the fact that the Spleen qi is failing to nourish the Lung qi. All of this contributes to the patient's disposition to catching cold.

Treatment strategy. The patient was treated for two years with Chinese herbs. The main aspect of the illness was the pattern of deficiency. Treatment consisted of strengthening the Spleen qi and yang, and regulating the qi mechanism of the middle burner by simultaneously eliminating the inner dampness and the remaining heat toxin. The digestive problems were much improved by the use of Pinellia Decoction to Drain the Epigastrium (*bàn xià xiè xīn tāng*).

After two years of treatment, the liver enzymes had been normalized. The viral activity, however, had only slightly decreased. The patient was much stronger and was not as exhausted as before. He rarely had colds, and experienced digestive problems only after eating fatty foods. Eight years later the patient feels fine. He has no digestive problems anymore; he reported weight gain and no increase of the liver enzymes.

Fig. 2.5.5. presents special tongue signs. The uneven sides to the tongue as well as the shifted midline signal possible obstruction of the channels and muscles by an underlying Spleen qi deficiency

Tongue description	**Chinese diagnosis**
Pale	Spleen qi deficiency → blood deficiency
Slightly swollen and uneven edges	Malnourishment of the channels
Yellow, thin coating at the root	No pathology

Fig. 2.5.5
Female
41 years old

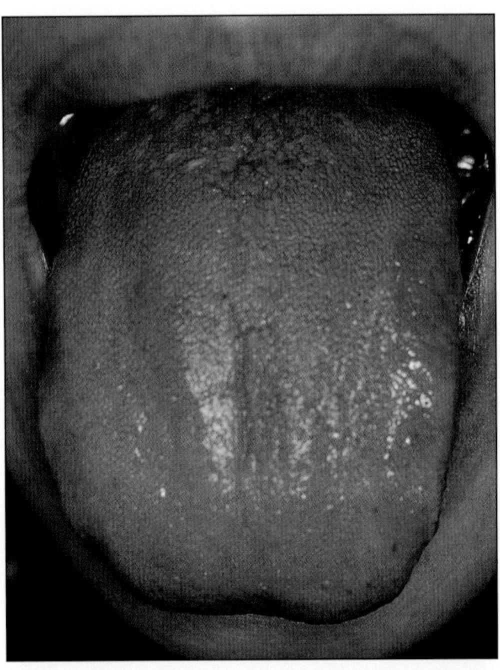

Symptoms

Difficulty walking, occasional numbness and paralysis of the left leg
Backache
Tiredness

Western diagnosis

Spina bifida

Background to disease

Congenital illness
Overexertion

CASE HISTORY The patient, a 41-year-old secretary, had been unaware of her bad posture for years, and this resulted in left-sided pain. At the age of six she was diagnosed with spina bifida. In her mid-thirties the left leg became increasingly numb, resulting in occasional bouts of mild paralysis. There was no clear pattern to the appearance of the symptoms, but the patient felt that the numbness and paralysis occurred more when she was under either mental or physical stress. She also had a dull, deep backache in the lumbar region, which could not be attributed to the weather, but which could be brought on by exhaustion. There were no other symptoms, and the patient otherwise enjoyed her life. Her pulse was tight, thin, and weak.

Analysis. The uneven sides to the tongue are obvious and are significant. In my experience, this tongue sign develops only after a chronic illness or traumatic injury that causes a one-sided body ache or weakness in the extremities. Uneven sides to the tongue are often an indication of insufficient nourishment in the channels, muscles, sinews, and tendons caused by underlying qi and blood deficiency.[14] In this particular case, the uneven sides are deemed

Pathomechanism

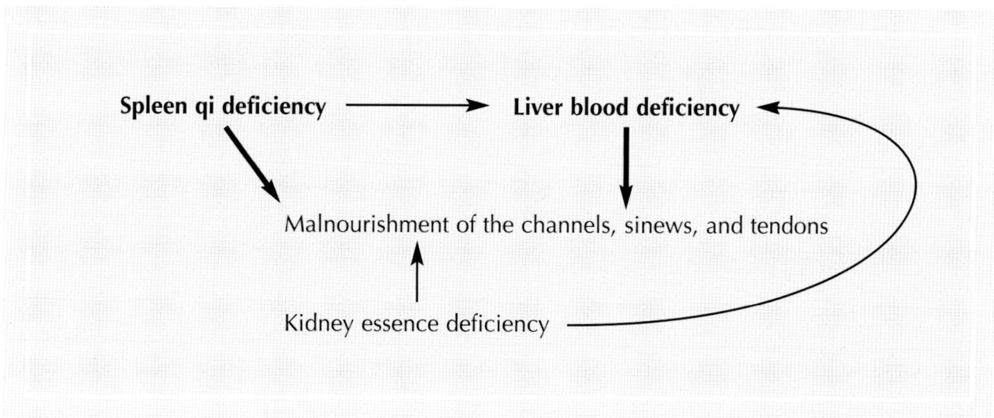

to be a constitutional sign. Therefore, the prognosis for a positive outcome is not favorable.

The patient has spina bifida, which Chinese medicine describes as an atrophy disorder stemming from weakness of the Kidney essence. The onset of numbness and paralysis occurred when the patient was in her mid-thirties. The pathomechanism centers on two factors:

- the congenital illness
- the reduction of qi and blood in the yang brightness channels

The extraordinary vessels also play an important role in the pathology of this patient since they transport Kidney essence to the different regions and tissues of the body.

The congenital weakness of Kidney essence has, in this case, affected the Governing vessel and resulted in undernourishment of the spine. The Girdle vessel is also involved since, as a result of its (inner) pathways, it enfolds the channels of the Stomach, Kidney, and Spleen as well as the Penetrating and Conception vessels. When the energy in the yang brightness channels is weak, the Penetrating vessel and aforementioned channels suffer from a lack of nutritive qi reaching the legs, leading to an overly loose Girdle vessel. "The Girdle vessel is not able to control [the other channels] because the Stomach channel is depleted. The outcome is atrophy and weakness of the leg muscles."[15] In women over the age of 35, there is a reduction in the qi and blood in the yang brightness channels (i.e., they are insufficiently fed),[16] which, together with the Penetrating vessel, are responsible for providing nourishment to the sinews, bones, and muscles.[17] Symptoms such as paralysis and/or difficulty in walking result from this energetic weakness. The Penetrating vessel is especially important, since it joins the pre- and postnatal essence.

In this case, only one side of the tongue body is noticeably swollen. A pale tongue body in conjunction with uneven sides indicates that the underlying Spleen qi deficiency has affected only the channels and muscles, but not the organs. Here, as a result of the deficiency, the nutritive qi and blood are depleted. Hence they cannot contribute to the nourishment of the muscles and flesh, which manifests in occasional feelings of numbness and paralysis.[18]

The sinew channel of the Spleen spreads in the chest, and from there, a branch adheres to the spine, thus adding to the supply of qi and blood. Consequently, Spleen qi deficiency can contribute to weakness and stiffness in the spine, especially if the deficiency is intensified by emptiness of the Governing vessel, evidenced here in the deficient nature of her back pains they are dull and deep and can be triggered by exhaustion.

Treatment strategy. Strengthen the Spleen, nourish the blood, regulate the yang brightness channels and the Governing and Girdle vessels.

The patient refused Chinese herbs and was treated with acupuncture alone. After 10 sessions, there was no improvement.

2.6 Case Histories: Pale and Swollen Tongues with a Depression at Their Root

The following case histories all present with pale, swollen tongue bodies with a depression or contraction at the root of the tongue. These tongue signs reflect a disturbance in the relationship between the Kidneys and the Spleen, and thus between pre- and postnatal essence.

The root of the tongue body reflects the condition of the Kidneys. A depression at the root of the tongue often mirrors a deficiency of essence, a 'lack of material' to replenish the root of the tongue. The same interpretation is valid for a contracted root (Figs. 2.6.1 and 2.6.2).

Patients exhibiting either of these tongue signs often have a weak constitution, which manifests as deep exhaustion (Figs. 2.6.1 and 2.6.2). Kidney essence deficiency can result in several different signs: tendency to catch colds, forgetfulness and lack of concentration (Fig. 2.6.2), or hair loss.

The dynamic and warming power of the gate of vitality (*mìng mén*) is very important in initiating all the processes of transformation in both the

- Spleen and middle burner, where the transformation of ingested food occurs
- Kidney and lower burner, where the transformation of turbid fluids occurs.

If, over a period of time, there is insufficient transformation of ingested food and drink, fluids accumulate and will eventually take the form of dampness. This pathological process will change the shape of the tongue body, resulting in pronounced swelling and increased wetness of the entire tongue body. The health of the yang corresponds to the degree of transformation and transportation of the fluids. As a rule, the extent of yang deficiency can be deduced from the degree of swelling of the tongue body (Fig. 2.6.1).

Pronounced qi and yang deficiency will lack the strength to transport sufficient blood to the tongue, and will result in a pale tongue body. Extreme paleness of the tongue body, as in Figs. 2.6.1 and 2.6.2, signifies yang deficiency, especially if accompanied by wetness (not present in these two cases).

Tongue description	**Chinese diagnosis**
Very pale, very swollen	Spleen and Kidney yang deficiency → accumulation of dampness → phlegm
Depression at the root	Kidney essence deficiency
Yellow, thin coating at the root	No pathology

Symptoms

Exhaustion, heavy sensation in the body
Soft, odorless stools, distended abdomen, dry mouth
Tinnitus, inability to concentrate

Western diagnosis

Chronic diarrhea of unknown origin

Background to disease

Overwork, irregular eating habits, too many raw foods

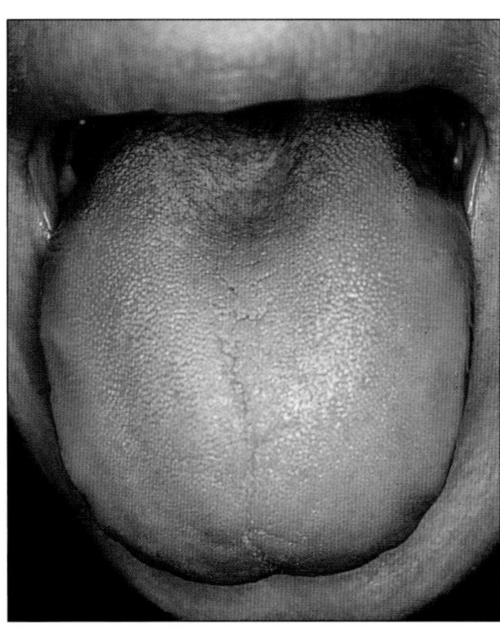

Fig. 2.6.1
Female
34 years old

CASE HISTORY For many years, this 34-year-old teacher suffered from loose, soft stools. She evacuated her bowels twice daily, mainly after breakfast, but her abdomen was extremely bloated. She often changed her dietary habits and had now become a vegetarian. In order to control her distended abdomen, she tried to eat as little as possible, although her appetite was good. While never feeling thirsty, she frequently suffered from dryness of the mouth.

For years she had felt tired, and after a day's work, would feel exhausted. A sensation of heaviness in the body, with a feeling of inner cold, accompanied the exhaustion. She experienced tinnitus, and had twice suffered a sudden loss of hearing, which she associated with the demands of work. Her pulse was deep and weak.

Analysis. The extremely swollen, pale tongue body reflects severe Spleen qi and yang deficiency and the onset of Kidney yang deficiency. Unformed stools, which occur in the early morning, are symptomatic of this type of deficiency. Irregular dietary habits, as well as excessive consumption of raw foods, have impaired the Spleen's transportive and transformative functions, which is compounded by injury to the yang qi of the middle burner (see below). If this pathomechanism continues over a long period of time, it will adversely affect the Kidney yang. In this patient, the onset of Kidney yang deficiency is reflected in her exhaustion and sense of inner cold.

The distended abdomen and accumulation of dampness are signs of blocked qi in the middle burner. The patient felt that only reduced food intake could relieve the bloating.

The patient's healthy appetite is considered a positive sign, as it shows that the Spleen still has vitality. However, the entire tongue body, especially its extreme swelling and the depression at the root, reflects the relatively weak constitution of the patient.

Although she never felt thirsty, the patient occasionally experienced some dryness of the mouth, and the body of the tongue did appear to be slightly dry. A pale and dry tongue body usually indicates a deficiency of blood. However, a pale and dry tongue can also reflect Kidney

Pathomechanism

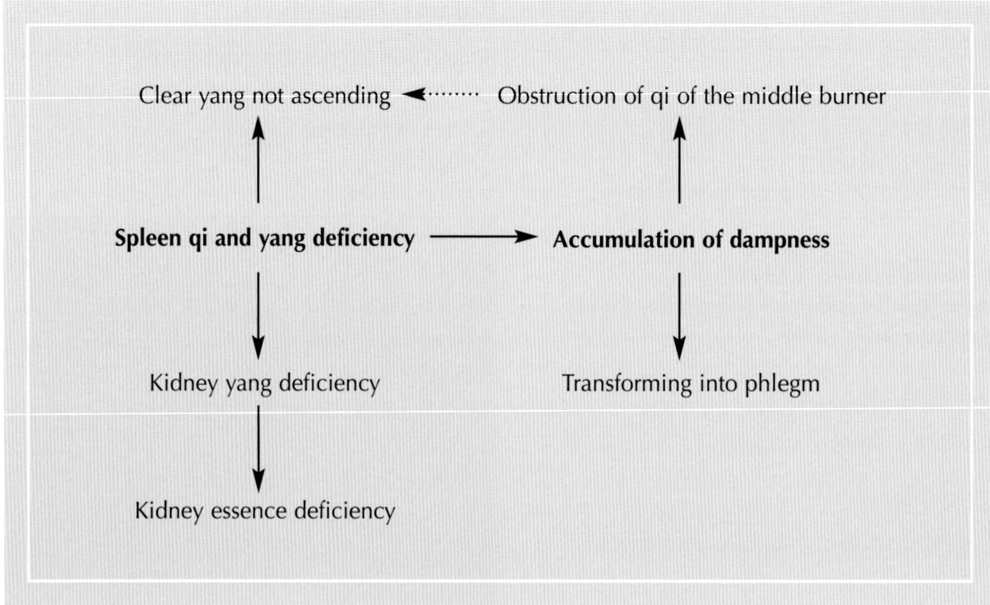

yang deficiency, especially if the tongue body is very swollen, which is the case here. When the Kidney yang is too weak, the upward transformation of fluids is impaired, resulting in fluids that do not reach the tongue and mouth; hence, the sense of dryness in the mouth and tongue. This symptom, together with the feeling of inner cold, soft stools early in the morning, and severe exhaustion confirmed the diagnosis of Kidney yang deficiency. Thus, the entire tongue with its pale, swollen, and slightly dry tongue body reflects the progression from Spleen yang deficiency toward Kidney yang deficiency. Because of the unusual nature of the latter tongue sign, it must be taken into account when formulating a treatment strategy.

When, as a result of long-standing Spleen qi deficiency, the fluids are not transformed, internal dampness will develop. In this case, some of the dampness collected in the muscles of the patient and produced the heavy sensation in the body.[19]

Sudden loss of hearing and tinnitus are often caused by ascending Liver yang or Liver fire, but in this case, neither the tongue body nor the pulse showed any sign of heat. The sudden loss of hearing occurred when the patient was under great physical or mental strain. Here, the weak Kidney essence and source qi reflected in the deep depression at the root of the tongue resulted in insufficient nourishment reaching the ears, leading to the short episodes of hearing loss and chronic tinnitus. In addition, the swelling of the tongue body should be noted. The large amount of swelling not only reflects the accumulation of dampness in the middle burner, but also its transformation into phlegm. The presence of phlegm prevents the clear yang from ascending, depriving the sensory organs of sufficient energy. When the clear yang is obstructed in this manner, the turbid qi becomes dominant. Here, it has led to a blockage of the ears, which contributed to the development of tinnitus.

Two patterns of deficiency are responsible for the lack of concentration: the impaired ascent of clear yang and the weakened Kidney essence. The Kidney essence fills the brain, and with improper nourishment, it will decrease one's ability to concentrate.

Treatment strategy. Strengthen the Spleen qi and yang, warm the Kidney yang, stop the diarrhea, and support the ears.

A modified form of Tonify the Middle and Augment the Qi Decoction (*bǔ zhōng yì qì tāng*) was prescribed. Alpiniae oxyphyllae Fructus (*yì zhì rén*) and Cinnamomi Cortex (*ròu guì*) were added to strengthen the Spleen and Kidney yang, and Acori tatarinowii Rhizoma (*shí chāng pǔ*) was added to open the ears.

After three months of treatment, the patient felt much stronger. She seldom had diarrhea, but the tinnitus had not improved. Six months later, the patient became pregnant. Both the pregnancy and birth were problem-free.

Tongue description	**Chinese diagnosis**
Very pale	Spleen qi and yang deficiency → blood deficiency
Swollen from the edges to the middle	Spleen qi deficiency
Contracted root	Kidney essence deficiency
Peeled, dry coating	Stomach qi and yin deficiency, onset of Kidney yin deficiency

Symptoms

Exhaustion, nausea, heartburn
Stomach pain and feeling of pressure, epigastric fullness, belching
Insomnia, sadness

Western diagnosis

Mammary gland carcinoma with lymph node involvement

Background to disease

Condition after chemo- and radiation therapy

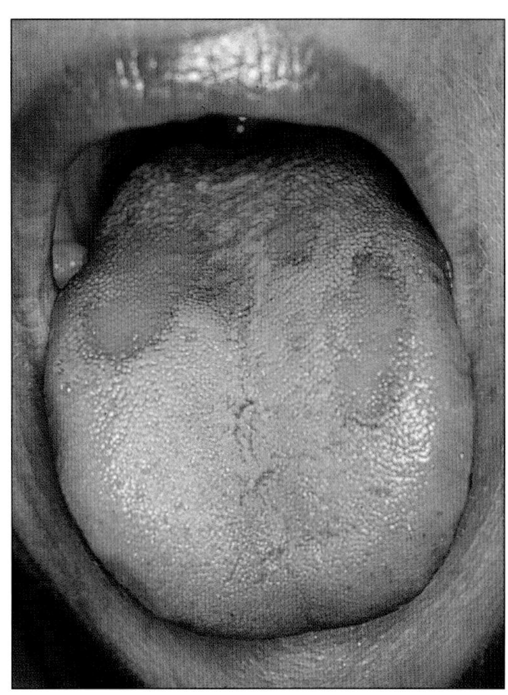

Fig. 2.6.2
Female
51 years old

CASE HISTORY Fifteen months prior, the patient had three cancerous lumps and twenty-one lymph nodes removed from her right breast. Since then she suffered from hot flushes and exhaustion. The hot flushes always occurred at night, interfering with her sleep, which aggravated her exhaustion.

Nine months prior, following a course of chemotherapy, the patient still had not recovered. She was tired and exhausted. Radiation therapy made her even more exhausted. She lacked a zest for life and was noticeably bitter and depressed.

Since the chemotherapy, the patient complained of stomachache and cramps. Occasionally, the cramps were so severe that the pain radiated to her shoulder. The symptoms almost always began after eating, when she also experienced frequent belching and heartburn. She often felt nauseous throughout the day. The nausea was not linked to eating, as it occurred randomly and had no recognizable pattern. Her appetite changed constantly: Sometimes she was ravenously hungry, and at other times completely lost her appetite. Her thirst and bowel movements were normal, and her pulse was deep and weak.

Analysis. The patient's tongue body reflects the energetic effects of the chemotherapy. Most important is the marked paleness of the tongue body, which indicates severe Spleen qi deficiency with ensuing blood deficiency. The peeled, dry tongue coating signals the injury to the fluids of the Stomach and to the Kidney yin. The root of the tongue is slightly contracted,

Pathomechanism

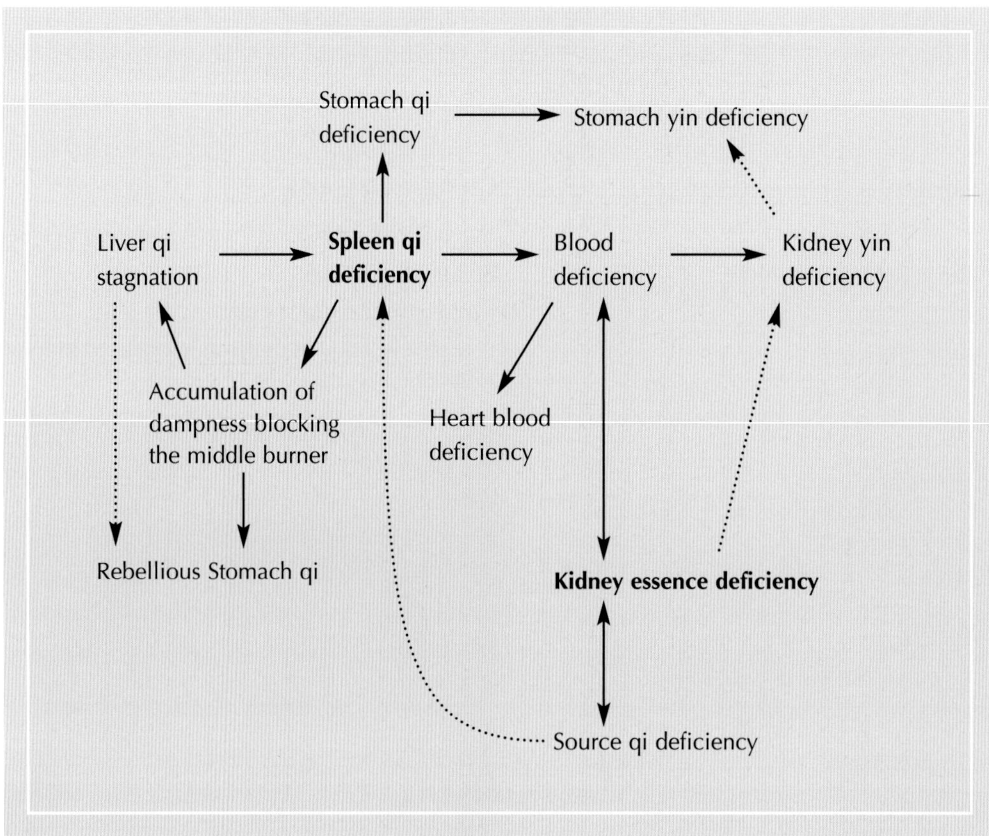

suggesting deficiency of Kidney essence. Overall, the tongue reflects the weakened constitution of the patient.

Chemotherapy affects people differently, depending on their constitution. The suppression of bone marrow activity generally reduces the production of (among other things) red and white blood cells. When toxic substances penetrate the bone marrow, they injure the marrow and also the blood. Radiation therapy acts like an external attack of heat toxin that injures the yin and fluids, which in turn causes dryness. All of this leaves patients feeling extremely fatigued.

In this case, the chemotherapy and radiation profoundly injured the postnatal essence, yin, and marrow,[20] which is built by the Kidney essence. Postnatal essence is closely related to the Spleen and Stomach, and is of paramount importance in the production of qi and blood. It also serves to replenish the Kidney essence.

Spleen qi deficiency, as well as diminished source qi, can result in a decline in the production of blood. The tongue body is dry. The pale and dry tongue body is an indication of serious blood deficiency (leading to yin deficiency) as well as a decline of the fluids in the Stomach. Both fail to adequately moisten the tongue. The ensuing Heart blood deficiency has led to insufficient nourishment of the spirit, as reflected in her insomnia and depressive moods. When this is accompanied by qi deficiency, the patient will show a lack of zest for life. The sadness as well as the Spleen qi deficiency have contributed to a deficiency of Lung qi. This pattern of deficiency compounds the tiredness of the patient.

The middle part of the tongue body is swollen, and the tongue body itself is very pale. These signs reflect an extreme weakness of Spleen qi, especially its ability to transform and transport. The accumulation of dampness, which occurs in the middle burner, obstructs the flow of Stomach qi. A passage in *Divine Pivot*[21] is apropos of this situation: "When clear and turbid [qi] are entangled with each other and [cause] restlessness in the Heart, then the patient is depressed, reticent, and withdrawn." This implies that entanglement of clear and turbid fluids and energies can affect the Heart. Perhaps this mechanism contributed to the patient's lack of drive and zest for life.

Nausea, heartburn, and belching are symptoms of rebellious Stomach qi. The blockage of the qi in the middle burner is caused by internally-accumulated dampness, which manifests here as epigastric fullness. Since the Stomach's ability to transform food is hampered, the food stagnates. Food stagnation is characterized by complaints that occur following eating. Stomach pains and occasional cramp-like sensations are here exacerbated by the Liver qi stagnation, which is the result of the patient's suppressed anger and bitterness.

The rootless coating of the tongue extends over a large area. This sign implies that blood, as part of the yin, is not sufficiently nourishing the yin and that the medical treatment has injured the fluids and yin of the Stomach.

The hot flushes and inability to sleep through the night are caused by the onset of Kidney yin deficiency, and can be attributed to the chemotherapy and radiation as well as the weakness of the postnatal essence and blood. Kidney yin deficiency is usually reflected in a red, dry tongue body or a red tongue body with a rootless or peeled coating. Here, it is the contracted root of the tongue and the peeled coating, despite the pale tongue body color, that suggest the onset of Kidney yin deficiency.

Treatment strategy. Strengthen the Spleen qi, nourish the fluids in the Stomach, the blood, and Kidney essence, promote the movement of qi in the middle burner, and reduce food stagnation.

Seven-Ingredient Powder with White Atractylodes (*qī wèi bái zhú sǎn*) was prescribed, with the addition of Astragali Radix (*huáng qí*) and Ganoderma (*líng zhī*). The digestive problems improved in a few weeks. Although the patient began to sleep better, her exhaustion was unchanged. She is continuing with the treatment and has started psychotherapy.

2.7 Spleen Yin Deficiency and Tongue Signs

Surprisingly, Spleen yin deficiency is discussed very little and has always played a secondary role in many of the different schools of Chinese medicine. This is all the more surprising since the other yin organs, which are also basically responsible for the storage and conservation of essences and fluids, commonly have specific pathologies attributed to their yin aspects. This omission may simply have arisen because Spleen qi and yang deficiency occur so readily in people. However, it is more likely a result of the influence of Li Dong-Yuan, author of the famous 13th-century book *Discussion of the Spleen and Stomach (Pi wei lun)*. Li and his followers strongly emphasized tonifying the Spleen qi and yang with warm, sweet foods and herbs. Nevertheless, there are other schools of thought which discuss in great detail the signs, symptoms, and treatment methods associated with pathologies of the Spleen yin.[22]

The yin of the Spleen has been important in Chinese medicine for some time. Consider, for example, the following passage from Ch. 8 of the *Divine Pivot:*[23]

> Nutritive qi is stored in the Spleen. ... It is the yin of the Spleen that forms the basis of the nutritive qi and blood. Stomach yin controls the body fluids and is regarded as the sea of fluids. The yin of the Spleen supports the production of blood and fluids, and thus has the ability to moisten and support Stomach yin.

Despite sharing many common symptoms, there are important differences between the Stomach and Spleen yin. Exhaustion of the Spleen yin develops very slowly, often over the course of years or during a serious illness. By contrast, Stomach yin deficiency can develop quite quickly; for example, through an externally-contracted illness with fever and sweating, or through poor eating habits. Typical symptoms of Stomach yin exhaustion include dry mouth and throat, constipation, stomach pains, and thirst that can only be sated in small sips.

Spleen qi deficiency that has existed for a long time serves as the foundation for Spleen yin deficiency. Because of this, symptoms will manifest primarily as digestive problems. Besides the well-known symptoms of Spleen qi deficiency (soft stools, lack of appetite, fatigue, weakness in the extremities), other symptoms that are specific to Spleen yin deficiency include dry lips, wasting or difficulty in gaining weight, and emaciation.[24]

Over a period of time, yin deficiency causes a loss of substance, which will manifest in the tongue as transverse cracks at the sides. If they appear in conjunction with a red tongue body and other symptoms just described, a diagnosis of Spleen yin deficiency would be justified.

Spleen and Stomach yin deficiency can also be responsible for the already described peeled tongue coating. In this case, the tongue is pale red or red, and shows an irregularly distributed coating. The peeled coating is shiny like a mirror and the tongue papillae in these areas are not visible (Fig. 4.1.4.4).

Tongue description	**Chinese diagnosis**
Slightly pale, thin	Spleen qi deficiency with blood deficiency
Pale, slightly curled-up edges	Liver blood deficiency, Liver qi constraint
Deep cracks at the sides	Long-standing Spleen qi deficiency

Symptoms

Severe mood swings
Depression
Exhaustion
Soft stools
Intense menstrual pains

Western diagnosis

Anorexia nervosa

Background to disease

Sexual abuse
Repressed emotions

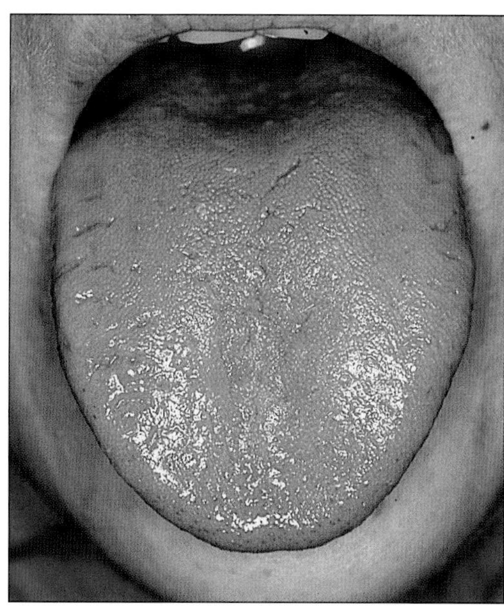

Fig. 2.7.1
Female
38 years old

Tongue description	**Chinese diagnosis**
Slightly pale, slightly thin	Spleen qi deficiency with blood deficiency
Thin, vertical crack at the center	Onset of fluid deficiency in the Stomach
Transverse cracks at the sides	Severe Spleen qi deficiency
Red points at the tip	Heat in the Heart

Symptoms

Pressure pain under the ribs
Depression
Constipation
Fatigue

Western diagnosis

Poisoning through pesticides

Background to disease

Pesticide poisoning

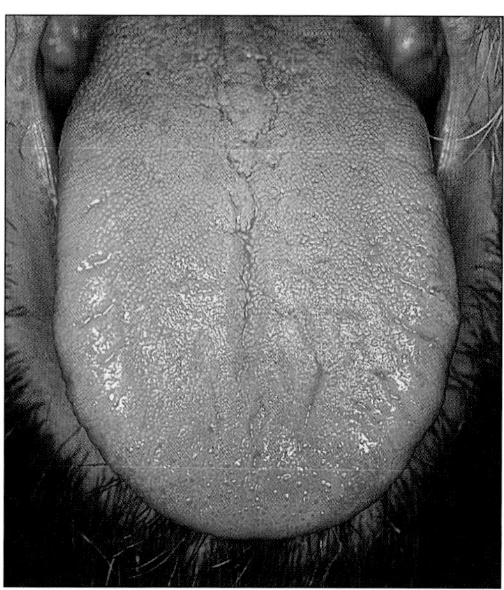

Fig. 2.7.2
Male
40 years old

Tongue description	**Chinese diagnosis**
Reddish, slightly swollen	Heat in the blood
Long vertical crack	Heat in the Heart
Cracks at the sides	Long-standing Spleen qi deficiency and onset of Spleen yin deficiency
Red spots at the side of the tongue	Ascending Liver yang

Fig. 2.7.3
Female
28 years old

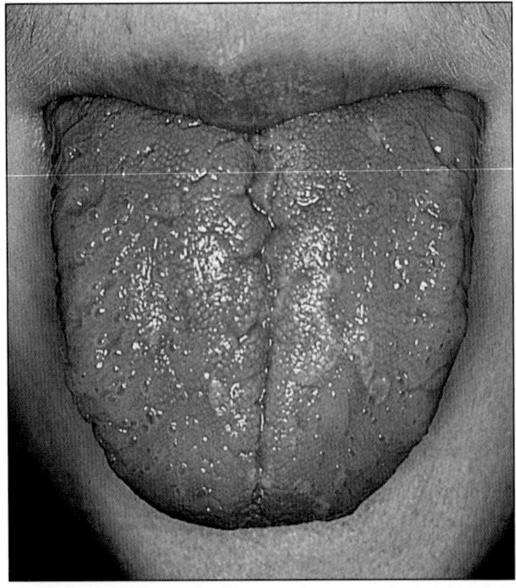

Symptoms

Severe migraines with the onset of menstruation
Shortened menstrual cycle (23 days) with profuse bleeding
Intense lower abdominal pain with menstrual bleeding
Severe thirst
Dry mouth
Inner restlessness

Western diagnosis

None

Background to disease

Irregular lifestyle
Alcohol and caffeine abuse
Overwork

Tongue description	**Chinese diagnosis**
Reddish	Normal
Deep transverse cracks at the sides	Long-standing Spleen qi and yin deficiency
Cracks in the anterior third	Lung yin deficiency
Curled-under tip	Heat from deficiency in the Heart
Slightly yellow coating without root	Accumulation of damp-heat in the lower burner, Stomach yin deficiency

Fig. 2.7.4
Female
78 years old

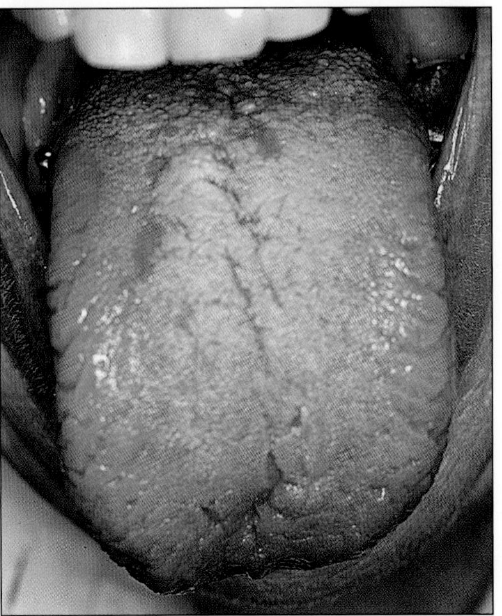

Symptoms

Intense pain and twitching of the left leg
Insomnia
Dizziness
Urgency of urination at night
Dry mouth
Cold hands and feet

Western diagnosis

Deafness
Irregular heartbeat

Background to disease

Shock during World War II (buried under rubble)

Endnotes

1 Frequent colds and flu must be considered within the context of weakening essence. It is often forgotten that the strength of the protective qi is not only dependent on the Lung qi but also on the Kidney yin and yang, the essence, and the source qi. The essence is responsible for the construction of the body while the source qi is vital in supplying the body with dynamic and warming qi. The source qi is a catalyzing force that underlies all energetic activity.

Kidney yang and the source qi supply the Bladder with qi in order to transform the pure part of the impure fluids. The transformed fluids flow to the skin and muscles and indirectly connect with the protective qi. If the Kidney yang is deficient, the fluids will not be transformed, resulting in malnourishment of the protective qi.

The distribution of the protective qi throughout the body is also influenced by the eight extraordinary vessels, especially the Governing, Conception, and Penetrating vessels, which partly act as a reservoir for the essence. The protective qi is thus rooted in the Kidneys, nourished by the essence, and supported in its circulation by the source qi. Frequent colds thus not only weaken the protective qi, they also affect the essence and source qi.

2 Unfortunately, while this is potentially a very important issue, the literature on the subject is limited.

3 Anonymous. *Nan-Ching, The Classic of Difficult Issues,* translated by Unschuld P. Berkeley: University of California Press, 1986: 417.

4 Anonymous. *Su wen* [Basic Questions], edited by He W-B et al. Beijing: China Medicine Science and Technology Press, 1996. See Ch. 1 for a description of a woman's seven-year cycle.

5 Anonymous. *Huang di nei jing ling shu yi shi* [Translation and Explanation of the Yellow Emperor's Inner Classic: Divine Pivot], edited by Nanjing College of Traditional Chinese Medicine, Traditional Chinese Medicine Department. Shanghai: Shanghai Science and Technology Press, 1997: 8:76.

6 *Basic Questions,* 22:140.

7 Ibid., 9:54.

8 Ibid., 80:513.

9 Maciocia G. *The Practice of Chinese Medicine.* Edinburgh: Churchill Livingstone 1994: See Ch. 9.

10 See Ch. 9 of this book.

11 *Basic Questions,* 10:62.

12 Ibid., 29:177.

13 Ibid., 44:249.

14 Ibid.

15 *Basic Questions,* 44:250.

16 Ibid., Ch. 1.

17 Ibid., 44:250.

18 Ibid., 34:199.

19 *Basic Questions,* 65:343.

20 In Chinese medicine it is thought that the Kidney essence serves as the basis for the formation of the bone marrow, among other things.

21 *Divine Pivot,* 34:238.

22 Clavey S. Spleen and Stomach yin deficiency: differentiation and treatment. *The Journal of Chinese Medicine* 1995,47:23-29.

23 See RenY-Q. *Huang di nei jing zhang ju suo yin.* Beijing: Peoples Medical Publishing House, 1986:291.

24 Clavey, ibid.

CHAPTER 3

Tongue Signs Associated with Kidney Disharmonies

This chapter focuses on tongue signs associated with Kidney yin deficiency. Tongue signs associated with Kidney yang deficiency are discussed in Ch. 2. It should be noted that a pale, swollen, wet tongue can occur in individuals who are either Spleen yang or Kidney yang deficient. The individual's symptoms must be investigated to distinguish between these two deficiencies.

3.1 Characteristics of Yin-Deficient Tongues

Everyone possesses a basic constitution that shapes and influences that individual. Assessing a patient's constitution is based on knowledge of the patient's previous illnesses and their course of development, as well as on observing the individual's 'being' or 'rhythm of life.' The constitution is also reflected in the face, pulse qualities, and tongue. In a person with a yang constitution the tongue is often reddish, long, and big, while with a yin constitution the tongue body tends to be pale and swollen. It is therefore sensible to take note of the tongue, especially its shape and consistency, when evaluating an individual's constitution.

The Kidneys house both yin and yang. Yin manifests in the body through the fluids, substance, and structural elements. Pure fluids and blood belong to the domain of yin. Yin nourishes and moistens all the tissues of the body. Each of the various yin organs controls and preserves specific aspects of yin. The nutritive qi, which nourishes the five yin organs and moistens the six yang organs, has its root in the Spleen. Blood is stored in the Liver and produced by the Heart. The Lungs distribute fluids, which originate in the Spleen and Kidneys, and nourish the skin and hair. However, the body's yin is rooted in the Kidneys.

Qi governs the movement of blood and fluids and transports them to the tongue. Thus, the tongue body color, shape, and moisture always reflect the condition of qi and yin in each of the yin organs. Malnourishment of the yin is reflected in the tongue body

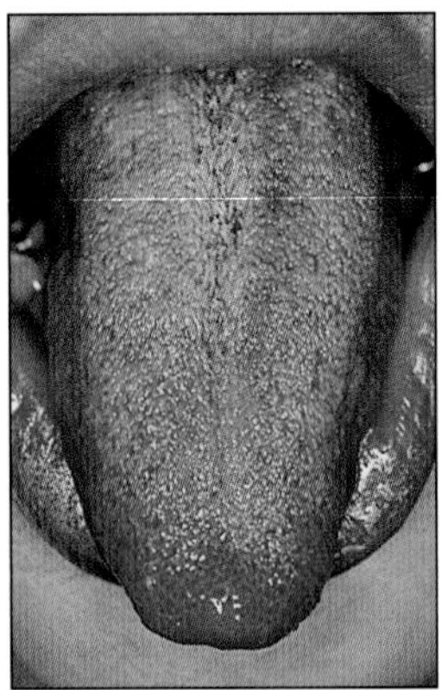

Fig. 6.2.1

color, shape, as well as consistency and nature of the tongue coating, for example, a red, dry, stiff, or (in severe cases) even shrunken tongue body, a red tongue body without or peeled coating, and/or cracks in the tongue body (Fig. 6.2.1).

Kidney yin and essence nourish each other and are mutually dependent, especially in maintaining the body structures and the quality of the fluids. The fluids and blood are yin in nature. Together, they supply the tongue with sufficient 'substantive energy' so that the tongue body achieves its normal volume, elasticity (softness), a fresh reddish color, and moisture. An excess of yin, however, for instance in the form of dampness, inevitably leads to a swollen tongue body.

3.2 Red Tongues with Kidney Yin Deficiency

A common result of Kidney yin deficiency is the development of heat from deficiency, which, over a long period of time, will dry the fluids and injure the blood. This implies that the blood is not nourished and moistened sufficiently by the clear fluids (*jīn* fluids). As a result the tongue appears red and dry, often only covered with little coating. The stronger the heat, the greater the injury to the blood and fluids, which in turn leads to a redder and drier tongue body.[1] Symptoms associated with Kidney yin deficiency with deficient heat are tinnitus, night sweats, hot palms and soles, dry mouth, and a flushed face.

In cases of constrained heat, smoldering fire or fire toxin can develop, the tongue body will be of an extremely red color and will be covered with a yellow coating, which constitutes an important difference to a tongue denoting Kidney yin deficiency. Symptoms associated with this excessive disorder include fever, irritability, a dry mouth and throat, thirst, and mouth ulcers. In order to evaluate the origin, degree, and intensity of the heat or fire and the resulting injury to the yin and fluids, the practitioner should observe not only the intensity of the red discoloration on the tongue body, but also its shape and coating.

Heat generated by deficient yin that smolders for a long time in the body can become uncontrollable. This will inevitably affect the essence. This energetic deficiency, which can develop over the course of years or be accelerated by a serious illness, may lead to a collapse of the yin, which thereby allows the yang to rise uncontrollably. The mildest expression of this energetic imbalance is the sudden loss of hearing, while its most severe form is cerebral stroke. In some cases, the burn-out syndrome, which is often followed by a nervous breakdown, is subject to the same pathology. A good visual image for what happens energetically is a candle burning at both ends. The candle wax is the substance, which corresponds to the yin and essence, while the flame corresponds to the yang. At the end, when the wax finally burns away, there is a short, intense flickering of the flame: the excessive yang. This upward-blazing fire in the body vents itself in such disorders as myocardial infarction, stroke, hypertensive crisis, or uncontrollable bleeding. The tongue body is commonly red, dry, contracted, or stiff (Fig. 3.6.6). The heat has injured the fluids and yin so severely that the muscles, sinews , and tendons, including those of the tongue, become malnourished. This condition can cause the internal movement of wind (see Ch. 7 for further discussion). A deep red discoloration of the tongue also arises when heat enters the nutritive and blood levels (see Ch. 9).

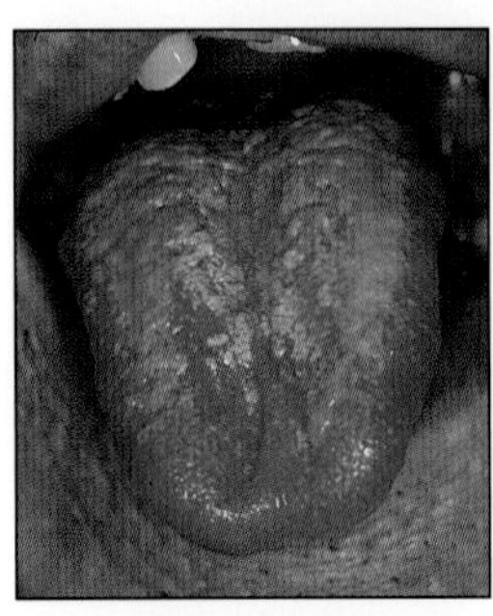

Fig. 3.6.6

Surprisingly, this pathology can also produce a soft red tongue, an indication of malnourishment of the sinews and tendons due to extreme heat. Patients with this tongue type often suffer from hemiplegia (following stroke), or from atrophy disorders. The soft red tongue is, accordingly, an unfavorable prognostic sign.

There are many levels of Kidney yin deficiency. Tongue diagnosis can be an important tool in reaching a prognosis for the illness and in formulating the correct treatment strategy. Individual tongue signs should only be used in conjunction with other methods of diagnosis and should be evaluated in the context of the patient's symptoms.

Manifestations of tongue signs denoting Kidney yin deficiency in correspondence with other patterns are shown in the following chart.

Tongue Signs	Other Patterns
Reddish tongue body, dry and cracked	Kidney yin deficiency and dryness (Fig. 3.5.3)
Large area of peeled tongue coating	Kidney and Stomach yin deficiency, exhaustion of fluids (Figs. 3.8.1 and 3.8.2)
Red, shiny tongue body	Severe exhaustion of Kidney yin (Fig. 3.4.3)
Reddish tongue body, deep cracks, and a peeled coating	Depletion of Stomach and Kidney yin (Fig. 3.2.3)
Reddish tongue body and a red tip	Kidney yin deficiency with Heart yin deficiency and heat from deficiency in the Heart (Fig. 3.2.5)
Reddish tongue body, swollen edges, and peeled coating	Kidney and Liver yin deficiency with ascending Liver yang (Fig. 3.6.3)
Red tongue body with vertical cracks in the anterior third	Kidney yin and Lung yin deficiency (Fig. 5.2.3)
Reddish, dry tongue body with a red, peeled center	Kidney yin deficiency with Stomach yin deficiency (Fig. 4.1.3.1)

It is worth noting that it may take years for a pattern of Kidney yin deficiency to develop. This process can be observed as the tongue body gradually changes colors. Different shades of red, and differences in the size of the peeled areas of the coating, suggest the possibility of pathology as well as deterioration in the condition of the patient.

The photographs in this chapter reflect tongue body colors and shapes in relation to long-standing deficiency of yin and essence, which often occurs in chronic diseases. The sequence of tongue photos is in order of severity of the underlying deficiency. Thus, the first photo represents only slight deficiency while the last one reflects very severe deficiency. In addition, there are photos that depict the mutual relationships among Kidney, Heart, Lung, and Stomach yin deficiencies. Tongues that show specific signs of individual yin organ deficiency will be discussed in later chapters.

Tongue description	Chinese diagnosis
Red, thin, cracked	Blood and Kidney yin deficiency
Coating without root	Stomach and Kidney yin deficiency

Fig. 3.2.1
Female
34 years old

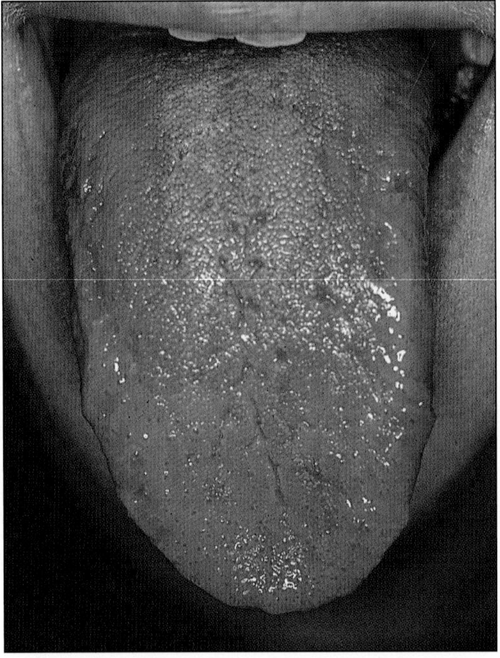

Symptoms

Severe exhaustion
Inner restlessness
Sore throat
Numbness of the left thigh
Frequent dizzy spells
Occasional night sweats

Western diagnosis

Multiple sclerosis
Chronic tonsillitis
Blindness due to optic nerve atrophy of the left eye

Background to disease

Irregular eating habits
Frequent bouts of influenza
Long-standing emotional problems

Tongue description	Chinese diagnosis
Reddish without coating	Kidney yin deficiency
Swollen	Spleen qi deficiency with accumulation of dampness
Numerous small cracks	Kidney yin deficiency
Cracks at the sides of the tongue	Spleen qi deficiency → Spleen yin deficiency
Slightly reddish tip	Heat from deficiency in the Heart
Depression at the root of the tongue	Kidney essence deficiency

Fig. 3.2.2
Female
67 years old

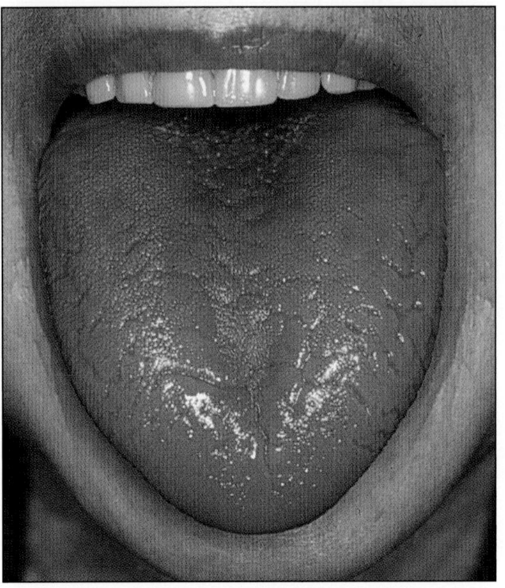

Symptoms

Dryness of the mouth, thirsty without desire to drink
Insomnia, night sweats
Constipation, constant weight gain
Occasional mouth ulcers

Western diagnosis

None

Background to disease

Lack of sleep over many years
Severe menstrual bleeding 20 years ago

Tongue description	Chinese diagnosis
Reddish, thin	Kidney yin deficiency
Cracks on the sides	Severe Spleen qi deficiency
Vertical cracks	Injury to body fluids
Peeled coating	Stomach and Kidney yin deficiency

Symptoms

Tinnitus, headache with numbness around the mouth
Lack of drive, exhaustion
Introverted
Impotence, no libido

Western diagnosis

Prolactinoma,[2] impotence

Background to disease

Taxing demands at work
Long-standing emotional problems

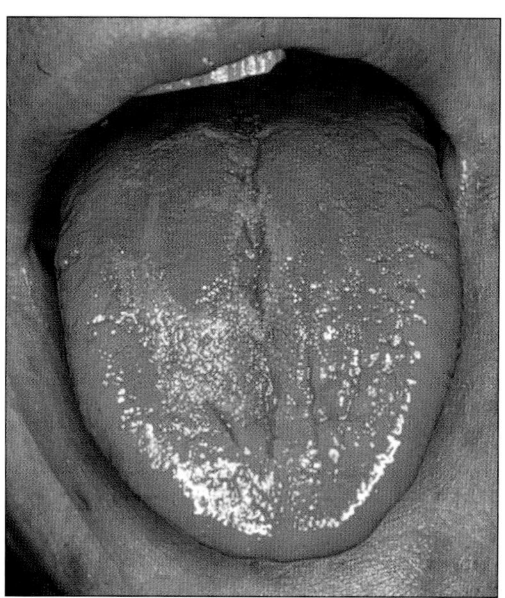

Fig. 3.2.3
Male
43 years old

Tongue description	Chinese diagnosis
Deep red, especially in the center	Kidney yin deficiency with Stomach fire
Wide shape	Internal heat and toxin due to alcohol
Deep red tip	Heart fire
Whitish, slippery coating at the sides, dirty yellow coating at the center	Long-standing accumulation of phlegm (phlegm-fire)

Symptoms

Severe heartburn, stomach pains
Insomnia, nightmares
Inner restlessness, panic attacks
Excessive sexual drive

Western diagnosis

None

Background to disease

Excessive use of alcohol, coffee, and nicotine
Excessive masturbation

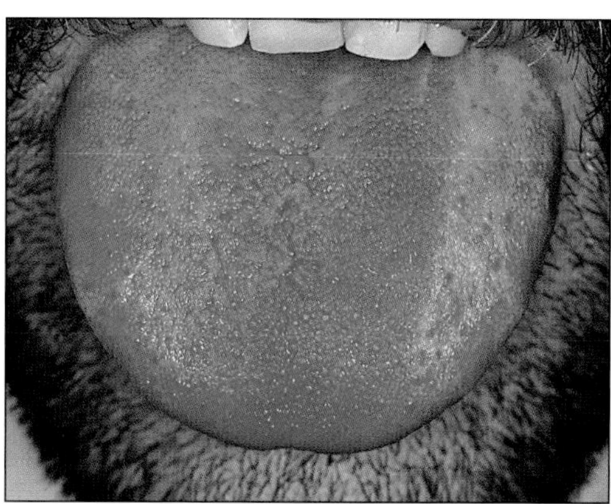

Fig. 3.2.4
Male
33 years old

3.3 Scarlet Red Tongues

This tongue body color is deep red with a slight pink hue. If the tongue is dry or without a coating, it is an indication of Kidney yin deficiency with vigorous internal heat. Occasionally only some areas of the tongue will present with this shade, most commonly the anterior third of the tongue. This discoloration corresponds to severe Lung yin and Stomach yin deficiency. Scarlet red tongues with coating are characteristic of warm-febrile diseases (see Ch. 9).

Tongue description	**Chinese diagnosis**
Scarlet red	Heat in the blood, slight Kidney yin deficiency
Dry, rough coating	Fluid deficiency
Notch at the tip	Slight Heart blood deficiency

Fig. 3.3.1
Female
22 years old

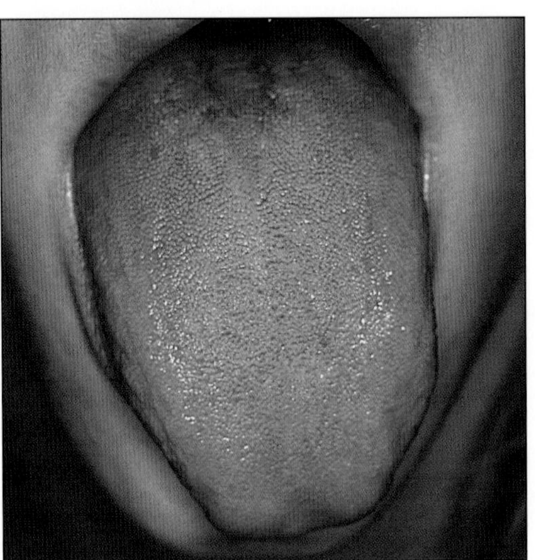

Symptoms

Dry, red, itchy skin
Fits of anger
Depression

Western diagnosis

Atopic eczema

Background to disease

Lack of sleep
Irregular lifestyle
Alcohol abuse

Tongue description	**Chinese diagnosis**
Scarlet red, slightly shiny	Kidney yin deficiency with heat from deficiency
Raw, reddish area in the center	Stomach yin deficiency
Swollen tongue sides, especially in the central part	Underlying Spleen qi and yin deficiency

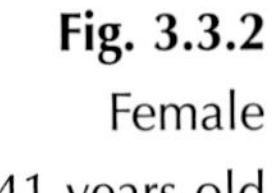

Fig. 3.3.2
Female
41 years old

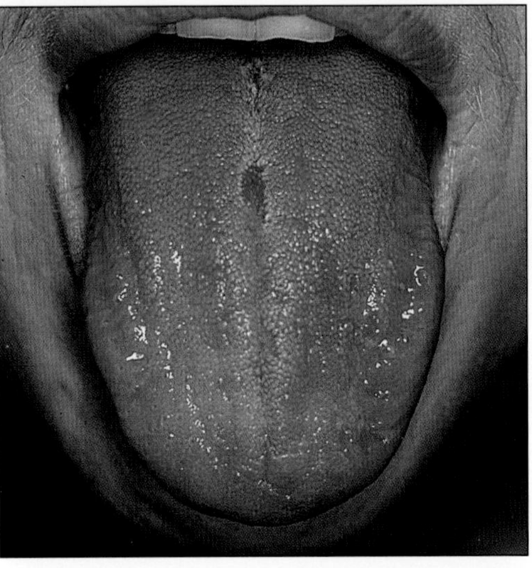

Symptoms

Exhaustion, inability to sleep through the night or restless sleep
Thirst
Depression
Heartburn

Western diagnosis

None

Background to disease

Pregnancy at a late age
Breastfeeding for too long

Tongue description	**Chinese diagnosis**
Scarlet red	Kidney yin deficiency
Raised, reddish dots distributed over the entire tongue	Heat in the blood
Long vertical crack	Constitutional weakness of the Heart, heat in the Heart

Symptoms

Inner restlessness
Tremor of the hands
Poor memory

Western diagnosis

None

Background to disease

Drug abuse (heroin, cocaine, ecstasy)
Lack of sleep
Overwork
Works with toxic substances

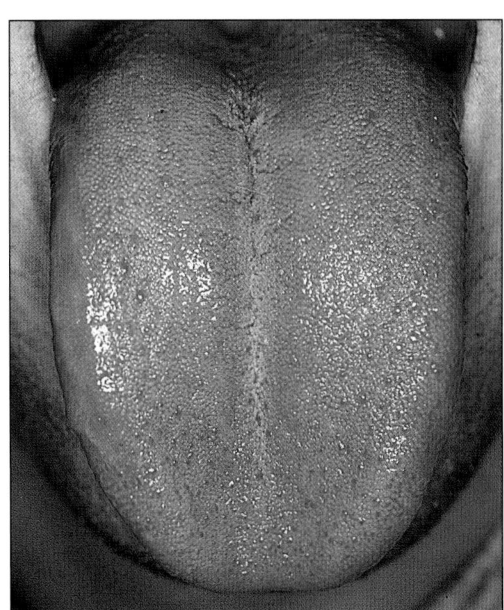

Fig. 3.3.3
Male
33 years old

3.4 Red, Short Tongues

This tongue type is indicative of severe exhaustion of the Kidney and Liver yin plus the development of vigorous heat. This can lead to very serious disorders as the extreme heat consumes the fluids and yin, the most serious being the internal movement of wind.

The tongue is short because the fluids, blood, and yin are not adequately nourishing the tongue muscles; the tongue thereupon loses its elasticity and its ability to move freely. If the tongue deviates to one side, this indicates the presence of internal wind.

Although this type of tongue is the result of severe yin deficiency, treatment with pure tonification is not indicated. The internal wind must be extinguished and the yang sedated.

Tongue description	**Chinese diagnosis**
Red, small, short	Kidney yin deficiency, onset of essence deficiency
Very pointed, prickles at the tip	Heart fire
Intense red edges	Heat in the Liver

Fig. 3.4.1
Female
19 years old

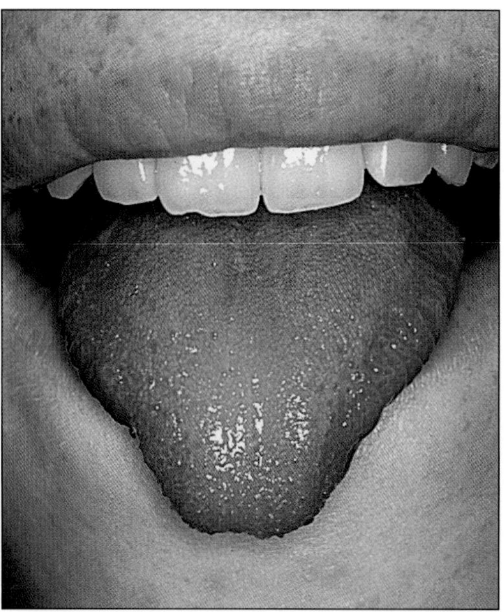

Symptoms

Lack of appetite
Constipation
Amenorrhea
Strong inner restlessness
Insomnia
Suicidal fantasies

Western diagnosis

Anorexia nervosa

Background to disease

Serious starvation
Divorce of parents

Tongue description	**Chinese diagnosis**
Deep red, thin, small, short	Kidney yin deficiency
Depression in the anterior third	Lung qi and yin deficiency
Redness in the anterior third	Heat in the Lungs

Fig. 3.4.2
Female
59 years old

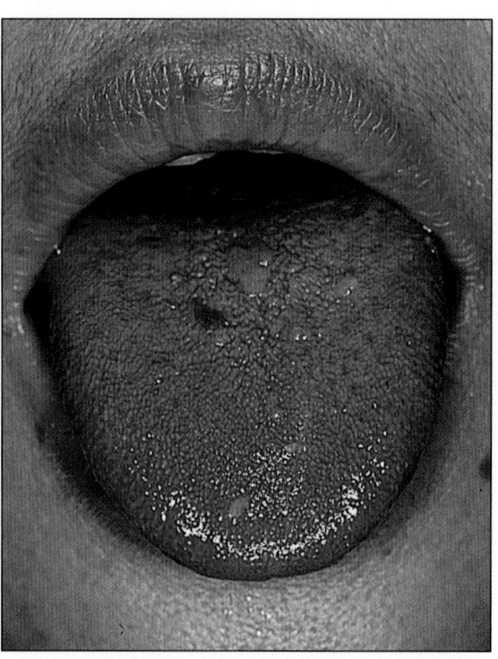

Symptoms

Dry cough
Dry mouth and throat
Pain in the chest
Hair loss
Lack of appetite

Western diagnosis

Metastasizing bronchial cancer

Background to disease

Possibly environmental factors
Chemotherapy

Tongue description --------------------------- **Chinese diagnosis**

Deep red, short, *shiny* — Stomach, Lung, and Kidney yin deficiency

Dry, without coating — Exhaustion of fluids

Symptoms

Cough with little phlegm
Night sweats
Low-grade fever, intense feeling of heat in the body
Shortness of breath
Exhaustion

Western diagnosis

Chronic bronchitis
Emphysema

Background to disease

Smoking for 60 years

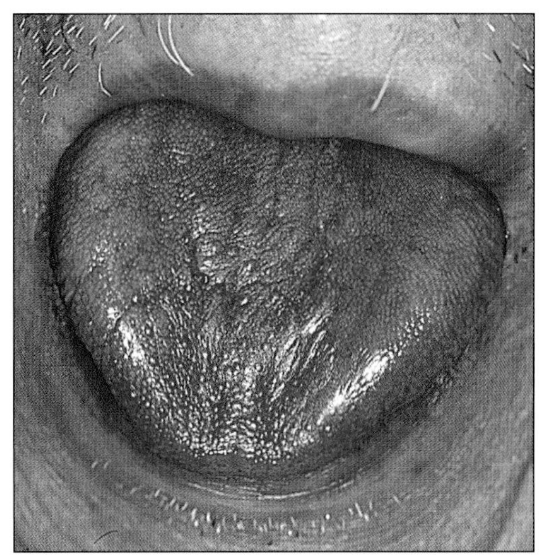

Fig. 3.4.3
Male
83 years old

Tongue description --------------------------- **Chinese diagnosis**

Deep red, wide, short — Severe Kidney yin deficiency with injury to fluids due to vigorous heat

Yellow, old, dry coating — Heat accumulation in yang brightness *(yáng míng)* organ stage

Symptoms

Fever
Constipation
Loss of memory
Wasting
Weakened vision

Western diagnosis

Stroke with hemiplegia

Background to disease

Smoking for 50 years
Alcohol abuse

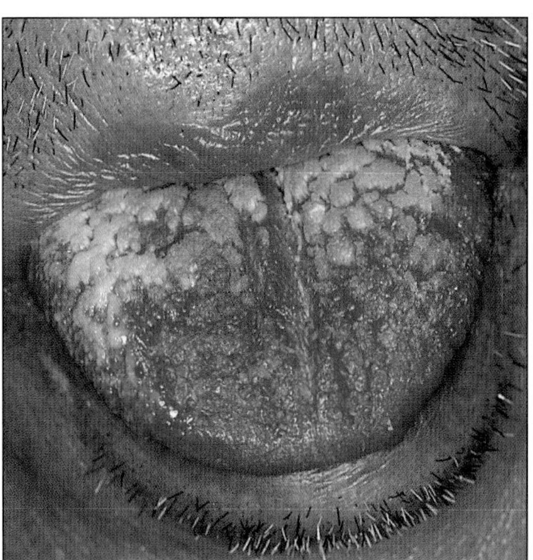

Fig. 3.4.4
Male
74 years old

3.5 Cracked Tongues

In general, there are no cracks in a normal tongue. The softness and suppleness of the tongue body shows that it is moistened by the fluids and nourished through the blood and yin. Heat and dryness account for the appearance of cracks in the tongue body. Thus, small, horizontal cracks are a sign of yin deficiency, especially when they appear on a red or slightly red tongue.

As a rule, injury to the substance does not occur unless the pathology has been present for a while. This is one reason why cracks are rarely seen in the tongues of children. In adults, they appear rather suddenly, for example, during a severe disease, after chemotherapy, or when yin-injuring habits (like cigarette smoking or frequent consumption of spicy foods) are indulged over a long period of time.

Cracks in a pale tongue body can originate from blood deficiency. If they are only superficial, this is an indication of Stomach and Spleen qi deficiency with blood deficiency. In the case of deep cracks, besides blood deficiency, there may also be injury to the fluids.[3]

In a red tongue, cracks are an unmistakable sign of the exhaustion of fluids or the onset of Stomach and Kidney yin deficiency, caused by injury from excessive heat in the nutritive and blood levels. A red, shiny tongue (see Ch. 4) with cracks indicates severe yin and fluid damage.

A single, small crack on the tongue body is less significant than cracks that are distributed over the entire body of the tongue. In modern China, cracks are differentiated according to the following three degrees of severity:

- *First degree:* Flat and short, that is, no longer than 0.55mm, and no more than three cracks.
- *Second degree:* Identical to the first degree except there are four or more cracks.
- *Third degree:* The cracks have a depth of at least 1mm and are longer than 1.5cm.[4]

The following photographs illustrate this pattern. They are presented in order of increasing degree of injury to the yin. The first photograph shows a slight deficiency of fluids and yin, while the last one shows a severe deficiency.

Tongue description	**Chinese diagnosis**
Pale red	Slight Spleen qi deficiency
Pale sides	Liver blood deficiency
Curled-up edges	Liver qi constraint
Horizontal cracks in the center	Lack of fluids, Stomach yin deficiency, onset of Kidney yin deficiency
Depression at the root	Onset of essence deficiency

Symptoms

Headaches
Pain in the shoulder girdle
Inner tension
Exhaustion
Poor memory
Depression
Toothache

Western diagnosis

Onset of periodontitis

Background to disease

Pregnancy at a late age
Breastfeeding for a long time
Lack of sleep

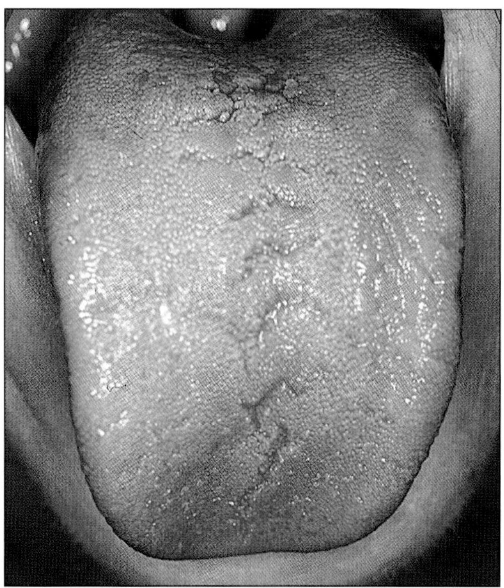

Fig. 3.5.1
Female
41 years old

Tongue description	**Chinese diagnosis**
Pale	Blood deficiency
Red in anterior third	Heat in the upper burner
Vertical crack with horizontal cracks branching out	Onset of Stomach and Kidney yin deficiency
Dry, reddish center	Lack of fluids in the Stomach
Thorns distributed over the entire tongue body	Internal heat

Symptoms

Exhaustion
Thirst
Severe palpitations
Headaches at the vertex
Night sweats

Western diagnosis

Iron deficiency anemia

Background to disease

Caffeine and nicotine abuse

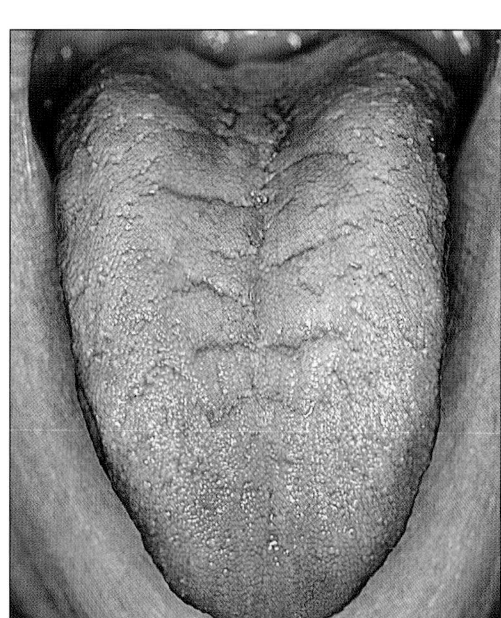

Fig. 3.5.2
Female
49 years old

Tongue description	**Chinese diagnosis**
Reddish	Slight Kidney yin deficiency
Cracks distributed over the entire tongue body	Stomach and Kidney yin deficiency
Center of the tongue red and without coating	Stomach yin deficiency
Yellow coating, thicker on one side	Slight retention of damp-heat in the Liver and Gallbladder

Fig. 3.5.3
Female
42 years old

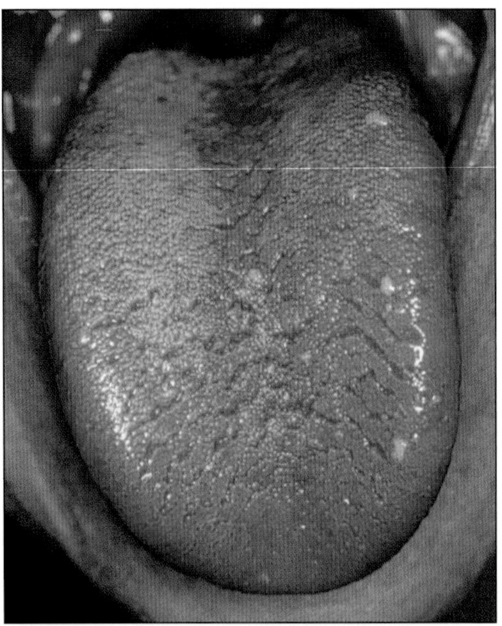

Symptoms

Burning sensation of the tongue
Night sweats
Palpitations
Insomnia
Frequent, smelly, loose stools
Pain under the right hypochondrium
Inner restlessness

Western diagnosis

None

Background to disease

Overworked
Caffeine abuse
Pregnancy at a late age

Tongue description	**Chinese diagnosis**
Slightly red, firm tongue body	Kidney yin deficiency
Slightly bluish	Blood stasis
Horizontal cracks over the entire tongue body	Kidney yin deficiency
Yellow, dry coating	Accumulation of damp-heat in the Liver and Gallbladder

Fig. 3.5.4
Male
48 years old

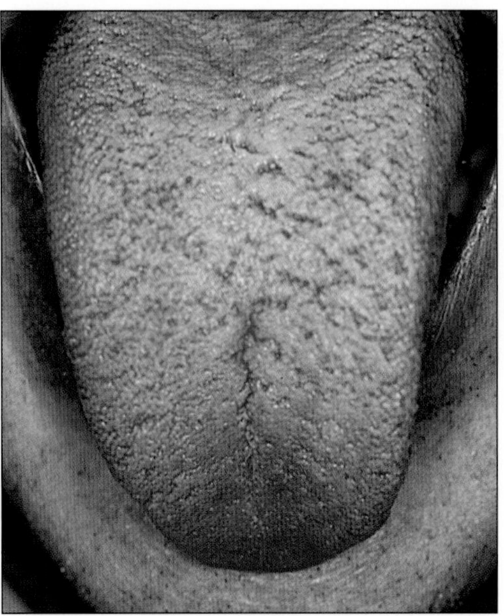

Symptoms

Pain in the ankle upon exertion
Smelly diarrhea
Chronic sinusitis
Itchy scalp

Western diagnosis

Sudeck syndrome

Background to disease

Alcohol and salt abuse
Trauma (fracture of the tibia with ensuing osteoporosis)

3.6 The Tongue Coating and Kidney Yin Deficiency[5]

A red tongue with a peeled coating is a definitive sign of Stomach and Kidney yin deficiency. This coating has lost its root. Due to the lack of fluids, insufficient material is available for the formation of the turbid 'steam' that contributes to the formation of the coating. The function of Stomach qi is to ferment the solids and liquids. In the normal course of things, during the process of digestion a little dampness rises to the tongue and forms the coating. However, where there is deficiency, too little moisture rises and this manifests in the peeled tongue or in an irregularly distributed coating.

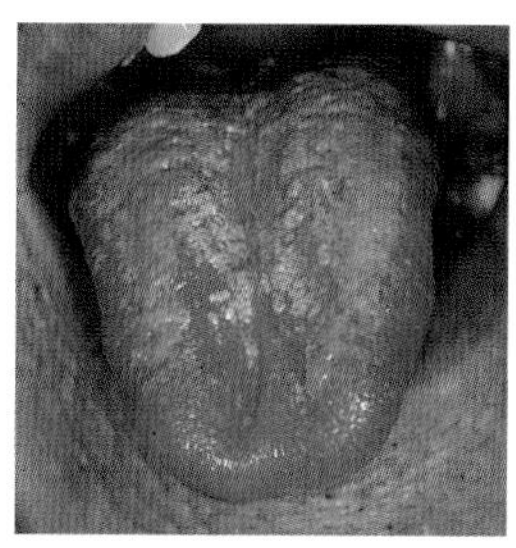
Fig. 3.6.6

The same energetic imbalance can create an old-looking coating, that is, it looks dry and gives the impression that it could be easily wiped off (Fig. 3.6.6). Where a new, fresh coating should have appeared, the old coating remains next to a raw or dry area (Fig. 4.1.3.1). The formation of new coating does not take place because of exhaustion of and injury to the fluids. The result is a tongue coating without root, which can evolve into a dry tongue or one without coating.

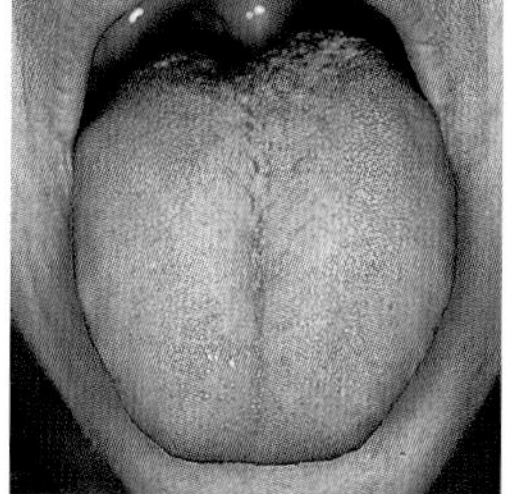
Fig. 4.1.3.1

A red tongue with no coating at the root, but which is red and dry, indicates extreme exhaustion of Kidney yin that has led to Kidney fire. Although it does indicate a less severe pathology, the same is true for a pale red tongue with no coating at the root, or a discolored, reddish root.

Tongue description	Chinese diagnosis
Slightly red, swollen	Accumulation of damp-heat
Peeled coating, especially in the anterior and posterior thirds	Stomach yin deficiency, lack of communication between Heart and Kidney
White, slightly greasy, thin coating in the center	Blockage of Stomach qi by damp turbidity

Symptoms

Panic attacks with tachycardia and pain in the chest
Inability to fall asleep, fatigue
Fits of rage
Feeling of heaviness in the body

Western diagnosis

Cardiac neurosis

Background to disease

Excessive anger and frustration
Unsatisfactory emotional relationships
Excessive consumption of sweets

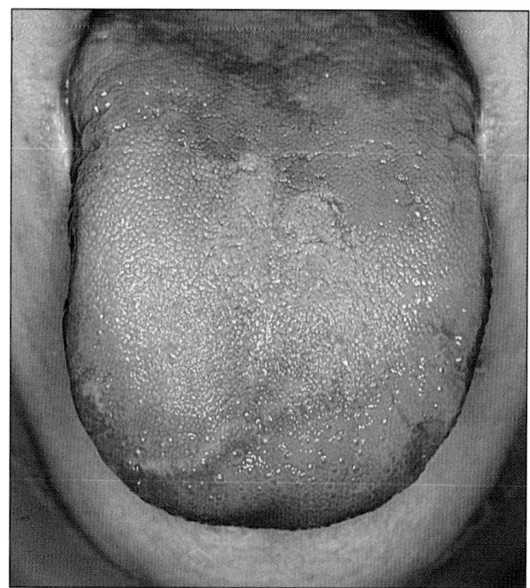

Fig. 3.6.1
Female
28 years old

Tongue description	**Chinese diagnosis**
Red, swollen	Kidney yin deficiency, accumulation of damp-heat in the Liver and Gallbladder
Peeled coating, especially in the posterior third	Kidney yin deficiency
Thorns in the posterior third	Kidney fire
Deep vertical crack with yellow coating	Phlegm-fire in the Stomach

Fig. 3.6.2
Male
25 years old

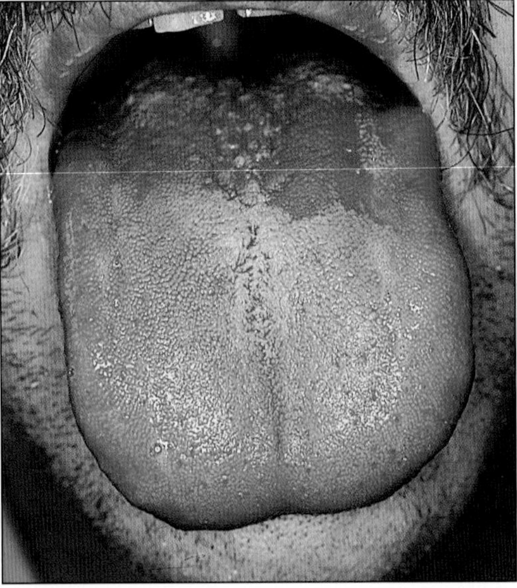

Symptoms

Inner restlessness
Feeling of heat in the body
Vertigo
Soft stools
Occasional night sweats

Western diagnosis

None

Background to disease

Improper treatment with Radix Aconiti lateralis praeparata *(zhì fù zǐ)*

Tongue description	**Chinese diagnosis**
Red	Kidney yin deficiency
Red, swollen sides	Ascending Liver yang
Slightly deviated	Internal wind
Swollen, red tip of tongue	Heart fire
Peeled coating, especially *in the posterior third*	Kidney yin deficiency

Fig. 3.6.3
Male
23 years old

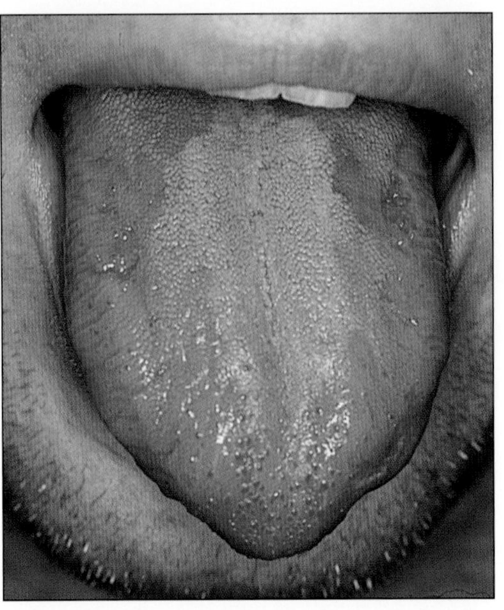

Symptoms

Intense dizziness
Feeling of heat in the head
Bad mood
Smelly, loose stools

Western diagnosis

Vertigo

Background to disease

Overwork
Caffeine abuse
Emotional problems

Tongue description	Chinese diagnosis
Pale red, swollen	Spleen qi deficiency (accumulation of dampness)
Red center with yellow, old coating	Stomach heat with phlegm-fire
Peeled coating and red root	Kidney yin deficiency with Kidney fire

Symptoms

Paranoiac panic attacks
Inner restlessness, nervousness
Night sweats
No drive

Western diagnosis

Manic depression

Background to disease

Unresolved emotional conflicts
Caffeine and nicotine abuse
Irregular eating habits
Excessive consumption of chocolate and sweets

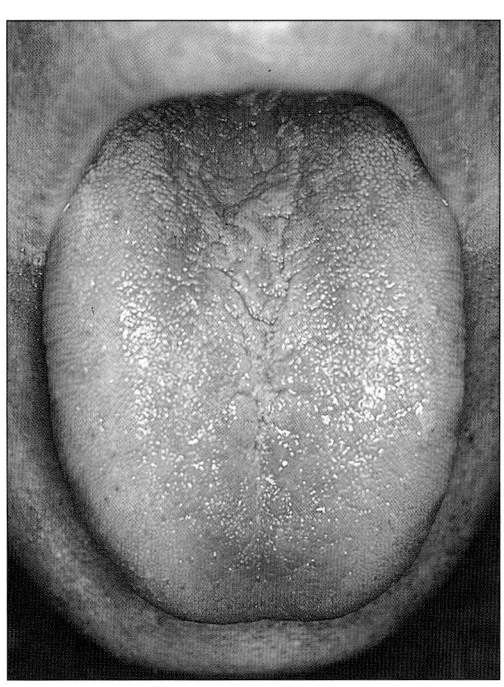

Fig. 3.6.4
Male
53 years old

Tongue description	Chinese diagnosis
Red, contracted	Severe exhaustion of Kidney yin and essence, heat in the blood level
Dry	Lack of fluids
Yellow, old, one-sided coating	Stomach yin and Kidney yin deficiency with clumping of damp-heat in the Gallbladder
Flattened and contracted tip	Heart yin deficiency

Symptoms

Extreme physical weakness
Night sweats
Chronic low grade fever
Dry cough
Mouth ulcers
Stomach pain

Western diagnosis

AIDS
Anemia
Kaposi's sarcoma

Background to disease

Viral activity

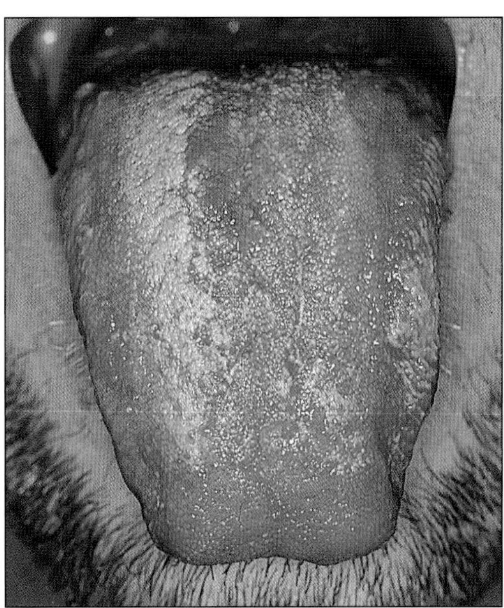

Fig. 3.6.5
Male
44 years old

Tongue description	Chinese diagnosis
Red, firm, stiff	Kidney yin deficiency with internal heat
Dry	Lack of fluids
Yellow, old, tofu-like coating	Stomach and Kidney yin deficiency with heat accumulation in yang brightness organ stage *(yáng míng fŭ zhèng)*

Fig. 3.6.6
Male
65 years old

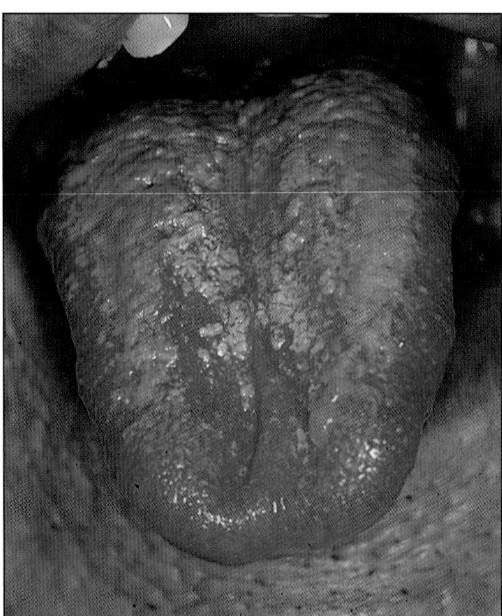

Symptoms

Loss of memory
Severe headache
Fever
Occasional night sweats
Constipation
Vertigo

Western diagnosis

Suffered stroke 3 days before

Background to disease

Smoking cigarettes for 30 years
Alcohol abuse

3.7 Special Tongue Shapes Associated with Kidney Yin Deficiency

A pale, hammer-shaped tongue represents severe exhaustion of qi in the middle burner. A red, hammer-shaped tongue is indicative of severe exhaustion of yin. Severe, long-term emotional problems, irregular eating habits, or excessive sexual activity can each lead to the exhaustion of qi and yin.

As discussed in Ch. 2, a deficiency of yin and essence may manifest as a depression at the root of the tongue. In red tongues this pathology shows itself occasionally in a contracted tongue root. This is a sign that the yin's strength is diminishing. It is important to remember that the root of the tongue represents the strength and vitality of the Kidney energy.

Tongue description

Pale red, *hammer-shaped*

Red on the anterior third with red points

Chinese diagnosis

Spleen qi, Kidney yin, and essence deficiency

Heart fire

Symptoms

Restless fetus, slight uterine bleeding (8th week of pregnancy)
Low-grade fever
Insomnia
Nervousness, inner restlessness, panic attacks
Pain around the kidneys
Lack of appetite

Western diagnosis

Habitual miscarriage, acute threatened miscarriage
Underweight

Background to disease

Unresolved emotions due to suicide of mother
Insufficient intake of food and drink
D & C twice

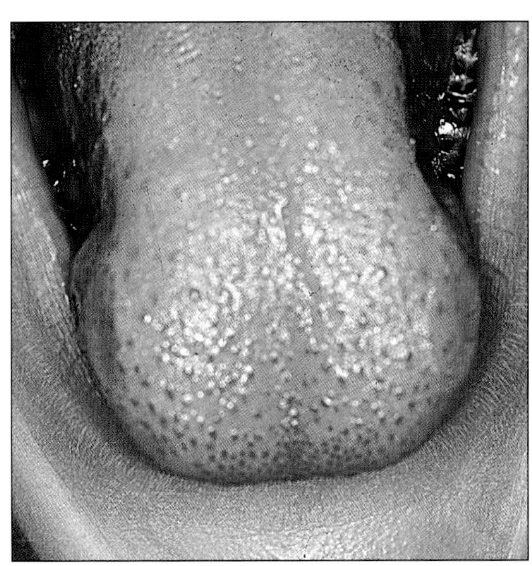

Fig. 3.7.1
Female
29 years old

Tongue description

Pale red, swollen edges

Contracted root with thin, yellow coating

Chinese diagnosis

Spleen qi deficiency

Kidney yin deficiency with accumulation of damp-heat in the Bladder

Symptoms

Frequent and urgent urination
Insomnia
Night sweats
Depression
Feeling of pressure in the stomach
Epigastric fullness

Western diagnosis

Chronic cystitis

Background to disease

Irregular eating habits
Lack of sleep
Overwork
Unresolved emotional problems

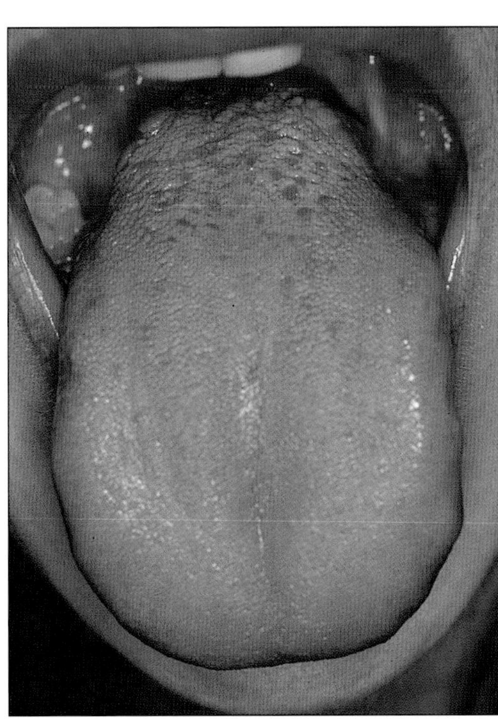

Fig. 3.7.2
Female
33 years old

3.8 Case Histories: Combined Patterns that Include Kidney Yin Deficiency

The case histories in this chapter are devoted exclusively to patterns of Kidney yin and/or Kidney essence deficiency, whether alone or as part of a combined pattern. Case histories in which Kidney yang deficiency is an integral part of the pathomechanism are discussed in other chapters.

Kidney yin deficiency patterns are characterized by a lack of body fluids and the development of heat from deficiency. Kidney yin deficiency can be caused by a number of factors, including:

- Chronic or serious illnesses (Figs. 3.4.1, 3.4.2, 3.8.2)
- Abuse of alocohol, recreational and medical drugs (Figs. 3.2.4, 3.3.3, 3.4.3, 3.4.4, 3.5.3, 3.5.7)
- Mental overwork and/or hectic lifestyle and stress (Figs. 3.8.2, 3.8.3)
- Lack of sleep (Figs. 3.2.2, 3.5.3)
- Aging (Fig. 3.2.2)
- Long-standing emotional problems, especially feelings of fear (Figs. 3.6.1, 6.1.4.7, 6.2.4)
- Serious blood loss (Figs. 2.5.2, 7.2.1.4)
- Injury to the body fluids as a result of patterns of heat (Fig. 3.3.1, 9.2.8)

"Kidney yin represents the essence and the fluids within the Kidneys."[6] Thus, Kidney yin deficiency can lead to weakness of Kidney essence. These two types of deficiency, however, have quite different manifestations. Kidney yin deficiency is characterized by heat from deficiency and its associated symptoms. By contrast, Kidney essence deficiency invariably deprives various body tissues—especially those of the brain, bones, teeth, and hair—of nourishment. Symptoms that characterize weakness of Kidney essence are decreased libido, premature ejaculation, weak bones, poor memory, and an inability to concentrate.

In some cases, a pattern of Kidney yin deficiency occurs alongside a pattern of Kidney essence and blood deficiency (Figs. 3.8.1, 3.8.2). Kidney yin deficiency can sometimes cause night sweats (Figs. 3.8.1, 3.8.3), while a pattern of Kidney essence and blood deficiency may be associated with hair loss (Fig. 3.8.1).

If Kidney yang and essence deficiency appear together, a whole range of symptoms including cold extremities, edema, impotence, infertility, weakness of the bones in the knees or lumbar region may present. Since the "Kidneys rule the bones and the marrow,"[7] exhaustion of the Kidneys will result in bones that are not properly nourished, which can appear as weakness in the lumbar region and knees (Fig. 8.1.1).

The Kidneys play an important role in the transformation and transportation of body fluids. Kidney yang supplies qi and heat to the Bladder, enabling it to transform the fluids and excrete impurities in the urine. The Kidneys also control the flow of urine. The balance between Kidney yin and Kidney yang controls the opening and closing of the urethra. A weakness of Kidney yin or yang may therefore lead to incontinence or anuria (Fig. 3.8.2).

As the following case histories illustrate, a pattern of Kidney yin deficiency rarely occurs by itself. It will usually engender additional disease patterns, especially in chronic illnesses. This type of deficiency may therefore have the following effects:

1. The Kidney yin and yang balance each other and are mutually dependent. Therefore, a pattern of Kidney yin deficiency can evolve into Kidney yang deficiency, and vice versa, and symptoms may develop that are characteristic of both patterns. Young or middle-aged individuals with these combined patterns will present with serious weakness as a chief symptom. In Fig. 3.8.2, the incontinence indicates deficiency of Kidney qi and yang, while the night sweats indicate a pattern of Kidney yin deficiency. In Fig. 3.2.3, the impotence reflects Kidney yang deficiency, while the tinnitus reflects Kidney yin deficiency.

   In the elderly, deficiency of source qi and essence, as well as Kidney yin and yang, are to be expected. The nature of the deficiency will depend on the constitution, state of health, and circumstances of the person. In old age it is common for symptoms to appear that signal Kidney yin as well as Kidney yang deficiency.

   It should be noted that the tongue cannot necessarily be used to deduce the history of these patterns, that is, the tongue cannot be used to determine if Kidney yin deficiency evolved into a combined pattern of Kidney yin and yang deficiency, or if Kidney yang deficiency evolved into the combined pattern. Nevertheless, tongue diagnosis is still very important since the tongue body color reflects the dominant deficiency underlying the current pathology.

2. The Kidney yin nourishes all the yin organs and supplies yin to the Stomach. Kidney yin deficiency may therefore lead to yin deficiency of the Liver, Heart, Lungs, Spleen, or Stomach.[8] The relationship between Kidney yin and the yin organs is briefly outlined here.

   a. If the Kidney yin fails to properly nourish the Heart yin, the close relationship between the Kidneys and the Heart is easily disturbed, leading to heat from deficiency in the Heart. This process is associated with inner restlessness, palpitations, and an inability to sleep through the night (Fig. 3.8.3).

   b. The Kidneys and Liver also have a special bond. It is said that the Kidneys and Liver have a common origin, that is, the Liver stores the blood while the Kidneys store the essence, and the Liver blood nourishes the essence while the essence contributes to the production of blood, which in turn nourishes the Kidney yin. According to the rules of 'mother-child', the Kidney yin generates and nourishes the Liver yin, and together they provide nourishment to the sinews, tendons, and bones (Fig. 3.8.3).

      In addition, if the Kidneys and Liver are weak, the eyes will lack proper nourishment, resulting in dry eyes or poor eyesight. Ascendant Liver yang may evolve from the combined pattern of Kidney and Liver yin deficiency and present such symptoms as dizziness, tinnitus, and/or headaches (Fig. 7.1.2.5).

   c. If Kidney yin deficiency affects the Lungs, the symptoms will include dry cough, dry mouth, dry throat, subfebrile temperatures, and night sweats (Fig. 5.2.3).

   d. The Kidneys and Stomach are also closely associated. If the fluids that originate in the Stomach are injured, the ensuing Stomach yin deficiency will, over the long term, engender Kidney yin deficiency. Symptoms associated with this condition are thirst with no desire to drink, lack of appetite, and constipation. There may be additional symptoms such as insomnia and night sweats (Fig. 4.1.2.8).

Tongue description	Chinese diagnosis
Pale	Spleen qi deficiency → blood deficiency
Long	No pathology
Peeled, red, dry coating	Stomach qi and yin deficiency with onset of Kidney yin deficiency

Fig. 3.8.1
Female
34 years old

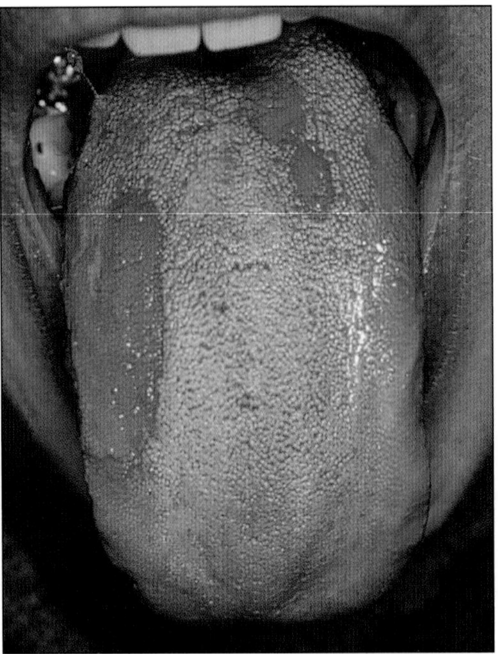

Symptoms

Severe exhaustion, weight loss
Nausea, lack of appetite, thirst, loose stools
Occasional night sweats
Hair loss, dry skin
Tendency to catch cold

Western diagnosis

None

Background to disease

Condition started after birth of first child six months earlier

CASE HISTORY Because of her baby's constant waking, the patient got very little sleep and became exhausted. She therefore had trouble looking after the baby. For example, although she enjoyed breastfeeding, it made her tired. In addition, although she was still nursing, she had two painless but heavy periods.

The patient was 5 feet 11 inches tall and weighed only 120 pounds. She never felt hungry, but occasionally felt nauseous. She was always thirsty but liked to drink just small amounts.

Over a three-week period she noticed that she was losing hair and also had unusually dry skin. During and since her pregnancy, she had developed a propensity for catching colds. She also experienced occasional night sweats. Her pulse was floating, thin, and tight.

Analysis. The patient's pregnancy, giving birth, and breastfeeding depleted her qi, blood, yin, and essence. Her symptoms are those of a marked deficiency of the Spleen and Stomach qi, as well as deficiency of Kidney yin and essence.

The tongue signs reflect the development of the different patterns that are responsible for the acute symptoms experienced by the patient. Uppermost is the Spleen and Stomach qi deficiency, which contributed to the weakness of the Kidney yin and essence. The pale tongue body reflects the Spleen qi and blood deficiency. The raw, red, and peeled areas indicate quite the opposite: the onset of Kidney yin deficiency.

The length of the tongue body often corresponds to the height of the patient. This patient is tall, so the length of the tongue here is not an indication of disharmony associated with the Heart.[9]

When ingested food is rotted and ripened by the Stomach qi, a turbid steam is created that rises and forms a coating on the tongue. In this case, a new coating is not being formed because the Stomach qi is so weak, and there is a lack of fluids caused by the Stomach and/or Kidney yin deficiency. Since the tongue appears to have peeled areas, the coating gives the

Pathomechanism

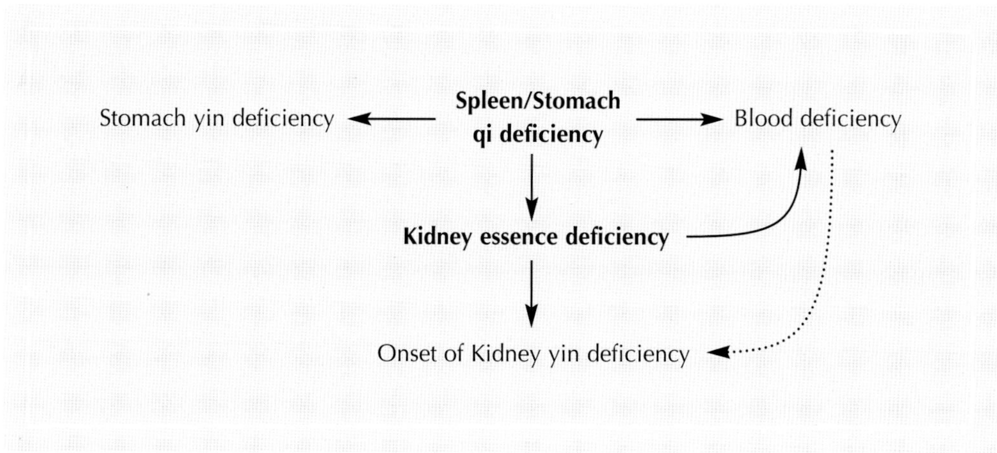

impression of being 'without root.' The coating will usually disappear from the center first;[10] this is the region of the tongue that corresponds to the Stomach. The color of the tongue body will indicate whether there is underlying Stomach qi or yin deficiency. In this case, the tongue coating is clearly peeled at the side and on the posterior third, which correspond to the Liver and Kidneys. It is therefore interpreted as a sign of Kidney yin deficiency.[11] This conclusion is based on both the extent of the peeled area and the red and raw appearance of the tongue. The rootless coating underlines the deterioration in the condition of the patient. The texture of the remaining tongue coating, which is thin and new, signifies that the deficiency has recently developed.

The night sweats are indicative of the development of a condition that has changed from qi deficiency to yin deficiency. The onset of Kidney yin deficiency manifests as sweating, which is caused by the heat from deficiency. The nature of the patient's thirst is another indication of yin deficiency: although she is thirsty, she only likes to drink small amounts of fluids.

Many factors contribute to the energetic weakness of this patient. A pregnant woman's Kidney essence nourishes the fetus during the months of pregnancy. Pregnancy can weaken the Kidney essence if the constitution or disposition of the mother is itself weak. In addition, the birthing process is characterized by severe pain and physical effort that can lead to a depletion of Lung and Spleen qi.

Breastfeeding may also reduce the blood and essence of the mother. Maciocia[12] cites a passage from the *Secret Records of Master Feng's Brocade Bag* that "menstrual blood and breast milk are both produced by the Spleen and Stomach. After being digested by the Stomach, the pure part of water and food goes to the Heart channel where it changes its color becoming red, thus forming blood. Soon after the delivery, the pure part of food then goes to the Lungs and then flows into the breasts to become milk, which is white in color, white being the color of the Lungs." Hence it can be seen that the Spleen and Stomach are pivotal during this time, and that deficiency should be considered when, following childbirth, a woman has symptoms of physical exhaustion, tiredness, and lack of appetite.

The blood deficiency in this case is not only attributable to the deficiency of Spleen qi and Kidney essence, but also to her menstruating twice while she was still breastfeeding. Breast milk arises from the transformation of blood in the Penetrating vessel. Menstrual bleeding does not usually occur during pregnancy or while nursing, and thus no excess blood is lost. Consequently, most healthy and strong pregnant or nursing women have a surplus of blood. If bleeding does occur during the time of nursing, blood deficiency will develop, which in turn may impair the function of the Penetrating vessel. Blood is an aspect of yin; thus if blood deficiency is present before the pregnancy, it may lead to a weakness of the yin and essence. The patient's blood and yin deficiency is reflected in her floating and thin pulse.

The hair loss here stems from a deficiency of blood and Kidney essence. "The flourishing of the Kidneys shows in the head hair."[13] The dry skin reflects insufficient moistening from the blood.

The Spleen and Stomach are the root of postnatal essence. Both organs are pivotal in the production of qi and blood. As previously noted, pregnancy, birthing, and breastfeeding reduce a woman's energy. Thus, this patient not only suffers from exhaustion caused by a lack of nutritive qi, she also experiences recurring colds as a result of the weakness of her protective qi.

The patient's continual weight loss and thin appearance can be attributed to her lack of appetite. She consumes just enough to cover her daily requirements, and thus her Stomach and Spleen do not have enough 'material' at their disposal to transform the ingested food and to transport the essence derived from the food. This aggravates her qi deficiency, and because her Spleen and Stomach qi are depleted, her Kidney yin and essence are not properly nourished. The combination of malnutrition and her pregnancy has aggravated her deficiencies, resulting in severe exhaustion.

Loose stools are another sign of Spleen qi deficiency. The Spleen qi sinks downward, which means that the clear yang cannot be lifted. However, the remaining tongue coating is slightly yellow and dry, which suggests stagnation of food, that is, what little food the patient does eat is barely digested. Together with her underlying Stomach qi deficiency, this results in the counterflow of the Stomach qi and is responsible for the occasional bouts of nausea.

Treatment strategy. Strengthen the Spleen and Stomach qi, and nourish the Kidney yin and Kidney essence.

A decoction of Six-Ingredient Pill with Rehmannia *(liù wèi dì huáng wán)* was prescribed, with the following additions: Polygonati Rhizoma *(huáng jīng)*, Polygonati odorati Rhizoma *(yù zhú)*, Polygoni multiflori Radix *(hé shǒu wū)*, and Codonopsis Radix *(dǎng shēn)*. After taking the decoction for two weeks, the patient's appetite returned and her weight remained stable. She felt slightly stronger. After four weeks, she felt much better, her appetite was normal, and she had gained weight. The hair loss stopped after taking the decoction for six weeks.

Tongue description	**Chinese diagnosis**
Slightly pale, cracked tongue body	Blood and Kidney yin deficiency
Peeled coating on the center and posterior third	Stomach and Kidney yin deficiency
Red spots on the anterior and middle thirds	Remaining heat factor

Fig. 3.8.2
Female
46 years old

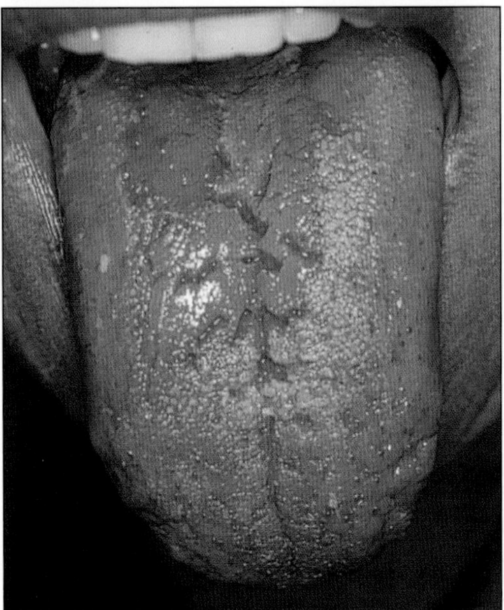

Symptoms

Incontinence of urine, dribbling of urine after urination
Night sweats
Bleeding gums, receding gums

Western diagnosis

Weak pelvic muscles, Morbus Hodgkin, periodontitis

Background to disease

Chemotherapy and radiation 12 months before
Birth of first child three years before

CASE HISTORY After giving birth to her first child at the age of 43, the patient's bladder became weak. She performed pelvic floor exercises daily, but there was still some slight dribbling following urination that developed into a greater loss at unexpected times. She breastfed for one year, which she enjoyed, but it left her feeling exhausted.

Eighteen months ago she was diagnosed with Morbus Hodgkin; as a result, she underwent chemotherapy and radiation therapy and is now in remission. However, since the treatment, her sleep is disrupted, and she suffers from severe night sweats and hot flushes. The patient attributes her exhaustion to lack of sleep.

Since the time of her chemotherapy, her gums receded and bled easily, and even after dental treatment, there was no improvement. Her pulse was floating and deficient.

Analysis. The patient's late pregnancy, at the age of 43, plus one year of breastfeeding, weakened her blood and Kidney yin and essence. The blood deficiency is reflected in the slightly pale tongue body, and the Kidney yin deficiency in the cracked tongue body and peeled coating. The deep cracks in the center and posterior third of the tongue underline this deficiency. It is important to note that the cracks are very pronounced and deep at the center of the tongue. Starting at this area, the coating is without root and extends to the posterior third of the tongue. There is no normal tongue coating because of the lack of fluids caused by the underlying Kidney yin deficiency. The extensive peeled coating and cracks suggest both Stomach and Kidney yin deficiency. The tongue body color is relevant to this analysis because it helps determine the treatment strategy, that is, both the yin and blood are in need of nourishment.

The patient's pregnancy, breastfeeding, and chemotherapy are responsible for the blood and yin deficiency. The Kidneys are the root of yin and yang in the body. They control the two lower orifices, the urethra and the anus. These orifices only open and close appropriately when the yin and yang are in harmony. Their dysfunction may be caused by deficiency of the Kidney yin or yang. In this case, the deficiency of Kidney yang is a result of diminished Kidney yin, which stems from the pregnancy, and, possibly, the chemotherapy. Since the Kidney qi cannot hold the urine, she has become incontinent.

The Kidney yin function of drawing the yang inside has been impaired, and thus the yang remains on the surface, where it is manifested in night sweats. Because these symptoms appeared during and after her chemotherapy, it can be assumed that the medication weakened the yin.

Pathomechanism

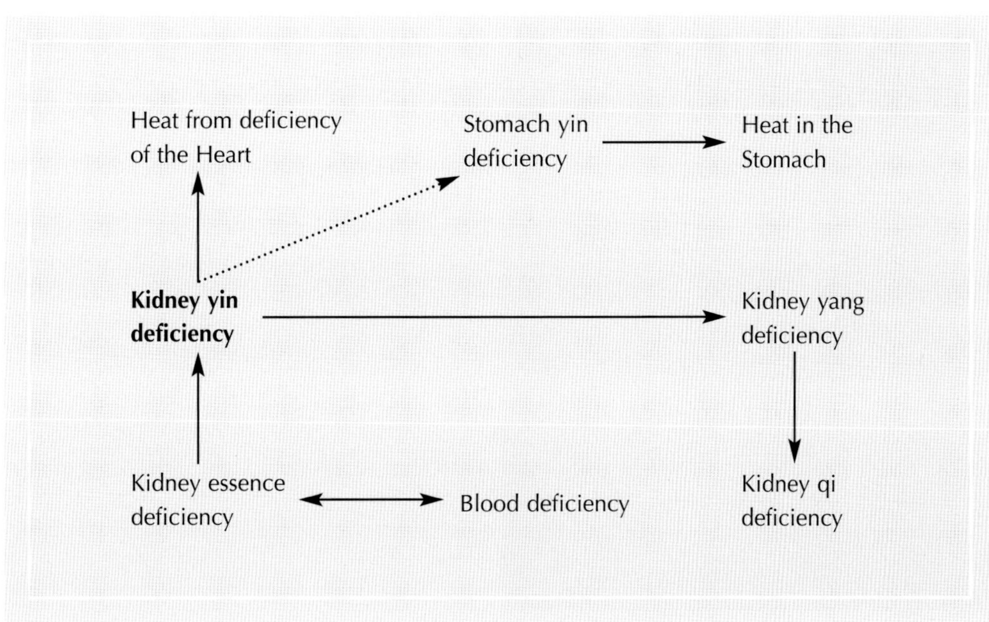

The deep cracks in the center of the tongue indicate injury to the Stomach yin and fluids, resulting in developing heat that affects the Stomach and yang brightness channels. Acute bleeding of the gums is a result of this condition. The Kidneys control the firmness of the teeth. It is said that the teeth are a surplus of the bones, and that the bones are governed by the Kidneys. In this case, loose teeth, a result of receding gums, is interpreted as another sign of Kidney yin deficiency. The floating and deficient pulse confirms the diagnosis of Kidney yin deficiency.

The red spots on the tongue body may denote an externally-contracted pathogenic factor or an accumulation of heat toxin from the chemotherapy and radiation. Since the patient could not remember an acute infectious illness, the first possibility can be eliminated. The radiation in this case was applied to the neck and chest area. Thus, the penetration and accumulation of heat toxin manifested as red spots.

Treatment strategy. Nourish the blood and the Stomach and Kidney yin, strengthen the Kidney qi, and drain heat from the Stomach.

The patient was treated with acupuncture once a week over a five-week period. The following point combination was very successful as she lost no urine for two weeks after the needling:

HT-6 *(yīn xī),* KI-5 *(shuǐ quán),* and CV-4 *(guān yuán)*

Other points used included KI-6 *(zhào hǎi)*, KI-7 *(fù liū)*, ST-36 *(zǔ sān lǐ)* and BL-23 *(shèn shū)*.

At the same time, a modified version of Mantis Egg-Case Powder *(sāng piāo xiāo sǎn)* was prescribed. Following this treatment, the incontinence, night sweats, and hot flushes rarely appeared. The patient felt much stronger and is continuing with the treatment.

Tongue description	**Chinese diagnosis**
Red with peeled coating	Kidney yin deficiency
Two parallel cracks in the anterior third	Constitutional weakness of the Lungs
Deep, vertical central crack in the anterior third	Lung yin deficiency

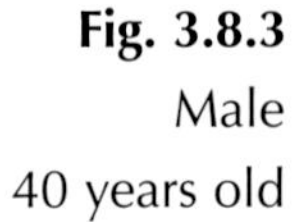

Fig. 3.8.3
Male
40 years old

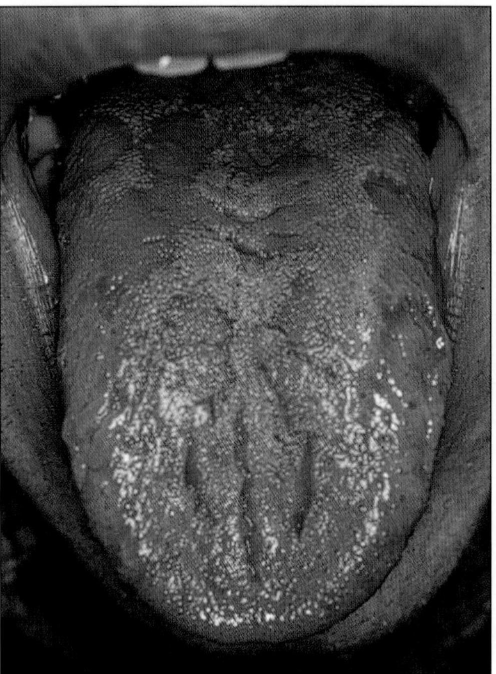

Symptoms

Weakness of the legs
Tingling and numbness of the left arm
Unclear speech, sight defect
Night sweats
Inner restlessness, inability to concentrate

Western diagnosis

Multiple sclerosis

Background to disease

Physical and mental overexertion

CASE HISTORY The first acute attack of multiple sclerosis occurred one year prior to visiting the clinic, with the sudden paralysis of the right arm and the inability to speak properly. The administration of cortisone was immediately successful, but the patient, although physically well, became severely depressed.

A week before the consultation the patient experienced weakness in the legs, accompanied by tingling and numbness of the left arm. His condition visibly deteriorated over the course of a few days. His speech became slurred and he was unable to concentrate. His visual acuity also declined, especially in relation to colors.

His sleep was very poor, which he attributed to his emotional state, and he sweated profusely at night. He refused a second cortisone treatment because he feared another bout of depression.

Prior to the onset of multiple sclerosis, he had never been ill. The only symptom he had experienced during the previous few years was night sweats.

Owing to his responsibilities at work, his family life had suffered, which burdened him both physically and emotionally. He ate irregularly and often missed meals. His pulse was rapid, floating, and deficient.

Analysis. In Chinese medicine, multiple sclerosis is characterized as an atrophy disorder. Its appearance is attributed to the following disease factors:

- Externally-contracted dampness
- Excessive consumption of raw foods and dairy products
- Excessive sexual activity
- Mental shock

After a thorough investigation it appeared that none of these factors applied to the patient. He stressed, again and again, that over the years many physical and mental demands had been made of him, which he had dealt with only through sheer willpower. Financial concerns, the education of four children, the lengthy construction of his house, and his exhausting workload had worn him down. These factors, plus the injury to his fluids as a result of frequent night sweats, may have been responsible for the depletion of his Kidney yin, which manifested in the reddish tongue body and rootless coating, and was confirmed by the rapid, floating, and deficient quality of his pulse.

The depletion of Kidney energy was caused by the taxing physical and mental demands made upon him, as well as the excessive use of willpower. ("The Kidneys house the will."[14])

Pathomechanism

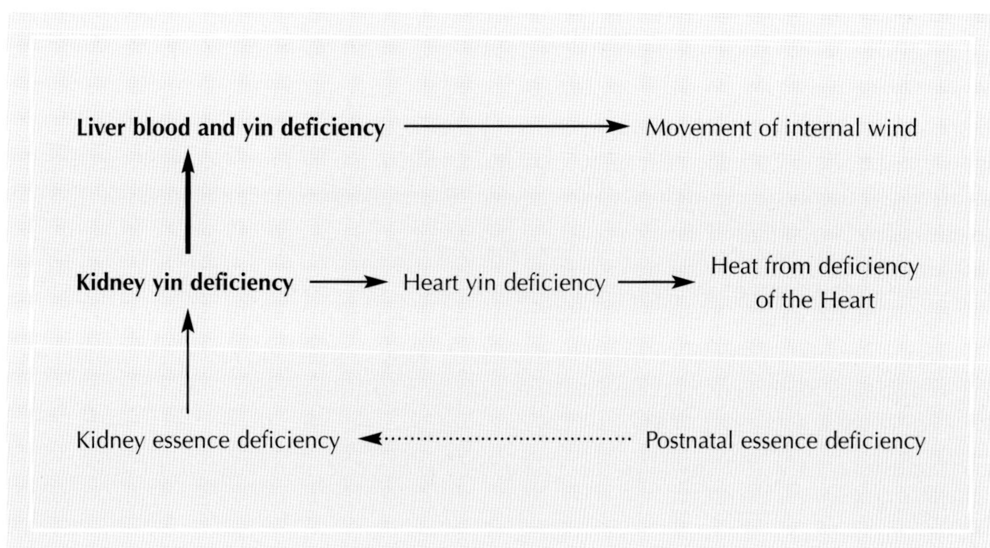

The will *(zhì)* bestows on man steadfastness, endurance, and decisiveness. But when it is abused, the result may be depletion of qi and essence. All of these factors resulted in a weakening of Kidney yin and essence. The patient's irregular eating habits injured his postnatal essence, which in turn failed to properly nourish the Kidney essence.

Insufficient nourishment of the sinews, tendons, and bones results from Kidney and Liver yin deficiency. This was experienced here as a lack of strength in his legs. Liver yin deficiency, which includes the pattern of Liver blood deficiency, contributed to a decline in visual acuity. At the time of the first multiple sclerosis attack, the extent of Liver blood and yin deficiency was enough to cause internal movement of wind. Tingling and a sensation of numbness in the arms were the first signs of this pathology.

The strong night sweats are the result of Kidney and Heart yin deficiency that led to the development of heat from deficiency. The slurred speech might have been caused by insufficient nourishment to the root of the tongue (attributable to the Kidneys), but since the tongue is an offshoot of the Heart, it is possible that the development of heat disturbed the Heart qi, which led to hesitant speech.

The weakness of the Kidney energy disrupted communication with the Heart. Indications of this are fear, inner restlessness, the inability to concentrate, as well as an inability to change his life even though he knew he must. This underlying disharmony may have been responsible for the serious depression that followed the administration of the cortisone, since the medication may have caused an imbalance of yin and yang in the Kidneys.

Treatment strategy. Extinguish the internal wind, nourish the Kidney yin, Liver yin and blood, and calm the spirit.

A large dose of Anemarrhena, Phellodendron, and Rehmannia Pill *(zhī bái dì huáng wán)* was prescribed, with the addition of Lycii Cortex *(dì gǔ pí)*, Trionycis Carapax *(biē jiă)*, and Taxilli Herba *(sāng jì shēng)*. After four days the tingling and numbness were very much reduced, and the patient felt calmer.

His night sweats, impaired vision, and speech did not improve. Therefore, Lycii Fructus *(gǒu qǐ zǐ)*, Acori tatarinowii Rhizoma *(shí chāng pǔ)*, and Polygalae Radix *(yuǎn zhì)* were added to the prescription. After two weeks, the night sweats were radically improved. The patient still felt exhausted and psychologically unstable, and the treatment therefore continued. However, herbal treatment over a period of nine months did not improve the condition of the patient. He had one more serious bout which led to paralysis of the extremities and confined him to a wheelchair.

Endnotes

1 In some rare cases a red, wet tongue is not indicative of yin deficiency, but quite the opposite: It reflects yang deficiency. For a discussion of red, wet tongues, see Maciocia G. *Tongue Diagnosis in Chinese Medicine*, rev. ed. Seattle: Eastland Press, 1995:47-48.

2 A pituitary tumor characterized by the hypersecretion of prolactin.

3 Over the past years of clinical practice I have come to pay less attention to the cracks, especially when they appear in combination with a pale tongue body color. I now deem them important if they are covered by a yellow coating or if around the crack a reddening can be seen. Both signs indicate that heat is present, contributing to or causing the formation or deepening of the crack.

4 Compare Li N-M. *Zhong guo she zhen da quan*. Beijing: Xueyuan Publishing Company, 1994:1196.

5 A pathological tongue coating caused by Stomach yin deficiency will be discussed in Ch. 4.

6 Maciocia G. *The Foundations of Chinese Medicine.* Edinburgh: Churchill Livingstone, 1989: 249.

7 Anonymous. *Su wen* [Basic Questions], edited by He W-B et al. Beijing: China Medicine Science and Technology Press, 1996: 44:249.

8 These disharmonies are discussed in more detail in the corresponding chapters.

9 See Ch. 6.

10 See Fig. 4.1.1.2.

11 Note that a peeled area does not always signify pathology in a corresponding organ.

12 Maciocia G. *Obstetrics and Gynecology in Chinese Medicine.* London: Churchill Livingstone, 1998: 14.

13 *Basic Questions,* 9:54.

14 *Basic Questions,* 3:147.

CHAPTER 4

Tongue Signs Associated with Stomach Disharmonies

4.1 Disease Patterns and Tongue Signs Associated with the Stomach

The Stomach plays a very important role in the production of energy and fluids. It is the only hollow (yang) organ that can present with a pattern of true yin deficiency; it has a close connection to the five yin organs.[1]

In the Chinese medical classics, the Stomach is described as the "sea of fluids and grains."[2] Solids and liquids are received, rotted, and ripened by the Stomach. In order to properly function, the Stomach needs a damp environment, hence the saying, "The Stomach loves dampness and dislikes dryness."[3] The Stomach condenses the impure part of the essence in food, which then forms part of the body fluids. The Stomach needs qi and fluids in order to digest food. The Stomach is filled with turbid dampness, a by-product of the rotting and ripening activity, and this turbid dampness 'steams upward' to the tongue, forming a healthy, white, thin, and slightly moist coating. The tongue coating reflects the quality of the Stomach qi and of the damp environment in the Stomach. A thin, white, and moist tongue coating is a sign of the harmonious working of healthy Stomach qi.

4.1.1 Stomach Qi

Stomach qi has a close relationship with the Spleen, and symptoms related to each organ may appear whenever there is Stomach and/or Spleen qi deficiency: tiredness, lack of appetite, weakness of the extremities, pale tongue body. An inappropriate diet is often the cause of this deficiency. Overconsumption of raw foods weakens the Spleen, while eating too little, as well as irregular eating, injure the Stomach qi (Fig. 2.1.3). Chronic illness may also deplete the Spleen and Stomach qi (Fig. 2.1.6).

Tongue signs

Pale with:

- thin coating in the center of the tongue
- peeled coating in the center of the tongue
- superficial cracks in the center of the tongue (Fig. 2.5.3). Occasionally, these cracks appear after an acute illness and will disappear over time; this is only true for small, superficial cracks. It should be noted that the presence of thin cracks on a pale or pale red tongue body is often inconsequential.

A chronic deficiency of Stomach qi may lead to deficiency of Stomach yin. In this case, the Stomach yin deficiency is often aggravated by irregular eating habits, a stressful lifestyle, or eating late meals (Fig. 4.1.5.1). If Stomach qi deficiency and Stomach yin deficiency occur simultaneously, symptoms of both conditions may occur: tiredness, soft stools, stomach pains, dry mouth, and/or a bloated feeling after meals (Fig. 4.1.2.5). In this instance, the center of the *tongue will be red and lack a coating*; the *tongue body* often remains *pale* or *pale red* (Fig. 4.1.2.5). This progression from Stomach qi deficiency to Stomach yin deficiency is often caused by inappropriate diet or malnutrition. In such cases, the injury to the Stomach yin is reflected by *cracks in the center of the tongue*, and the Spleen and Stomach qi deficiency is reflected in the pale tongue body color.

4.1.2 Stomach Yin

The yin of the body is rooted in the Kidneys. All the organs and tissues are nourished by this constructive energy. A general deficiency of yin will eventually lead to malnourishment of the Lungs, Liver, Heart, Stomach, and, to a lesser extent, the Spleen. Depending on the patient's constitution, Kidney yin deficiency may lead, for example, to Lung or Heart yin deficiency. However, a single yin organ can suffer from yin deficiency without the participation or involvement of Kidney yin. For example, an 'isolated' yin deficiency of the Stomach does not necessarily mean that the yin of the Kidneys is automatically affected. However, over the long term, deficiency of Stomach yin will lead to Kidney yin deficiency.

When taken in excess, fried or toasted foods, hot spices (curry, chili, pepper, mustard), or hot drinks (coffee) have a drying effect on the fluids in the Stomach. After a while, the continuous intake of such foods will injure the Stomach yin. This development is reflected in different signs on the tongue. First, a dry tongue center is visible, which is a sign of slight deficiency of fluids. If this area becomes redder, it reflects the development of Stomach heat. The typical feeling of hunger that accompanies this pathology is described as follows in Ch. 20 of the *Divine Pivot:* "When the pathogen is located in the Stomach and Spleen, a person will suffer from pain in the muscles and flesh. When the yang qi [Stomach] has a surplus and the yin qi [Spleen] is insufficient, there will be [a sensation of] heat in the center and the person will be constantly hungry."[4]

One who suffers from Stomach yin deficiency will experience constipation, dry mouth and throat, and thirst (but without a desire to drink). Stomach yin deficiency frequently occurs in combination with other disease patterns, especially heat in the Stomach, Liver qi stagnation, and Kidney yin deficiency. They are all represented in the case histories.

At first, deficiency of Stomach yin will not affect the Kidney yin and there will only be symptoms associated with a disharmony of the Stomach. In this case the tongue body itself will not necessarily be red or reddish. With Stomach yin deficiency, tongue signs will appear at the center of the tongue, that is, *a reddening in this area.*

Tongue signs

- rootless or no coating in the center (Fig. 4.1.2.2)
- short, small, irregular cracks in the center (Fig. 4.1.2.3)
- deep, vertical crack in the center (Figs. 4.1.2.9). In these cases, the cracks are limited to the center of the tongue and are not necessarily accompanied by a red discoloration of the tongue body, which would be the case if the condition were acute or severe.
- dry, cracked tongue body (Figs. 4.1.2.8). When there is a lack of turbid steam (due to a lack of fluids) the tongue becomes dry and usually signals dryness in the Stomach, which over time leads to insufficient coating.

If the Stomach yin deficiency is severe, the tongue body will take on a *red color with deep cracks in the center* (Fig. 4.1.2.8). These cracks are often an indication of an inappropriate diet or other habit, such as too much spicy foods, alcohol, or drugs. Too much of these things will injure the yin; as a result, the tongue body will lack sufficient moisture or nourishment and form small cracks. Acquired cracks are irregular and of different depths, which may indicate injury at different times, while a single deep, often wide, crack in the center of the tongue independent of the tongue body color points toward a constitutional weakness of the Stomach.

If, however, Stomach and Kidney yin deficiency do occur simultaneously, signs and symptoms of both will appear: night sweats, feelings of heat in the body, heat in the five centers, sparse, dark urine, and

- a red, dry tongue body (Fig. 3.6.6); or
- a red, dry tongue body with deep cracks in the center (Fig. 4.1.2.8)
- red tongue without a coating (Figs. 4.1.2.8)
- rootless, irregular-looking, widespread coating in connection with a red or reddish tongue body (Fig. 3.6.3).

Tongue description	**Chinese diagnosis**
Pale red, slightly swollen	Slight Spleen qi deficiency
Slightly peeled, red center	Onset of heat in the Stomach
Yellow coating with red points at the root	Damp-heat in the Intestines

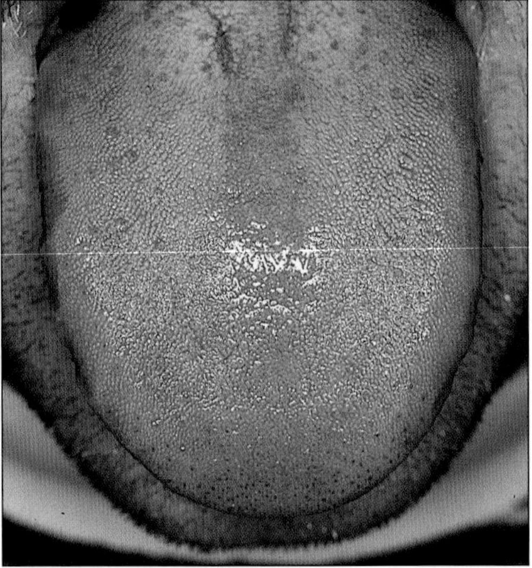

Fig. 4.1.2.1
Male
26 years old

Symptoms

Heartburn, regurgitation
Stomach pain with stress
Diarrhea after intake of dairy products

Western diagnosis

None

Background to disease

Stress due to examinations
Excessive intake of dairy products

Tongue description	**Chinese diagnosis**
Pale red	Normal
Peeled, red, cracked center	Stomach yin deficiency with heat in the Stomach
Yellow, greasy coating at the sides	Accumulation of damp-heat in Stomach and Large Intestine
Reddish in the anterior third	Heat in the upper burner, especially in the Heart

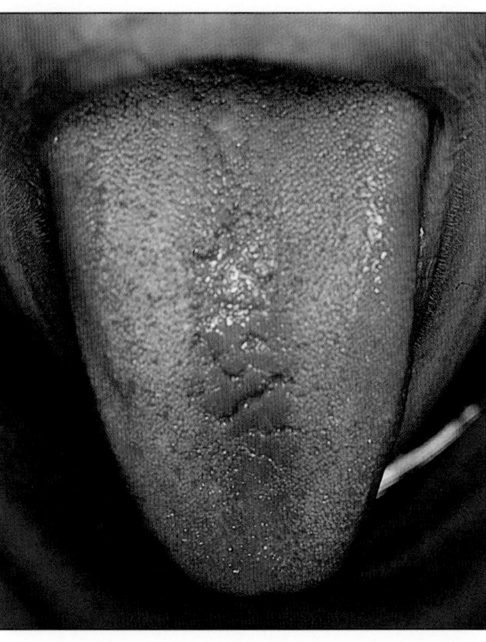

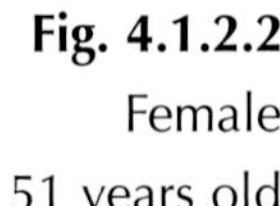

Fig. 4.1.2.2
Female
51 years old

Symptoms

Bleeding gums
Mouth ulcers
Dry stools
Vaginal discharge
Red face
Lumbar pain

Western diagnosis

None

Background to disease

Physically overworked
Late evening meals
Caffeine abuse

Tongue description	Chinese diagnosis
Pale red, slightly thin tongue body, edges slightly pale	Spleen qi deficiency (slight Liver blood deficiency)
Vertical crack with small horizontal cracks branching off, without coating	Stomach yin deficiency
Slightly reddish center to the tongue	Heat in the Stomach

Symptoms

Heartburn
Stomach pain
Hot feeling in the stomach
Fatigue, inability to fall asleep

Western diagnosis

Reflux esophagitis

Background to disease

Irregular eating habits
Strong demands at work

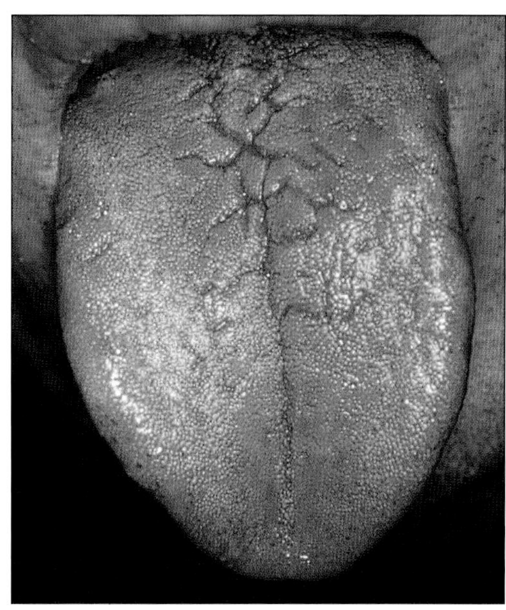

Fig. 4.1.2.3
Male
44 years old

Tongue description	Chinese diagnosis
Pale red	Normal
Slightly pale edges	Liver blood deficiency
Swollen	Spleen qi deficiency with accumulation of dampness
Reddish center without coating	Stomach yin deficiency
Cracks in the center	Stomach yin deficiency
Deep cracks at the sides of the tongue	Severe Spleen qi deficiency
Slightly reddish tip	Heat in the Heart

Symptoms

Stomach pain, especially on an empty stomach
Numbness, sensitivity of the thigh, feet, and small finger of right hand
Spasticity and weakness of the thigh muscles
Lack of appetite and thirst
Inner restlessness

Western diagnosis

Multiple sclerosis, duodenal ulcer

Background to disease

Cold working conditions, overconsumption of dairy foods, side effects of glucocorticoids

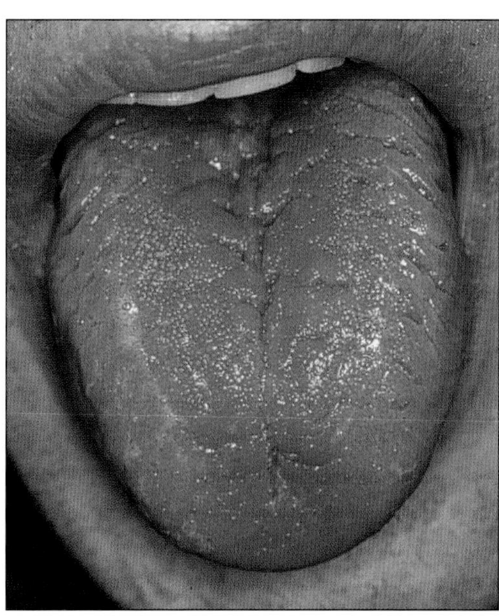

Fig. 4.1.2.4
Male
35 years old

Tongue description	Chinese diagnosis
Red, wide, thin	Injury to fluids due to heat
Peeled, red, cracked center	Stomach yin deficiency with heat in the Stomach
Curled-up, slightly swollen edges	Liver qi constraint with heat in the Liver
Reddish, curled-down tip	Heat from deficiency in the Heart
Yellow, slightly thick coating with red points at the root	Accumulation of damp-heat in Large Intestine

Fig. 4.1.2.5
Male
37 years old

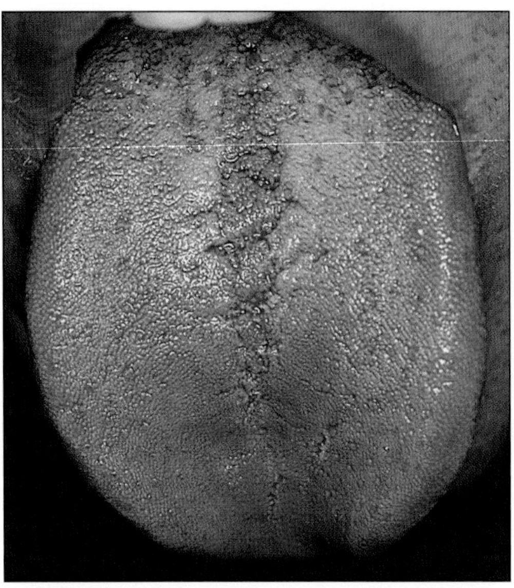

Symptoms

Constant headache, migraines
Inner restlessness
Occasional stomach pains
Smelly, loose stools

Western diagnosis

None

Background to disease

Trauma (fracture of the skull 2 years ago)
Alcohol abuse in the past
Excessive consumption of spicy foods
Emotional problems

Tongue description	Chinese diagnosis
Pale red, swollen	Spleen qi deficiency with accumulation of dampness
Thick, greasy coating on the left side	Accumulation of damp-heat in the Liver and Gallbladder
Coating without root	Stomach yin deficiency
Deep crack in the center with yellow, greasy coating	Stomach yin deficiency with accumulation of phlegm-fire in the Stomach

Fig. 4.1.2.6
Female
54 years old

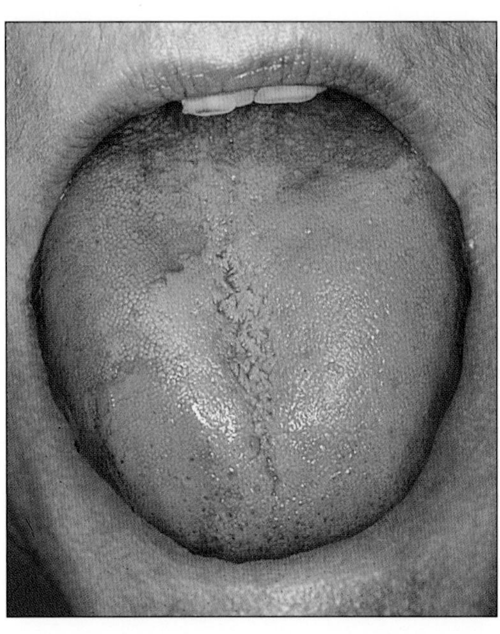

Symptoms

Loss of hearing in left ear
Tinnitus and earache
Panic attacks
Inner restlessness, nervousness
Dizziness in the morning
Headaches
Insomnia
Occasional night sweats

Western diagnosis

Acute loss of hearing

Background to disease

Excessive demands at work
Emotional problems

Tongue description

Reddish

Curled-up, slightly indented edges

Cracks in the center

Yellow, greasy coating with red points on the posterior third

Chinese diagnosis

Developing heat

Liver qi stagnation

Stomach yin deficiency

Food stagnation with developing heat

Symptoms

Difficulty in swallowing
Constipation with hard, pellet-like stools
Distended abdomen, fullness of the epigastrium, belching
Dryness of the mouth at night
Headaches with occasional vomiting of bile

Western diagnosis

Reflux esophagitis, hiatus hernia

Background to disease

Irregular diet
Frequent late evening meals
Long-standing emotional problems

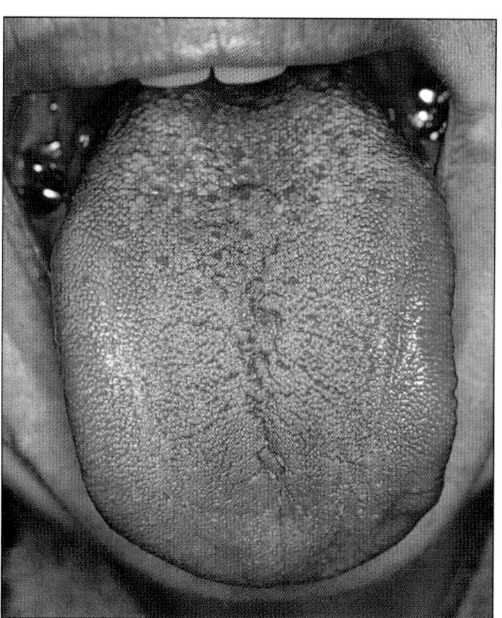

Fig. 4.1.2.7
Female
66 years old

About these case histories

These case histories are devoted to patterns in which Stomach yin deficiency is a major causative agent in the overall pathomechanism. Additional factors that play an important role in these case histories include other patterns of deficiency, such as yin deficiency of the Kidney and Heart blood deficiency.

Tongue description	Chinese diagnosis
Reddish, rough surface	Kidney yin deficiency
Wide	Possible Spleen qi deficiency
Pale edges	Liver blood deficiency
Red, dry center with deep cracks and yellow, old, sparse coating	Stomach yin deficiency with heat in the Stomach
Depression and slightly contracted root	Kidney yin and essence deficiency
Rootless coating	Kidney yin deficiency

Fig. 4.1.2.8
Female
62 years old

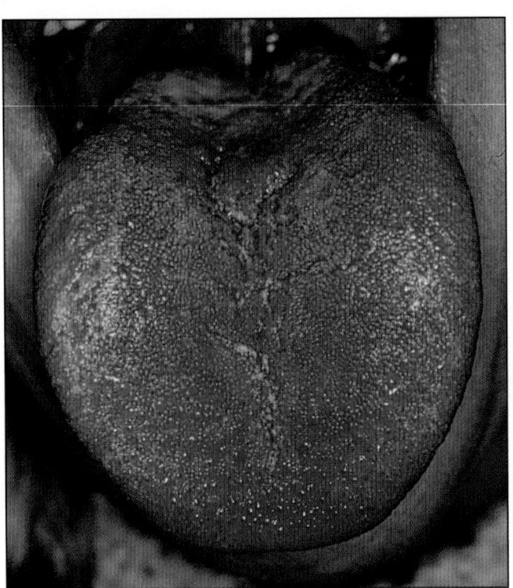

Symptoms

Toothache, bleeding of gums, loose teeth
Lack of appetite, extreme thirst
Insomnia, depressive moods
Hair loss
Severe exhaustion

Western diagnosis

Periodontal disease

Background to disease

Condition began two years after removal of right kidney due to benign tumor; unhappily married for 30 years

CASE HISTORY One year prior to visiting the clinic the patient had three teeth removed as a result of inflammation of the gums. The dental treatment, which included long-term administration of antibiotics, had not reduced or stopped the inflammation. She still had four loose teeth, and she suffered from severe toothache, which she tried to assuage with painkillers.

For 30 years she had suffered from insomnia and regularly took sleeping pills. Despite the medication, she woke many times during the night. She attributed her sleeping problems to her unhappy marriage. In addition, she suffered from dryness of the mouth and extreme thirst at night.

Since the removal of her right kidney, she had lost her appetite. She weighed 114 pounds, having lost 22 pounds since the surgery. She was 5 feet 9 inches tall. Both her depressive moods and extreme exhaustion made her antisocial, and she appeared weak and haggard. Her hair had become very thin and over the previous six months had started to fall out. Her pulse was floating, rapid, and tight.

Analysis. The rough surface of the tongue body combined with the rootless coating is very significant. These tongue signs are indicative of Stomach and Kidney yin deficiency as well as injury to the fluids. The cracks in the tongue body are especially pronounced on the posterior third of the tongue and signal injury to the Kidney yin. Overall, the tongue signs reflect an exhaustion of yin and point toward the patient's weak constitution.

The cracked, dry center of the tongue denotes underlying Stomach yin deficiency. Apart from the redness of the center, the remaining yellow, old, and sparse coating is an indication of developing Stomach heat that is transforming into fire and then injuring the fluids, particularly the Stomach yin; this process is inhibiting the formation of a new coating.

Pathomechanism

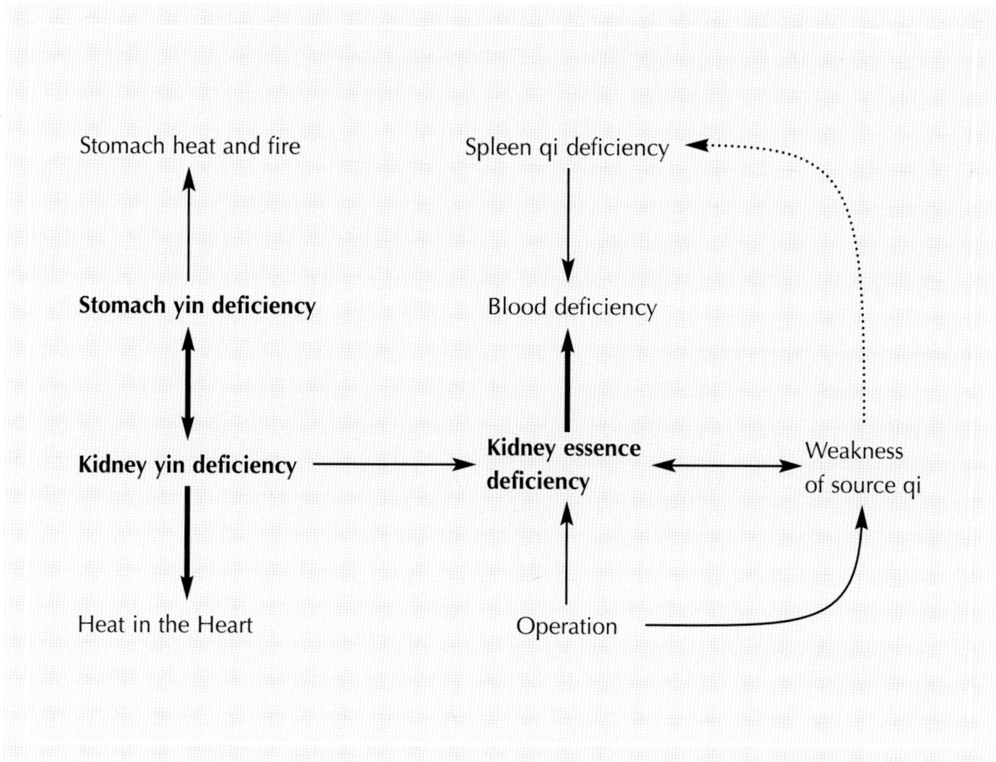

Severe toothache, bleeding gums, and loose teeth basically correspond to a pattern of Stomach heat with an underlying deficiency of Stomach yin; the yin deficiency and developing heat are also reflected in the floating and rapid pulse. The heat in the Stomach obstructs the flow of qi in the yang brightness Stomach and Large Intestine channels, which results in toothache. The patient's acute pain results in a tight pulse. Fire develops from the heat, causing injury to the blood vessels and thereby resulting in bleeding gums.

The Kidneys nourish the teeth; deficient Kidney yin cannot supply sufficient nourishment, which leads to loosening of the teeth. The dryness of the mouth and extreme thirst at night occur when the patient's yin reaches its maximum and is a manifestation of the lack of bodily fluids and yin. These symptoms are another expression of the Kidney yin deficiency, while the lack of appetite is a sign of Stomach yin deficiency. The slightly pale edges to the tongue also point to another deficiency, that of Liver blood.

The patient's general condition is very poor and her body and mind are exhausted. The long-standing disharmony of fire and water is responsible for her depression and severe sleeping problems. Fear of her husband's outbursts, and years of unhappiness, have contributed to an exhaustion of the yin. The areas of the tongue which reflect the condition of the Heart and Kidney show pathological changes. The root of the tongue is not only depressed, it is also slightly contracted. In addition, there is hardly any coating, which indicates a deficiency of Kidney yin and essence. The tip of the tongue is slightly red and signals heat in the Heart. Weakened Kidney yin allows heat in the Heart to develop, which in turn agitates the spirit and causes the insomnia.

The weakened constitution is manifested in the patient's air of resignation, tiredness, and lack of 'sparkle.' After an operation two years earlier, her general condition deteriorated. The tumor in the right kidney had not caused any symptoms and was found by chance. However, the operation had left her severely exhausted and with no appetite. Her weight loss suggests a decrease in source qi and Kidney essence. The source qi supports the Spleen's transportive and transformative functions. Inadequate nutrition, as well as Spleen qi deficiency, have weakened the postnatal essence, which in turn has failed to nourish the Kidney essence; this aggravates her severe tiredness. The tongue, however, does not show any signs of Spleen qi deficiency. Only, perhaps, the excessive width of the tongue body would suggest this. However, this sign is not very distinct; it cannot be interpreted with certainty, and is therefore not emphasized here.

As a rule, wide, swollen tongues reflect an accumulation of dampness. Here, however, the tongue is slightly thin and wide. In a red tongue, a slightly thin shape denotes deficiency of blood and yin. Here, the deficiency of Kidney essence and blood manifests as thinning hair accompanied by hair loss.

Treatment strategy. Drain heat from the Stomach, nourish the Stomach and Kidney yin, supplement the Kidney essence, and enrich the blood.

Over a period of many weeks the patient took Clear the Stomach Decoction *(qīng wèi tāng)*. Both her bleeding gums and toothache disappeared. However, four loose teeth had to be extracted. She then decided to have implants. During the course of her dental treatment (which progressed without complications) she continued to take Chinese herbs, which nourished her Stomach and Kidney yin.

Tongue description	**Chinese diagnosis**
Reddish, slightly dull	Spleen yin deficiency with development of heat
Swollen	Accumulation of phlegm
Deep vertical crack in the center	Stomach yin deficiency
Red center without coating	Stomach yin deficiency
Deep cracks at the sides of the tongue	Spleen yin deficiency
Reddish anterior third	Heat in the upper burner
Slight indentation of the tip	Heart blood and yin deficiency

Fig. 4.1.2.9
Female
25 years old

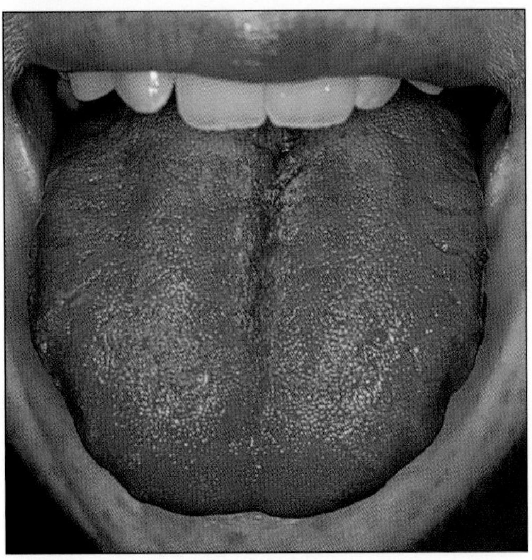

Symptoms

Lack of appetite, weight loss
Thirst with drinking of lots of water
Constipation
Insomnia
Swelling of the cervical lymph nodes

Western diagnosis

Hodgkin's lymphoma, splenomegaly

Background to disease

Anorexia nervosa between the ages of 11 and 14
Recurring tonsillitis
Chemotherapy and radiation

CASE HISTORY Hodgkin's lymphoma was diagnosed three years prior to meeting the patient. After nine months of chemotherapy and radiation, the patient was in remission. The swollen lymph nodes in the neck region, which were still present, were hard, fixed, and coarse. The enlarged spleen did not cause any problems.

Although the patient generally felt well, she was very worried about her continual weight loss; at 5 feet 5 inches tall, she weighed only 92 pounds. Her face seemed puffy and her connective tissue was very soft, all of which made her feel very unattractive.

She never felt hungry but she was thirsty and drank a lot of water. Her stools were hard and formed but she had a bowel movement only every second or third day.

She did not sleep well, waking once or twice in the night, but she did not feel particularly tired. Her periods stopped after the chemotherapy. She frequently suffered from tonsillitis, both before and after the onset of the illness. Her pulse was slightly rapid, thin, and short.

Analysis. As is amply shown in the tongue body, this case is one of emaciation caused by Spleen and Stomach yin deficiency with the development of heat. The reddish tongue with cracks at the edges reflects the deficiency of Spleen yin and heat in the interior, while the deep, vertical midline crack indicates Stomach yin deficiency.

The swollen tongue body reflects an accumulation of dampness, a condition of excess, due to the underlying Spleen qi deficiency. The dampness manifests in the patient's puffy face. The congenital weak connective tissue suggests a constitutional weakness of Spleen qi since the Spleen governs the muscles and flesh.[5] During her years of puberty, the patient was anorexic, which probably severely injured her postnatal essence. A pale, swollen tongue body is usually

Pathomechanism

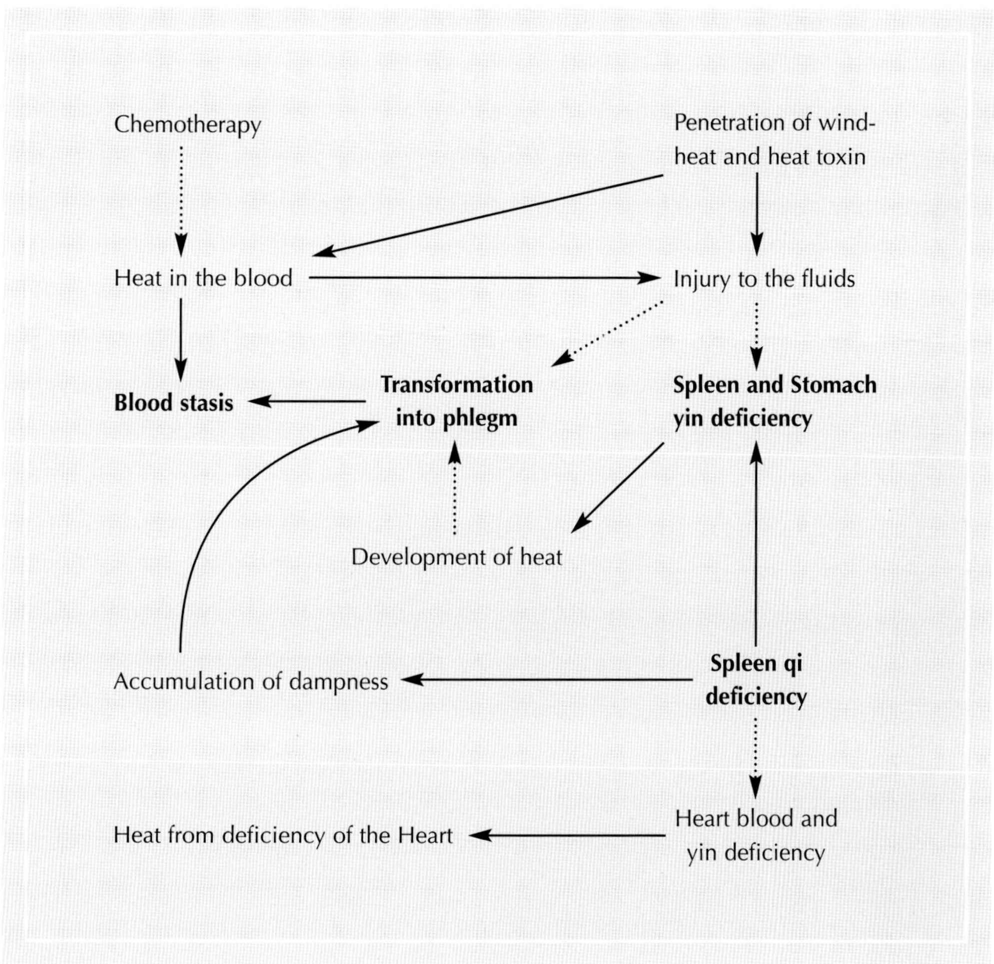

indicative of Spleen qi deficiency and accumulation of dampness. Here, the tongue is red, a significant sign of developing heat that has injured the yin. The color of the tongue body is highly relevant to diagnosing and formulating a treatment strategy.

When the transportive and transformative functions of the Spleen are impaired, accumulation of dampness ensues, and the dampness may transform into phlegm. If heat or fire is present, the clumping of phlegm will accelerate and intensify. Over the long term, the clumps of phlegm may congeal and form knots (see below).

The patient's Spleen and Stomach qi and yin have been severely injured by the course and treatment of her illness, as reflected in the long-standing lack of appetite and weight loss. All of these symptoms point toward Spleen yin deficiency, which is confirmed by the deep cracks on the sides of the tongue. "If the qi of the Spleen is hot, the Stomach is dry [the fluids of the Stomach have dried up]. The patient is thirsty, muscles and flesh are numb, and the flesh loses its function."[6]

The deep, vertical midline crack is a result of Stomach yin deficiency. The absence of coating in the center of the tongue indicates a lack of fluids and Stomach yin. Both engender dryness and deprive the Large Intestine, which is closely connected to the yang brightness Stomach channel, of sufficient moisture. The dryness, and the developing heat in the Stomach, obstruct the sinking of the Stomach qi, resulting in constipation.

Prior to the onset of Hodgkin's lymphoma, the patient frequently suffered from tonsillitis. The repeated penetration of externally-contracted wind-heat led to the formation of heat toxin. The frequency of the bouts suggests that pathogenic heat had accumulated and remained in the throat, manifesting in recurrent tonsillitis. The entrapped heat brewed slowly, injuring the fluids and contributing to the congealing of the blood. If congealed blood unites with phlegm, it gathers and forms knots.[7] This pathomechanism may have contributed to the onset of the illness, and to the appearance of the swollen, hard, fixed, and coarse lymph nodes. The enlargement of the spleen is also the result of blood stasis and the accumulation of phlegm.

After the Hodgkin's lymphoma was treated with chemotherapy and radiation, it went into remission, but left her with weight loss and a complete lack of appetite. In addition, her menstruation ceased. Radiation induces an accumulation of heat toxin and causes dryness and injury to the fluids and yin.[8] Chemotherapy often injures the qi, fluids, and yin, especially if the treatment induces severe vomiting. Over the long term, both forms of treatment may lead to injury of the yin and the development of heat, which is seen here in the red tongue body and very little tongue coating. Heat injures the body fluids and the blood, which can thicken and congeal. The resulting stasis of blood is possibly involved here in the cessation of menstruation. The blood stasis may be reflected in the dull color of the tongue.

The tip of the tongue shows a slight indentation, indicative of slight Heart blood and yin deficiency. Heat from deficiency of the Heart can unsettle the spirit and thereby prevent good sleep. The rapid, short, thin pulse denotes the development of heat from the underlying qi and yin deficiency.

Treatment strategy. Transform the phlegm, soften the knots, cool the heat, eliminate the remaining heat, nourish the Spleen yin and Stomach yin, strengthen the Spleen qi, and improve the appetite.

The patient was prescribed a modified version of Reduce Scrofula Pill (*xiāo luǒ wán*), with the addition of Prunellae Spica (*xià kū cǎo*), Hedyotis diffusae Herba (*bái huā shé shé cǎo*), Forsythiae Fructus (*lián qiào*), Forsythiae Fructus (*lián qiào*), Moutan Cortex (*mǔ dān pí*), Pseudostellariae Radix (*tài zǐ shēn*), Setariae (Oryzae) Fructus germinatus (*gǔ yá*), and Gigeriae galli Endothelium corneum (*jī nèi jīn*).

Her weight loss stopped after taking the decoction for four weeks. Her appetite improved, and she had daily bowel movements, although the stools were still very hard. After an additional six months with different decoctions, the patient's appetite improved still further, and she felt very good. The lymph nodes had shrunk in size and were considerably softer. There has been no recurrence of the tonsillitis, and the patient is continuing with herbal treatment.

4.1.3 Stomach Patterns and the Vertical Midline Crack

A reddish or red tongue with a vertical crack along the midline and within the center of the middle third of the tongue body is typical of Stomach yin deficiency. This is especially true when the center is dry. A diagnosis of Kidney and Stomach yin deficiency is confirmed when, in addition to the *midline crack, the tongue body color appears very red* and presents with either a *peeled coating or none* at all.

In clinical practice, this midline crack is often seen in patients with pale or pale red, swollen tongues. In such cases, the pathogenesis is complicated. The swollen tongue body denotes accumulation of dampness, which arises from a deficiency or weakness of Spleen qi. Spleen and Stomach qi deficiency often appear together. Spleen qi deficiency reduces the organ's function of transport; there is thus a lack of transport through the Stomach qi. Reduced appetite, loose stools, or weakness of the extremities are common symptoms of this pathology. Over the long term, however, Spleen and Stomach qi deficiency can evolve into yin deficiency. Now, in addition to qi deficiency symptoms, yin deficiency symptoms will also appear, for example, epigastric pain, dry mouth and throat especially in the afternoon, and intense thirst with no desire to drink. This yin deficiency is reflected in the vertical crack along the midline of the tongue.

If, however, a vertical crack along the midline appears with normal tongue body color and shape as well as a normal coating, it can be ignored, especially if the patient does not show any symptoms relating to the functions of the Spleen and Stomach. This is quite frequently witnessed in adults who, in puberty or early adulthood, experienced symptoms of Stomach yin deficiency and developing heat, but are currently free of such symptoms as their lifestyles became more regulated with advancing age. This sign may also indicate a *constitutional weakness of the Stomach*, provided that it is localized exclusively in the center of the tongue (Fig. 4.1.2.9). Another interpretation of this tongue sign can be found in the literature: A pale or pale red tongue with a vertical crack along the midline is interpreted as an indication of Stomach qi deficiency.[9]

Tongue description	Chinese diagnosis
Slightly red, swollen	Slight Kidney yin deficiency with accumulation of dampness
Thin, vertical crack	Onset of Stomach yin deficiency
White, new, thin coating in the center	Regeneration of Stomach yin and Spleen and Stomach qi
Slight depression at the root of the tongue	Slight deficiency of essence

Fig. 4.1.3.1
Female
37 years old

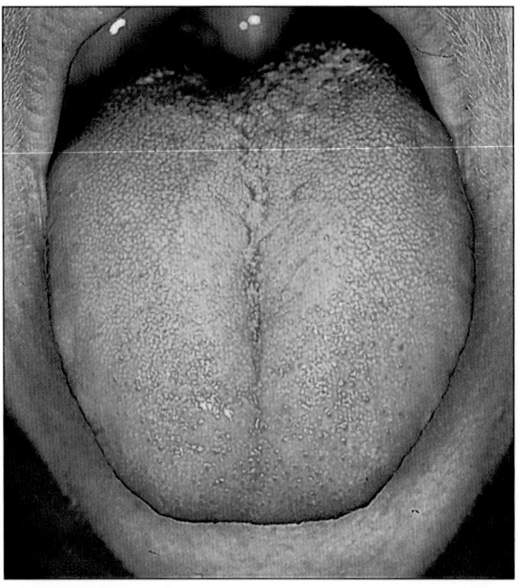

Symptoms

Night sweats
Severe exhaustion
Panic attacks
Sore lower back

Western diagnosis

None

Background to disease

Severe loss of blood following a traumatic injury to the underside of the leg, with subsequent amputation

Tongue description	Chinese diagnosis
Pale, slight teeth marks	Spleen qi deficiency with accumulation of dampness
Deep, vertical crack with small amount of yellow, greasy fur	Stomach yin deficiency with accumulation of damp-heat

Fig. 4.1.3.2
Female
43 years old

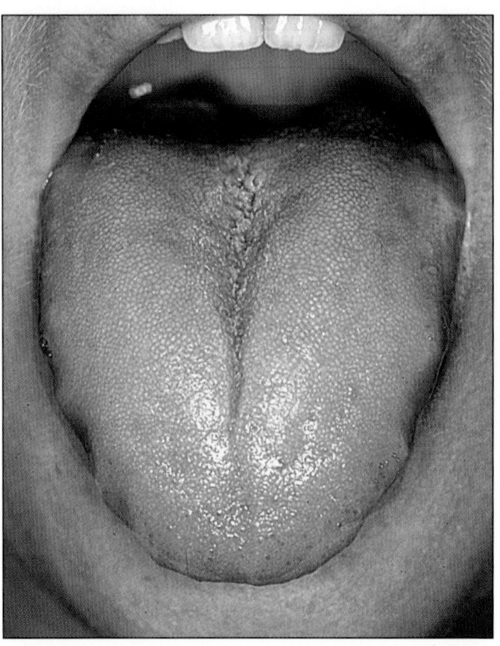

Symptoms

Frequent mucoid stools with undigested food
Tenesmus
Flatulence
Weight loss
No appetite
Fatigue

Western diagnosis

Ulcerative colitis for 10 years
Allergic rhinitis

Background to disease

Long-standing emotional problems

Tongue description	Chinese diagnosis
Reddish with red edges, slightly swollen	Accumulation of damp-heat in the Liver and Gallbladder
Vertical crack with greasy, yellow coating	Stomach yin deficiency with accumulation of phlegm-heat
Yellow, greasy coating at the root of the tongue	Accumulation of damp-heat in the lower burner

Symptoms

Back pain with numb feeling in the left leg
Inner restlessness
Insomnia
Nervousness
Panic attacks
Smelly, soft stools
Feeling of fullness after eating

Western diagnosis

Protruding disc between the 4th and 5th lumbar vertebrae

Background to disease

Alcohol abuse
Irregular eating habits
Suppressed emotions
Too much sitting

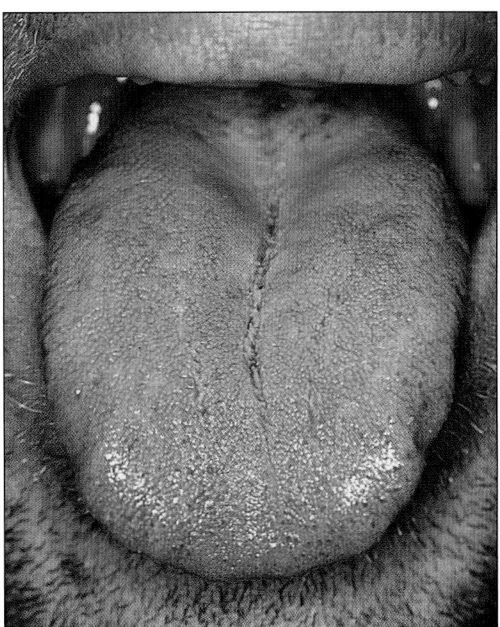

Fig. 4.1.3.3
Male
32 years old

Tongue description	Chinese diagnosis
Pale, swollen	Spleen qi deficiency with accumulation of dampness and blood deficiency
Deep, vertical crack and rootless, peeled coating	Stomach yin and Kidney yin deficiency
Peeled coating at the tip of the tongue	Heart yin deficiency

Symptoms

Severe attacks of fear and panic
Feeling of pressure in the head
Inner restlessness
Cold hands and feet

Western diagnosis

None

Background to disease

Mental overwork
Menopause

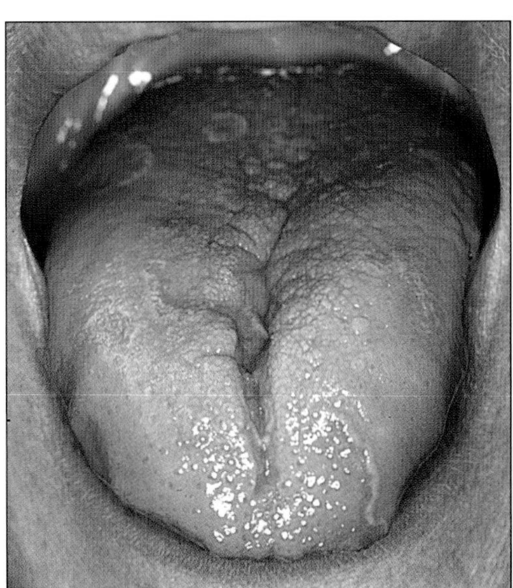

Fig. 4.1.3.4
Female
52 years old

4.1.4 Stomach Patterns and Shiny Tongues

These tongues have no coating. The entire tongue body appears very smooth, as if the skin has been peeled off. This gives the impression of a sheen due to the fact that the tongue papillae have atrophied, but in reality the tongue is dry. The tongue body, accordingly, often shows cracks and dryness and may even be contracted. This tongue type is characterized by the fact that the tongue papillae completely disappear, thus making it look like a mirror. The papillae on the tongue depend on the true qi (*zhēn qì*) and the fluids and yin of the internal organs for nourishment. If the fluids and yin dry up, qi also diminishes, and the tongue, particularly the papillae, will not be properly nourished. The papillae become smaller and smaller, and then disappear altogether until the tongue surface is shiny like a mirror.[10]

It is thus clear that the origin of this type of tongue is not only a deficiency of fluids and yin, but also of qi. The shiny tongue accordingly represents a combined pattern of qi and yin deficiency. As expected, the tongue body color and coating (if there is one) will then show which pathology predominates.

Tongue signs

- pale shiny or mirror tongue: severe deficiency of blood due to a long-standing deficiency of Spleen and Stomach qi.[11] In this case, the Stomach qi is too weak to build a new coating, and the blood deficiency is so severe that the tongue is no longer moistened.
- pale red, dry, and shiny tongue body: deficiency of qi and yin in addition to the presence of heat
- center of the tongue is visibly shiny: Stomach yin deficiency
- red or dark red, shiny tongue: Stomach and Kidney yin deficiency as well as a severe lack of body fluids. This tongue type is often present in the terminally ill, that is, in the terminal stages of cancer, liver cirrhosis, or tuberculosis. This stage of an illness is characterized by severe deficiency of fluids and yin, which is reflected in the shiny tongue. If this type of tongue develops during an illness, the condition of the patient can be expected to deteriorate.
- red and painful mirror tongue: deficiency of yin with blazing fire
- dark and purple mirror tongue: stagnation and obstruction of qi and blood

Tongue description	**Chinese diagnosis**
Pale red, *shiny tongue*	Severe Spleen and Stomach qi deficiency with deficiency of fluids
Slightly red, swollen sides	Heat in the Liver
Tofu-like, thin coating on the left side of the tongue	Dangerous exhaustion of yin

Symptoms

Shortness of breath
Severe exhaustion
Weight loss
Lack of appetite

Western diagnosis

Breast cancer

Background to disease

Unknown

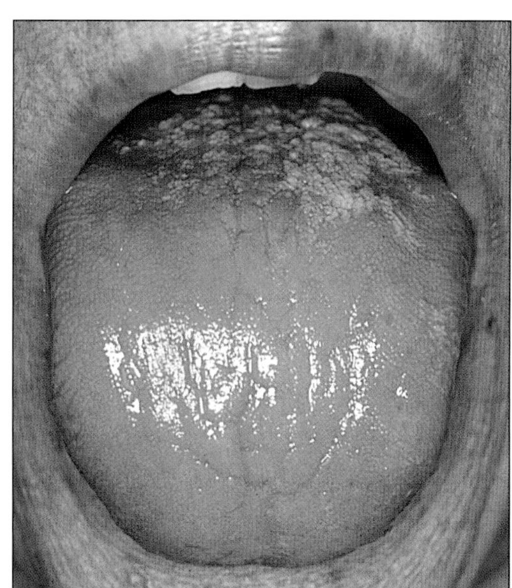

Fig. 4.1.4.1
Female
72 years old

Tongue description	**Chinese diagnosis**
Reddish, shiny tongue	Lung qi and yin deficiency, Kidney yin deficiency
Small cracks in the anterior third	Lung yin deficiency
Tofu-like, thin coating on the left side of the tongue	Dangerous exhaustion of yin

Symptoms

Shortness of breath
Dry cough
Pain in the chest
Intense thirst
Night sweats
Headache
Exhaustion

Western diagnosis

Bronchial cancer

Background to disease

Cigarette smoking for 40 years

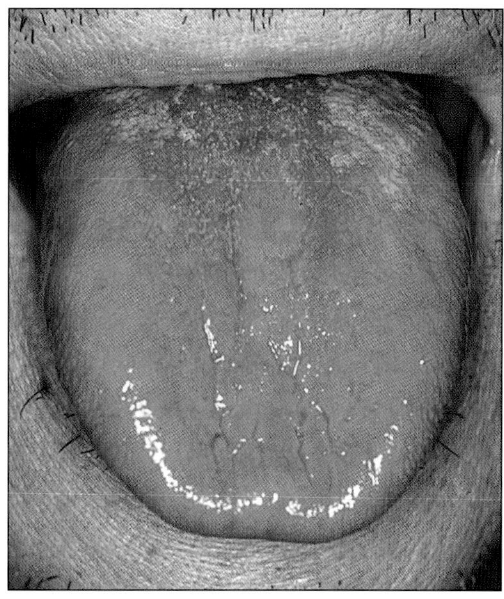

Fig. 4.1.4.2
Male
73 years old

Tongue description ------------------------- **Chinese diagnosis**

Reddish, *shiny, without coating* — Severe Stomach and Kidney yin deficiency

Swollen anterior third — Accumulation of phlegm-heat in the Lungs

Fig. 4.1.4.3
Female
75 years old

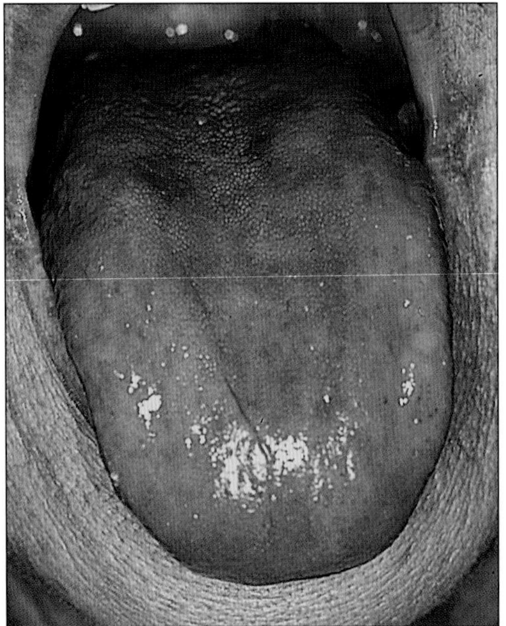

Symptoms

Shortness of breath
Chronic cough with expectoration of scant, thick, yellow sputum
Dry stools
Belching
Lack of appetite

Western diagnosis

Chronic bronchitis
Emphysema

Background to disease

Cigarette smoking for over 40 years

Tongue description ------------------------- **Chinese diagnosis**

Dark red, *shiny,* slightly thin, without coating — Severe Stomach and Kidney yin deficiency

Fig. 4.1.4.4
Male
83 years old

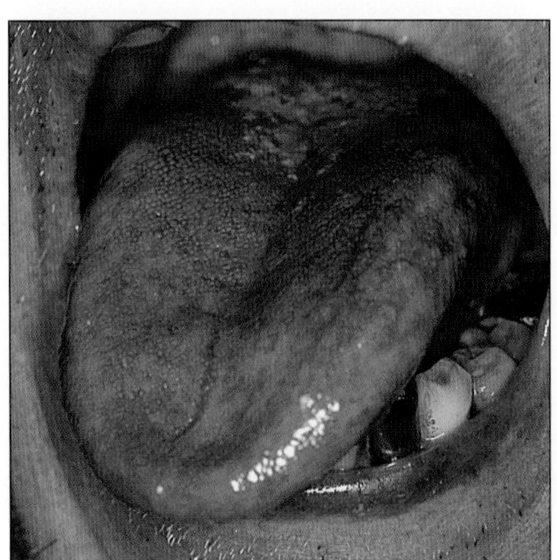

Symptoms

Insomnia
Frequent urination at night
Acute back pain

Western diagnosis

None

Background to disease

None known, except perhaps old age

4.1.5 Patterns of Excess Relating to the Stomach and the Tongue

Heat in the Stomach—often caused by an overconsumption of spicy or fatty foods, abuse of alcohol, caffeine and nicotine, or the taking of certain medicinal or hallucinogenic drugs like glucocorticoids, antiphlogistic agents (which counteract inflammation and fever), or cocaine—will injure the fluids in the Stomach. Over the long term, this will injure the Stomach yin (Fig. 4.1.2.5). Stomach heat can evolve into Stomach fire. Both of these injure the fluids in the Stomach and thus the Stomach yin. Intense heat in the Stomach can brew the fluids, promoting the development of phlegm-fire in the Stomach. The formation of this pattern is exacerbated by smoking and frequent eating of hot, spicy foods.

Tongue signs

- thick, greasy, and yellow coating
- very dry, thick, greasy, and yellow coating: If fire is the dominant aspect of phlegm-heat, there will be excessive heat and injury to the fluids. Because of the close connection between the Stomach and Large Intestine, the heat will affect bowel movements, resulting in dry and hard stools and constipation. Excessive heat in the yang brightness Stomach and Large Intestine channels is also responsible for bleeding gums, toothache, and facial pain (Figs. 4.1.5.1 and 4.1.2.8).
- very thick, greasy, and yellow coating: If phlegm is the dominant aspect of the pathology, a feeling of fullness or tightness in the stomach may be experienced, and thirst will be less pronounced. Phlegm-fire in the Stomach can agitate the Heart, which in mild cases will manifest as insomnia and in severe cases as mental illness (Fig. 4.1.5.2).
- midline crack covered by a yellow, dry, greasy coating (Fig. 4.1.5.3).
- furry coating that is either grain-like or thick (Fig. 4.1.5.3) occurs when phlegm and fire combine in the Stomach. The intensity of the phlegm-fire in the Stomach and the ensuing injury to the fluids will be reflected in the nature of the coating.
- greasy, white, grayish, or yellow coating, usually located in the center of the tongue: This type of coating suggests food stagnation.
- a white, thick, and, in more serious cases, black and wet coating reflects the penetration of externally-contracted cold to the Stomach. This sign is generally accompanied by acute digestive problems (Fig. 4.1.5.4). An attack on the Stomach by externally-contracted cold can result in vomiting, diarrhea, and stomach cramps. External cold blocks the normal descent of the Stomach qi, which causes the nausea and vomiting. The resulting stagnation of qi in the middle burner, particularly in the Stomach, causes severe stomach cramps.
- a bluish color at the center of the tongue reflects impaired circulation of the qi and blood in the Stomach (Fig. 8.2.3). It is characterized by a piercing, stabbing pain in the epigastrium.

Tongue description	Chinese diagnosis
Reddish	Interior heat
Curled-up, slightly reddish edges	Stagnation of Liver qi with developing heat
Cracks in the center	Dryness in the Stomach, Stomach yin deficiency
Reddish tip	Heat in the Heart
Yellow, greasy, thick coating at the root	Retention of damp-heat in the Large Intestine

Fig. 4.1.5.1
Male
62 years old

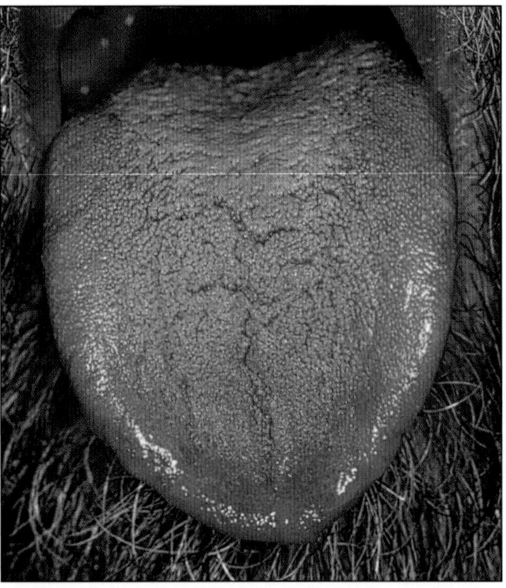

Symptoms

Facial pain, constipation with hard, dry stools
Dryness of the mouth, lack of appetite
Inner tension, outbursts of anger, sadness
Inner restlessness

Western diagnosis

Trigeminal neuralgia

Background to disease

Irregular eating habits, late evening meals, death of son seven years before

Tongue description	Chinese diagnosis
Pale	Spleen qi deficiency
Deep vertical crack in the center with yellow, dry coating	Onset of phlegm-heat in the Stomach
Reddish tip	Heat in the Heart
Whitish, slippery coating	Accumulation of dampness
Yellow coating with red points at the root	Retention of damp-heat in the lower burner

Fig. 4.1.5.2
Female
35 years old

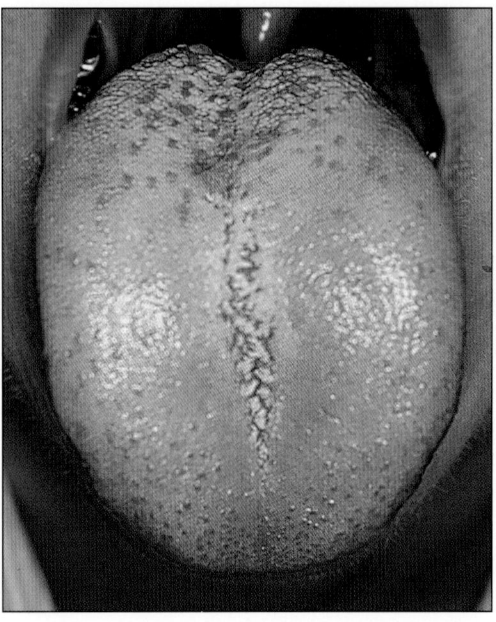

Symptoms

Bad breath
Heartburn, pain, and feeling of fullness in the epigastrium
Voracious appetite
Itchy vaginal discharge
Insomnia
Tiredness
Mood swings

Western diagnosis

None

Background to disease

Taxing demands at work, frequent travel, irregular diet

About these case histories

The first case below is a very good example of phlegm-heat in the Stomach causing halitosis as well as insomnia. By contrast, the second case describes how externally-contracted cold causes an acute digestive problem.

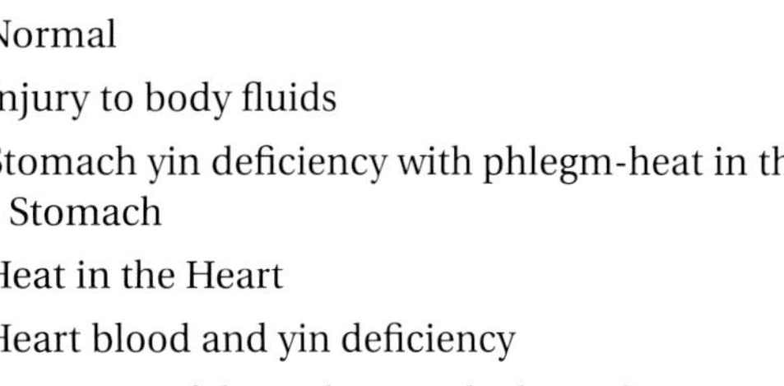

Tongue description	**Chinese diagnosis**
Pale red	Normal
Firm, narrow tongue body	Injury to body fluids
Deep, vertical crack in the center with yellow, greasy coating	Stomach yin deficiency with phlegm-heat in the Stomach
Reddish tip	Heat in the Heart
Slight indentation at the tip	Heart blood and yin deficiency
Yellow, greasy coating at the root	Retention of damp-heat in the lower burner

Symptoms

Bad breath
Heartburn, fullness of the epigastrium, belching
Insomnia with occasional night sweats
Lumbago
Exhaustion

Western diagnosis

Reflux esophagitis, primary infertility

Background to disease

Emotional problems, overwork, caffeine abuse

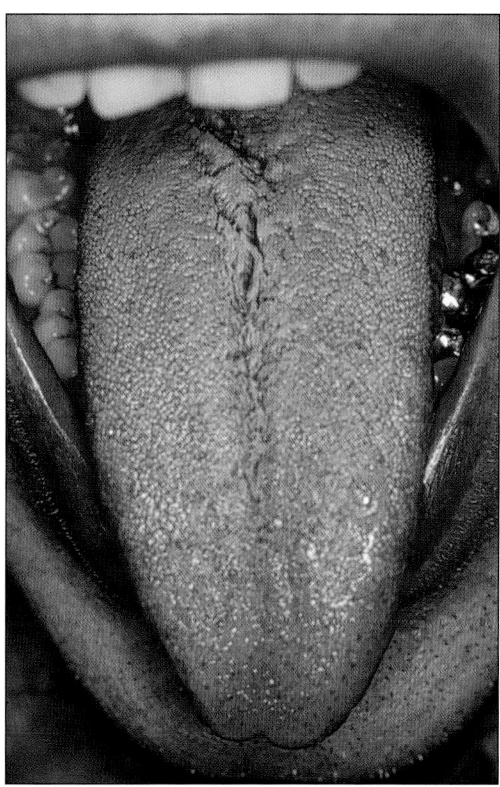

Fig. 4.1.5.3
Male
46 years old

CASE HISTORY The patient was deeply concerned about his bad breath. He changed his diet and abstained from eating cheese, meat, and fried spicy foods. Nevertheless, his bad breath and stomach problems persisted. He suffered from heartburn and belching every day and he often had a feeling of fullness and pressure in the stomach area.

His work was very demanding and he felt stressed from the work and fearful that it would disappear. His marriage was unhappy because his wife longed for a baby and he was infertile; inevitably, they ceased to have a sexual relationship. Because of his guilt, the patient never stood up to his wife's reproaches. If they quarreled, he could not sleep, and when he did, his dreams were often confused.

He felt weak and exhausted. His tiredness was often accompanied by a feeling of weakness in the lumbar region, which often felt cold. The impression he gave was that of a frail, unhappy

Pathomechanism

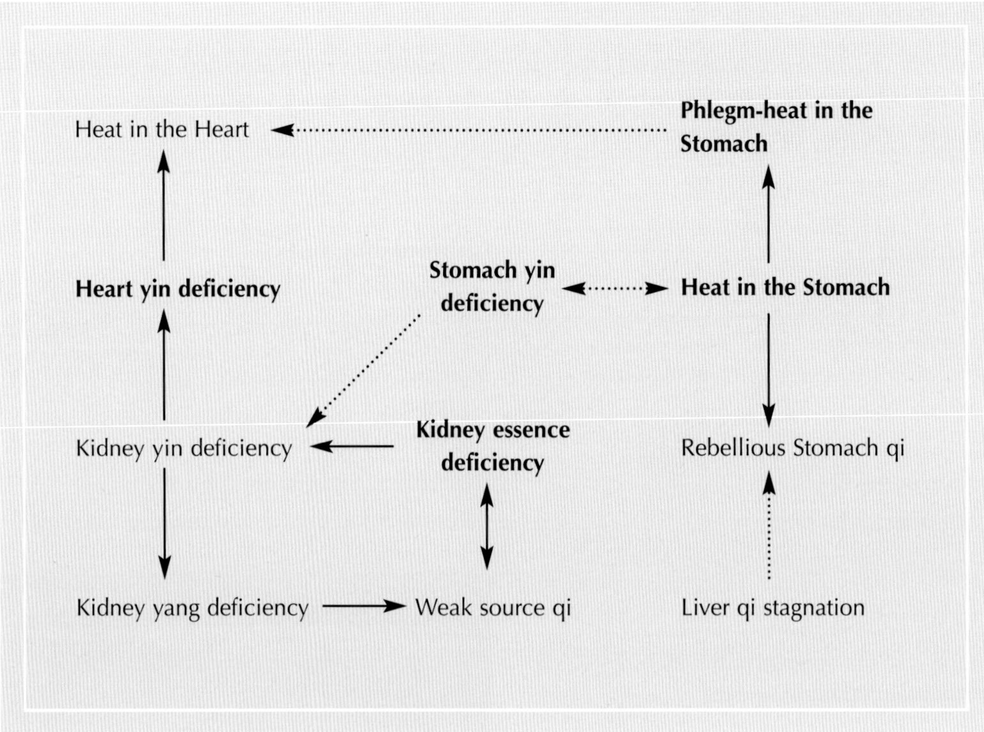

man. His thin body did not help, for while he was 6 feet 4 inches tall, he only weighed 172 pounds. His appetite, thirst, and bowel movements were normal. His pulse was thin and very tight.

Analysis. The presence of a crack in the center of the tongue with an absence of coating does not necessarily imply an abnormal condition. However, a central crack with coating is indicative of excess. The depth of the crack here signals long-standing injury to, or deficiency of, Stomach yin, which may be caused by eating late or by the overconsumption of spicy foods. The central crack may also indicate a constitutional weakness of Stomach yin, which may be true in this case since the patient has been unable to gain weight for many years. His tall, thin build denotes a constitution characterized by a dominance of yang and a weakness of yin.

Heat has developed in the middle burner and this is leading to a slow brewing and clumping of the fluids in the Stomach. The result is an accumulation of phlegm-heat in the Stomach, which is reflected in the dry, yellow coating in the central crack. This disease pattern obstructs the normal flow of qi in the Stomach. When the Stomach qi stagnates, there is a feeling of fullness and pressure in the abdomen and impairment of the Stomach's downward-directing function. If the Stomach qi is rebellious, turbid qi will rise and cause belching and bad breath. However, the development of heat in the Stomach here has not affected this patient's appetite or thirst.

Apart from the disharmony of the Stomach, an imbalance of the yin of the Heart and Kidney has developed. The patient's sterility, sleeping problems, and night sweats are clear signs of this imbalance. This pattern of deficiency is also clearly signaled by the narrow shape of the tongue body. However, since the color of the tongue body is normal, injury to the yin and blood from heat cannot be assumed to have occurred. Nor is injury to the yin and blood responsible for the reduced width of the tongue. Instead, this sign is a reflection of a constitutional weakness of the fluids and yin. In other words, the narrow tongue body shape, in conjunction with the central crack, suggest a deficiency of fluids and yin that has existed for years.

The patient's impotence reflects a deficiency of yin, yang, and essence. These energies are the basis for the formation of sperm. Apart from the reduced sperm count, the heads of the sperm are deformed and only show limited motility. The laboratory report described the diminished ejaculation as extremely viscous. The reduced quantity of sperm, and possibly their shape, are an indication of Kidney essence deficiency. The limited motility of the sperm shows Kidney yang deficiency. The sticky consistency of the ejaculate signals the presence of damp-heat in the lower burner, which is reflected in the yellow, thick coating at the root of the tongue. The damp-heat may also contribute to the diminished motility of the sperm.

The Kidneys influence the lower lumbar region. The deficiency of Kidney essence and Kidney yin has caused a weakening of the Kidney yang. If Kidney yang deficiency is caused by a decrease in Kidney yin, there are often no specific tongue signs. (However, if this pattern is the primary cause of the disease it will be reflected in a pale, swollen, and often wet tongue body; see Fig. 2.2.3.) Kidney yang deficiency affects the circulation of yang in the Governing vessel, which controls the spine and back. In addition, the circulation of yang and protective qi strengthens and warms the spine and back. Weakness of the lower back and a cold sensation in the lumbar region is, therefore, a sign of diminished Kidney yang, which in turn weakens the Governing vessel.

Despite psychotherapy, the patient was unable to resolve his guilty feelings about his sterility and marital problems, leaving him very unhappy. Unresolved feelings of guilt tend to constrain the flow of qi and lead, on a physical level, to symptoms of pain, distention, or feelings of pressure in the body. Feelings of guilt can constrain not only the Liver qi, but also the Heart qi. Despite the emotional history of the patient and the presence of a wiry pulse, Liver qi stagnation was not judged to be a primary factor in the patient's pathomechanism. This factor was deemed secondary, since characteristics associated with Liver qi stagnation—irritability, anger, or nervous tension—were missing. In addition, the tongue does not show any specific signs suggesting Liver disharmony, which is important when formulating a treatment strategy.

The patient is unable to sleep through the night, has confused dreams, and occasionally experiences night sweats. His constant fearfulness has weakened his Kidney yin; as a result, the Kidney yin is not strong enough to sufficiently nourish the Heart. The ensuing Heart yin deficiency, aggravated by the long-lasting emotional problems, has led to the development of heat from deficiency, which disturbs the spirit. This process is reflected in the red tip of the tongue, while the Heart blood and yin deficiency is signaled by the indentation of the tip. Phlegm-heat in the Stomach also aggravates the condition of the spirit and supports the described pathomechanism.

Treatment strategy. Drain the heat from the Stomach, transform the phlegm, harmonize the Stomach and regulate the flow of qi, harmonize and nourish the Heart and Kidney yin, strengthen the Kidney essence, and calm the spirit.

The patient received a modified version of Tangerine Peel and Bamboo Shavings Decoction (*jú pí zhú rú tāng*). After two weeks of taking this decoction, the patient's bad breath had disappeared. Whenever the complaint flared up again, he again took the decoction and his breath quickly improved. His sleeping problems also improved. Regular treatment with acupuncture alleviated his emotional state and his backache. Frequently used points included HT-5 (*tōng lǐ*), KI-3 (*tài xī*), KI-7 (*fù liū*), and BL-60 (*kūn lún*).

Tongue description	**Chinese diagnosis**
Pale, swollen, teeth marks	Spleen qi deficiency with accumulation of dampness
Bilateral black stripes with moist coating	Penetration of externally-contracted cold into the Stomach

Fig. 4.1.5.4
Female
27 years old

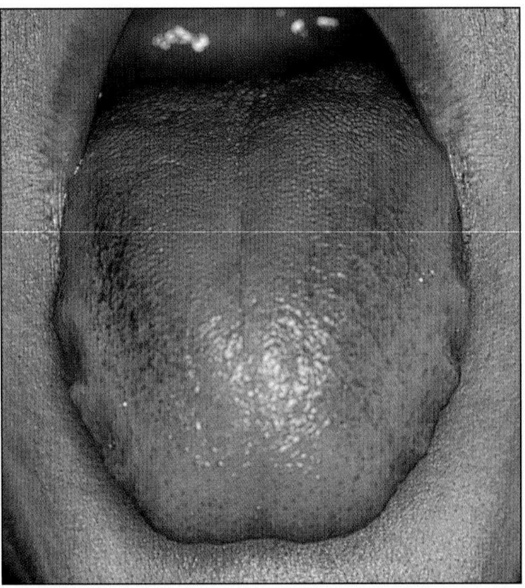

Symptoms

Watery stools
Abdominal cramps
Nausea, vomiting
Shivering

Western diagnosis

Acute enteritis

Background to disease

Excessive consumption of salads with mayonnaise

CASE HISTORY The patient requested a home visit because of the acuteness of her symptoms. She suffered from watery diarrhea accompanied by strong abdominal cramps. She felt nauseous, and even though she had no temperature, she shivered and felt very weak. She had attended a summer garden party, ate grilled meat and salads with mayonnaise, left late, and then a few hours later came down with diarrhea. Her pulse was floating and thin.

In the past the patient had received acupuncture and Chinese herbs for chronic diarrhea. Three years before, she had suffered from a hepatitis A viral infection, resulting in digestive problems. Her stools were always very soft and she had many daily bowel movements, which made her very tired. She had little stamina and needed long periods of recuperation.

Analysis. The primary culprit in this case is acute externally-contracted cold during the summer. The black, bilateral stripes together with the moist tongue body reflect the penetration of the pathogenic cold and its encounter with an interior condition of dampness. The pathogenic factor was so strong that it blocked the middle burner.

As a result of the blockage, the transportive and transformative functions of the Spleen and Stomach were impaired. The Spleen qi sank, causing the watery diarrhea. The flow of Stomach qi was equally obstructed, hence the nausea and vomiting. The patient's underlying interior dampness, reflected in the swollen tongue body, and the externally-contracted cold congealed in the abdomen and thereby caused the intense abdominal cramps.

The shivering, aversion to cold, and the black, moist tongue coating are unmistakable signs of external cold. Shivering is the result of the constraint of yang qi by cold, which in this case was exacerbated by the pre-existing internal dampness. The patient's exhaustion resulted from the impairment of the Spleen's function of circulating the nutritive qi as well as from injury to the qi and fluids from the severe diarrhea.

The tongue body is pale and swollen and has teeth marks. This indicates a combination of Spleen qi and yang deficiency and cold from deficiency in the middle burner. The patient had been suffering from soft stools and exhaustion for many years as a result of the chronic evacuation of soft stools.

Pathomechanism

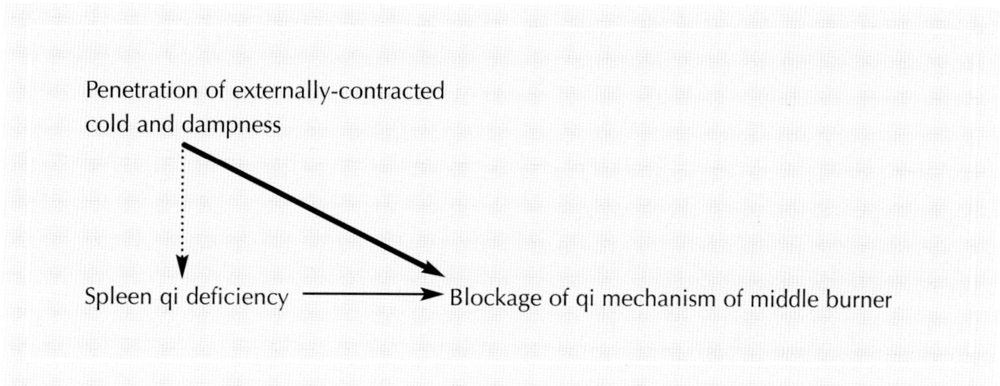

Treatment strategy. Release the exterior, transform the dampness, and strengthen the Spleen qi.

The patient took Ten-Ingredient Decoction with Mosla (*shí wèi xiāng rú yǐn*) for two days in order to release the exterior, transform the dampness, and strengthen the Spleen qi. In addition, CV-8 (*shén què*) was treated with moxibustion placed on a slice of ginger, and ST-25 (*tiān shū*) was needled, in order to stop the diarrhea and warm the Spleen qi. Her shivering and nausea disappeared after one day. After three days, the stools were less frequent and were also less soft and watery. The patient is continuing with treatment, the purpose of which is to warm the patient's Spleen qi and yang, as well as the middle burner, and to stop the chronic diarrhea.

Endnotes

1 Larre C, Rochat de la Vallée E. *Spleen and Stomach.* Cambridge: Monkey Press, 1990:135.

2 Ren Y-Q. *Huang di nei jing zhang ju suo yin.* Beijing: Peoples Medical Publishing House,1986:37. See also *Spleen and Stomach,* 134.

3 Maciocia G. *Foundations of Chinese Medicine.* Edinburgh: Churchill Livingston, 1989:113.

4 See Ren, 332.

5 Anonymous. *Su wen* [Basic Questions], edited by He W-B et al. Beijing: China Medicine Science and Technology Press, 1996: 44:249.

6 Ibid.

7 Zhu D-X. *The Heart and Essence of Dan Xi's Methods of Treatment,* translated by Yang S-Z. Boulder, CO: Blue Poppy Press, 1993: 19:77.

8 Liu L and Wang J-H. "Überblick über Chinesische Arzneimittel, die Tumorzellen gegen über Radioaktiver Bestrahlung Sensibilisieren." *Zeitschrift für Traditionelle Chinesische Medizin,* 2000;1:47-50.

9 Maciocia G. *Tongue Diagnosis in Chinese Medicine,* rev. ed. Seattle: Eastland Press, 1995:79.

10 Compare Li N-M. *Zhong guo she zhen da quan.* Beijing: Xueyuan Publishing Company, 1994:1190.

11 Ibid. The text cites an investigation undertaken in Inner Mongolia and states that the mirror tongue reflects conditions of deficiency as well as excess, or cold as well as heat patterns. With a heat disorder, the tongue body is red and dry, and with a cold disorder, the tongue body is pale and wet.

CHAPTER 5

Tongue Signs Associated with Lung Disharmonies

5.1 Tongue Signs Associated with Lung Qi Deficiency

The Lungs establish the foundation of qi.[1] They govern breathing. A disharmony or weakness of the Lung qi may cause an illness that affects the respiratory tract. Depletion of Lung qi will impair its descending function, which manifests as coughing, breathing difficulties, or shortness of breath on physical exertion. The Lung qi supports the Heart's function of controlling the circulation of blood. Lung qi deficiency contributes to a slackening in the circulation of blood, which, in mild cases, manifests as cold extremities, and in serious cases, as heart pain (Fig. 5.4.2). This manifests in a pale tongue body, which, however, is similar to the paleness of the tongue body in Spleen qi deficiency. Therefore, Lung qi deficiency can only be diagnosed within the context of the symptoms and other clinical signs of the patient.

There are, however, a few distinctive tongue signs that point to a disharmony of the Lungs, and they are all localized on the anterior third of the tongue: a pale tongue body with a depression in the anterior third of the tongue (Fig. 5.1.1). This reflects weakness in the gathering qi *(zōng qì)*. This energy controls the strength of the voice and influences speech as it supports the qi of the Heart and Lungs. Overuse of the voice may lead to a weakening of this energy and is common among teachers, singers, and actors. Such individuals may also have a tendency to catch colds or have trouble with their voice. Deficiency of the gathering qi is often accompanied by symptoms indicating Heart and Lung qi deficiency. Occasionally, this tongue sign appears in people who suffer from long-standing sadness and grief. Sadness disperses Lung qi and weakens Heart qi. If sadness and grief remain unresolved for many years, the Lung qi deficiency may evolve into Lung yin deficiency.

A deficiency of Lung qi can engender other patterns, for example, the Lungs' descending function will become hampered. Qi will then accumulate in the chest, resulting in the collection and accumulation of fluids. If there is also Spleen qi deficiency, this may result in an accumulation of phlegm in the Lungs, further impairing their descending function. Since phlegm originates in the Spleen but may be contained in the Lungs, this pattern involving both yin organs can result in chronic cough with white phlegm or tightness of the chest.

Swelling in the anterior third of the tongue signifies retention of phlegm in the Lungs (Fig. 5.3.1). This sign is only significant when it occurs in conjunction with other signs and symptoms, such as shortness of breath or coughing. If there are no other indications of Lung disharmony, this sign may be discounted.

Swelling that involves one-half of the tongue body[2] (Fig. 5.1.4) signifies Lung qi deficiency (an extremely rare sign). In this case, the Lung qi deficiency will cause shortness of breath with any physical exertion.

Tongue description	**Chinese diagnosis**
Pale red, swollen, with teeth marks	Spleen qi deficiency (accumulation of dampness)
Depression in the anterior third	Deficiency of gathering qi and Lung qi

Fig. 5.1.1
Male
32 years old

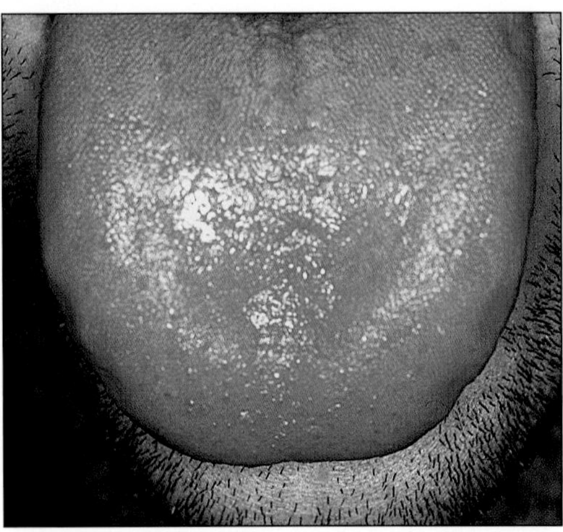

Symptoms

Runny nose
Sneezing fits
Tightness of the chest
Cough
Occasional difficult breathing
Tendency to catch colds

Western diagnosis

Allergic rhinitis
Allergic asthma

Background to disease

Family history of allergies
Overuse of voice (opera singer)
Overworking
Irregular eating habits

Tongue description	**Chinese diagnosis**
Pale with slight teeth marks	Spleen qi deficiency with blood deficiency
Depression in the anterior third	Deficiency of gathering qi and Lung qi
Yellow, thin, greasy coating	Slight accumulation of damp-heat in the lower burner

Symptoms

Dry throat
Dry cough
Tendency to catch colds
Constipation
Insomnia
Exhaustion

Western diagnosis

Prolapse of the uterus

Background to disease

Overwork
Lack of sleep

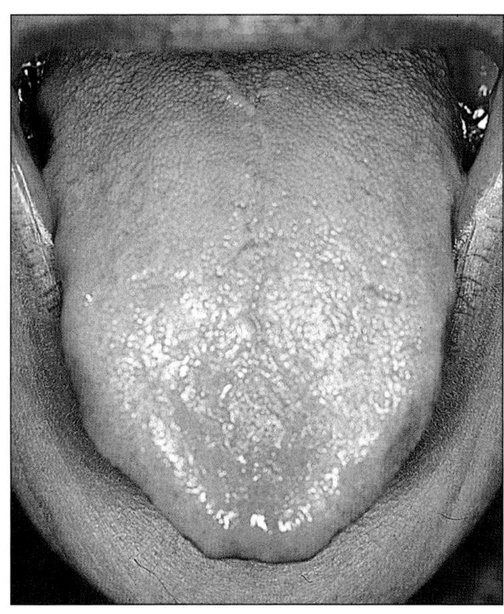

Fig. 5.1.2
Female
56 years old

Tongue description	**Chinese diagnosis**
Pale red, very swollen	Underlying Kidney yang deficiency (accumulation of dampness in the middle and upper burners)
Swollen, dry, and cracked in the anterior third and center of the tongue	Blockage of Lung qi due to accumulation of dampness, blockage of water pathways (onset of Lung yin deficiency)

Symptoms

Frequent colds with cough
Shortness of breath
Swollen lower legs
Dizziness
Intense inner feeling of cold

Western diagnosis

Edema of the lower legs
Chronic bronchitis

Background to disease

For years, her work required that she stand
Overwork

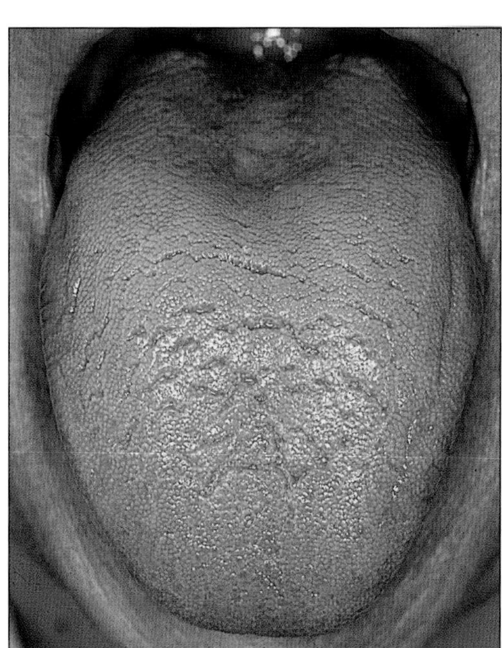

Fig. 5.1.3
Female
58 years old

Tongue description	Chinese diagnosis
Pale	Spleen qi deficiency → blood deficiency
Swollen	Accumulation of dampness
Pale edges	Liver blood deficiency
Swelling of left longitudinal half[3]	Lung qi deficiency
Thin, vertical crack in the center	Stomach qi deficiency

Fig. 5.1.4
Female
45 years old

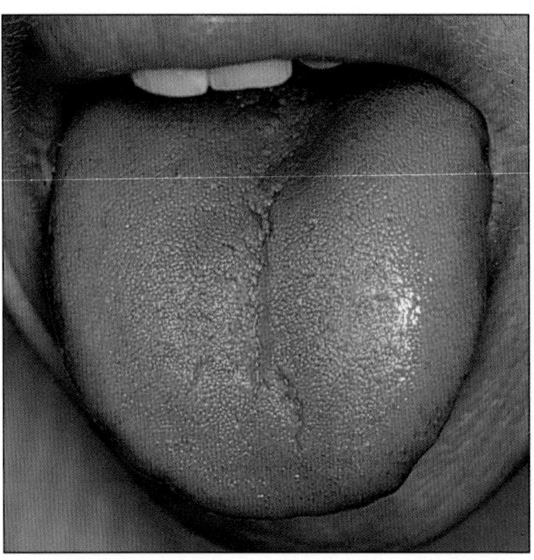

Symptoms

Shortness of breath on exertion, exhaustion
Difficulty falling asleep
Dry eyes
Lack of appetite

Western diagnosis

Chronic bronchitis

Background to disease

Vegetarian diet
Overwork

About these case histories

The case histories in this chapter are concerned exclusively with chronic illnesses and complaints of the Lung. The sequence of cases is structured to show the development from a pattern of Lung qi deficiency to one of Lung yin deficiency, not the severity of the condition.

CASE HISTORY Two years prior to treatment the patient suffered from chronic bronchitis after contracting a cold. The cough was productive with thick, white mucus, and she also experienced an increase in shortness of breath on exertion. Her symptoms worsened in the autumn and winter and the cough became stronger in cool, damp conditions. In addition, both of her thumb joints became painful when the weather turned cold and damp.

She was about 20 pounds overweight. She loved eating, particularly rich foods. After meals she often experienced a feeling of fullness in the epigastric region. To lose weight, she changed her eating habits, but her diet mainly consisted of low-fat yogurt. In general, the patient felt very well and suffered from no other complaints. Her pulse was slightly frail and slightly slippery.

Analysis. While the entire tongue is swollen, the anterior third in particular is quite swollen, indicating the retention of phlegm in the Lungs. Here, this tongue sign is significant as it points to a long-standing disease pattern. The cough began after the patient caught a cold. The penetration of externally-contracted pathogenic factors led to obstruction of Lung qi. If the Lung and protective qi are strong, pathogenic factors will be eliminated after a few days. If, however, the pathogenic factor is strong and the protective qi is weak, then the pathogenic factor may seriously impair the circulation of Lung qi.

The patient's underlying Spleen qi deficiency is reflected in the overall swollen, pale body of the tongue. This deficiency led to an accumulation of dampness, which was fueled by the excessive consumption of dairy foods. A famous axiom in Chinese medicine is applicable here: "The Spleen produces phlegm and the Lungs store it."

Tongue description	Chinese diagnosis
Pale	Spleen qi deficiency
Swollen	Accumulation of dampness
Swollen anterior third	Retention of phlegm in the Lungs
Light red spots on the anterior third	Attack of external pathogenic factor in the past
Thin vertical crack between the anterior third and center	Stomach and Lung qi deficiency
Whitish, thin, slippery coating	Accumulation of dampness

Symptoms

Cough with thick, white mucus
Shortness of breath on exertion
Feeling of fullness in the epigastrium
Pain in the carpal-metacarpal joint
Weight gain

Western diagnosis

Chronic bronchitis

Background to disease

Excessive consumption of dairy foods
Living in a cold, humid region

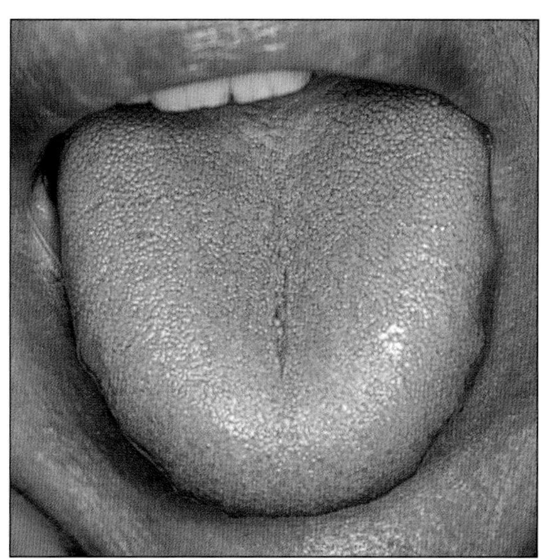

Fig. 5.1.5
Female
63 years old

Pathomechanism

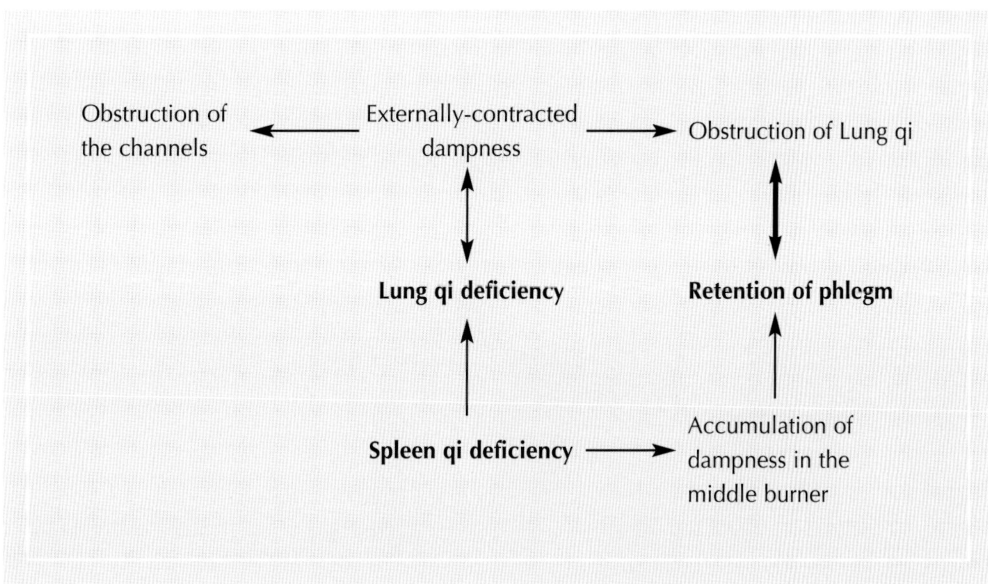

The ensuing dampness strained the Spleen, as it dislikes dampness. Accumulated dampness impairs the Spleen's functions of transforming and transporting food and drink. Phlegm arises from the accumulated dampness and gathers in the Lungs. Thus the root of the illness here lay in the Spleen qi deficiency, which caused Lung qi deficiency. Specifically, it manifested in the shortness of breath on physical exertion. Under these conditions, the patient's right distal pulse was frail, reflecting the deficiency of qi.

The manifestation of the disease appeared as a pattern of fullness produced by an accumulation of phlegm in the Lungs; the presence of phlegm can be discerned from the slippery pulse and swelling of the anterior third of the tongue. The presence of dampness is reflected in the slippery tongue coating. The cough with mucus resulted from damp-phlegm obstructing the Lung qi and impairing its ability to spread and descend. When it is expectorated, the mucus is thick and white. Its consistency reflects a condition of excess, and its color points to the presence of cold. External cold and dampness exacerbated the Lung qi's ability to descend, which gave rise to the strong coughing fits.

Red points are visible on the anterior third of the tongue and denote heat in the Lungs or in the upper burner. Because they are very light in color, they do not reflect an acute penetration of the pathogenic factor. Also, since they are not bright red or raised, they are not regarded as an important diagnostic sign; they merely point to a previous infection.

The vertical crack localized between the anterior third and the center of the tongue signals an injury to the Lung or Stomach qi. The Stomach qi is affected by the accumulation of dampness in the middle burner, which manifests here in the feeling of fullness in the epigastric region. The pain in her thumb joints is triggered by damp, cold weather, which obstructs the qi and blood in the channels of the Lung and Large Intestine. This pattern may be aggravated by the patient's tendency to accumulate dampness.

Treatment strategy. Drain the dampness, transform the phlegm, regulate the Lung qi, and strengthen the Spleen.

The patient was prescribed a combination of Two-Cured Decoction *(èr chén tāng)* and Three-Seed Decoction to Nourish One's Parents *(sān zǐ yǎng qīn tāng)*.[4] After taking this combination for two weeks, she felt better: her cough had improved and there was less phlegm. She abstained from eating dairy products. After a treatment period of three months, she was free of complaints. Her tongue, however, had not changed, implying that the patient remained susceptible to cold and dampness.

Tongue description	**Chinese diagnosis**
Pale	Spleen qi deficiency → blood deficiency
Swollen	Accumulation of dampness
Swollen anterior third	Retention of phlegm in the Lungs
Horizontal cracks on the anterior third	Lung yin deficiency
Whitish coating turning yellowish at the root	Stomach qi deficiency and the onset of Stomach yin deficiency

Fig. 5.1.6
Female
32 years old

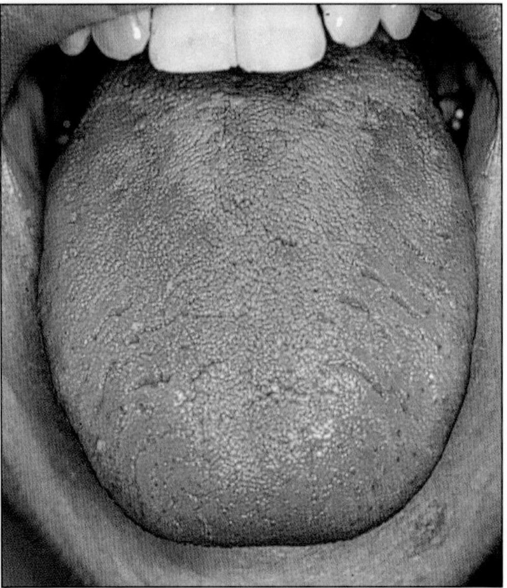

Symptoms

Cough with white mucus
Shortness of breath on exertion
Tiredness
Lack of appetite
Feelings of heat in the afternoon and evening
Night sweats

Western diagnosis

Sarcoidosis, iron deficiency anemia

Background to disease

Overwork

CASE HISTORY For several years the patient had been very exhausted. Laboratory tests found iron deficiency anemia. She felt slightly better after taking iron supplements, but without this medication the tiredness returned fairly quickly. She was very short of breath, especially when exercising. At the same time, she noticed a cough with the expectoration of sparse, white, thick mucus. Her work as a lawyer was very exhausting, and she thought that her tiredness stemmed from constant overwork. Six months later, her condition had not improved. Medical examination found sarcoidosis with enlargement (granulomas) of the two sides of the hilus pulmonsis. It was suggested that she start a treatment based on taking glucocorticoids, but this had not proved effective in other patients and she therefore refused.

The patient slept well but suffered occasionally from night sweats. Basically, she always felt cold, but in the few weeks prior to her first visit, she had noticed a feeling of heat in the afternoon and evening. She experienced this as a "floating feeling." The patient's weak voice was very noticeable. Her appetite was diminished but there were no digestive problems. Her menstruation was normal. Her pulse was slightly floating, frail, and soft.

Analysis. In this case the pathology is characterized by Lung qi and yin deficiency with an accumulation of phlegm in the Lungs. The pale, swollen tongue body reflects Spleen qi deficiency that led to an accumulation of dampness. The anterior third of the tongue is slightly swollen, denoting the presence of phlegm in the Lungs.

The patient's workload contributed to a deficiency of Spleen qi. This pattern of deficiency has far-reaching consequences. The Spleen qi sends food qi to the chest where it combines with air in order to form gathering qi, which supports the Lungs in their function of controlling breathing. Here the weakness of the gathering qi is manifested in her low, weak voice. The weakness in the gathering qi has also affected the normal qi, which originates in the Lungs; this has contributed to the tiredness of the patient.

The Spleen is too weak to nourish the Lungs (law of 'mother-child'), adding to the exhaustion of the patient. This connection between the Spleen and Lungs is readily seen on the tongue: the pale, swollen tongue body accompanied by swelling of the anterior third. The frail, soft pulse confirms the pattern of deficiency. The Spleen qi deficiency is responsible for the formation of phlegm that is being stored in the Lungs. Since, as a result of the phlegm, the Lung qi cannot descend, it becomes obstructed. This mechanism is responsible for the cough. Generally, the purpose of a cough is to release phlegm so that the Lung qi can again descend freely. But since the clearing of mucus is only a short-term solution and not a real transformation, the coughing quickly returns, and, in this case, has become chronic.

Pathomechanism

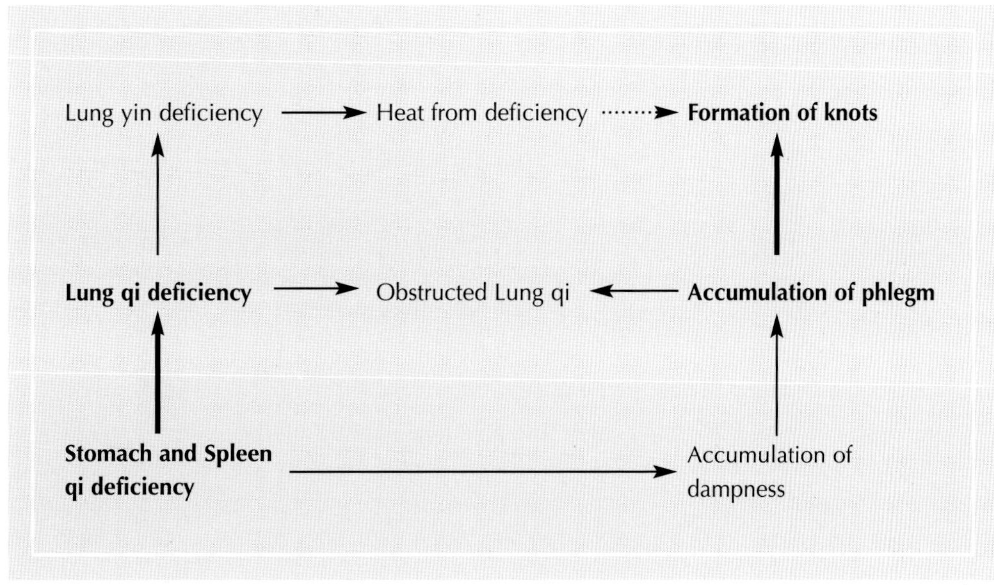

Physical exertion increases the circulation of Heart and Lung qi. If either yin organ is weakened, the circulation of qi and blood, especially in the thorax, may slacken because of the physical demands. In this case, the underlying deficiency of Lung qi and the accumulated phlegm in the Lungs has obstructed the Lung qi, which accounts for the severe shortness of breath on physical exertion.

From the perspective of Chinese medicine, the accumulation and congealing of phlegm is responsible for the benign granulomatosis found in the Lungs. When the phlegm thickens and congeals, it can form knots, especially when heat or blood stasis is part of the disease mechanism. Therefore, the swollen anterior third of the tongue requires further evaluation.

The tongue body shows relatively deep, horizontal cracks in the anterior third. These may indicate Lung yin deficiency that has arisen from the chronic Lung qi deficiency. Cracks in the tongue body are formed when excessive heat injures the yin. As a rule, the cracks are accompanied by a red, dry tongue body. By contrast, cracks on a pale tongue often signal underlying Stomach qi or blood deficiency: because the tongue, as a result of the blood deficiency, is not sufficiently moistened, cracks will appear.

In this case, the chronic pattern of qi and blood deficiency has injured the Lung yin. The pale, cracked tongue body is interpreted to be an indication of long-standing Lung qi deficiency that is evolving into Lung yin deficiency. This pattern manifests as a stubborn cough and in the feelings of heat in the afternoon, which trigger what the patient described as a "floating" sensation. In the afternoon, the yang should start to retract as the yin gathers and begins to grow. However, since the yin is deficient, the yang floats upward instead. At midnight the yin should reach its zenith. Night sweats result when heat, caused by the deficiency of yin, pushes the fluids outward in the form of sweat. The presence of heat is also reflected in the floating pulse.

An alternative diagnosis can be offered based on the ideas of Li Dong Yuan.[5] This diagnosis is based on the actions of the clear yang, which should normally rise. However, because the clear yang is blocked and constrained, it transforms into heat, which is evidenced by the cracks on the body of the tongue. This implies that the heat has not developed from a deficiency of yin, but is the result of Spleen qi deficiency that is impairing the rise of the clear yang. It is the ascent of the 'yin fire' toward the upper burner that is responsible for the heat. Accordingly, this symptom and the marked tiredness and exhaustion of the patient are more important than the presence of night sweats when determining the treatment strategy.

It should be noted that the tongue body, apart from the cracks on the anterior third, does not show any other sign of heat or yin deficiency. In addition, there are a small number of red points on the left side of the tongue. The source of the red points is not entirely clear, but several explanations are possible:

- An externally-contracted pathogenic factor. The patient, however, could not remember any recent colds or other infections.
- Ascending Liver yang or Liver fire. The patient has no other signs or symptoms to corroborate this diagnosis.
- The development of heat in the Spleen and/or Stomach.[6] Red points in the *middle* of the tongue body might support this diagnosis, but here they are found only on the left edge of the tongue, and there are no other corresponding symptoms.

The red points on the left edge of the tongue are the only sign of heat, and they are interpreted to mean an accumulation of heat in the upper burner.

The tongue coating is slightly peeled. The pale tongue body and peeled coating are here indicative of a weakness of Stomach qi. The lack of appetite, together with the rootless coating, suggests Spleen and Stomach qi deficiency with the possible onset of Stomach yin deficiency. In this case, the Spleen qi deficiency is causing blood deficiency that is contributing to the anemia of the patient.

Treatment strategy. Strengthen the Lung and Spleen qi, transform the phlegm, and nourish the Lung and Stomach yin.

The patient was given a decoction of Six-Gentleman of Metal and Water Decoction *(jīn shuǐ liù jūn jiān)*, with the addition of Platycodi Radix *(jié gěng)*, Benincasae Semen *(dōng guā zǐ)*, and Fritillariae thunbergii Bulbus *(zhè bèi mǔ)*. This eased the cough, and the patient began to expectorate copious white mucus. However, her strength did not improve.

The prescription was therefore modified, with the addition of Atractylodis macrocephalae Rhizoma *(bái zhú)*, Codonopsis Radix *(dǎng shēn)*, Lycii Cortex *(dì gǔ pí)*, and Mori Cortex *(sāng bái pí)*. The prescription was regularly modified, and after three months, the patient's symptoms had disappeared and she felt well. Six months later, an X-ray revealed that the sarcoidosis had disappeared. Her tongue, however, had not changed.

5.2 Tongue Signs Associated with Lung Yin Deficiency

Chronic and serious deficiency of Lung qi may lead to Lung yin deficiency. A Lung yin deficiency can develop during the course of an illness, or, depending on the individual's constitution, from Kidney yin deficiency. However, Lung yin deficiency may develop independently of Kidney yin deficiency. An important causative factor of an 'isolated' Lung yin deficiency is smoking. Over the long term, smoking generates heat in the Lungs, which gradually leads to a clumping of Lung fluids. The pathology is characterized by smoker's cough, which typically occurs in the morning and causes the expectoration of thick, discolored phlegm. Many years of smoking leads to a dry or irritating cough, a result of the phlegm drying up. The heat in the Lungs shows itself in the anterior third of the tongue, which will be red. In the case of a more advanced stage of injury to the Lung yin, this area of the tongue will present with small, thin cracks (Fig. 5.2.1).

Years of working in dry, dusty conditions can also cause Lung yin deficiency. Bakers and miners, for instance, often suffer from this condition. The Lung yin can also be injured by external dryness, either from extremely dry weather or central heating and air conditioning. Dryness in the Lungs manifests as a dry cough and dry throat or mouth. When Lung yin deficiency has manifested, additional symptoms such as hoarseness, itchiness of the throat, occasional blood-tinged sputum, and a feeling of heat in the body or of subfebrile temperatures in the afternoon will also appear.

Tongue signs

- red on anterior third of tongue: heat in the Lungs
- red on anterior third with small, thin cracks: heat in the Lungs and Lung yin deficiency
- red, dry tongue body with small, thin cracks on the anterior third: Lung yin and Kidney yin deficiency

Cracks and swelling of the anterior third of the tongue are only significant when they occur in conjunction with other signs and symptoms, such as shortness of breath or coughing. If there are no other indications of a Lung disharmony, these signs may be discounted. Cracks in the anterior third of a pale or pale red tongue body may be the result of past illness (Fig. 5.2.5), including a severe bout of bronchitis, or the result of smoking (Fig 5.2.3), even if the individual has not been smoking for several years. Again, they do not always denote an acute or active disease process. Rather, they may reflect past injuries to the fluids and yin. If, however, the cracks are present and the disease process is active and is accompanied by Lung-related symptoms, then the overall pathomechanism would include Lung qi deficiency progressing to Lung yin deficiency.

Serious Lung infections, like pneumonia or tuberculosis, are characterized by the development of extreme heat in the Lungs. This will always injure the fluids of the Lungs and may produce, in a short space of time, cracks on the anterior third of the tongue. At the onset of the illness, the cracks will be thin and superficial. However, if the heat is very intense and the Lungs are attacked for a prolonged period, the cracks will become deeper and wider.

A red discoloration on the anterior third of the tongue reflects heat in the upper burner or Lungs (Fig. 5.2.3) or an acute illness caused by externally-contracted pathogenic factors (Ch. 9). By contrast, redness on the tip of the tongue signals disharmonies associated with the Heart (Ch. 6).

Tongue description	Chinese diagnosis
Reddish, slightly thin	Slight blood and yin deficiency
Curled-up, slightly red edges	Liver qi constraint with heat in the Liver
Cracks in the anterior third[7]	Lung yin deficiency with heat in the Lungs
Yellow, thin, greasy coating	Slight accumulation of damp-heat in the lower burner

Fig. 5.2.1
Male
41 years old

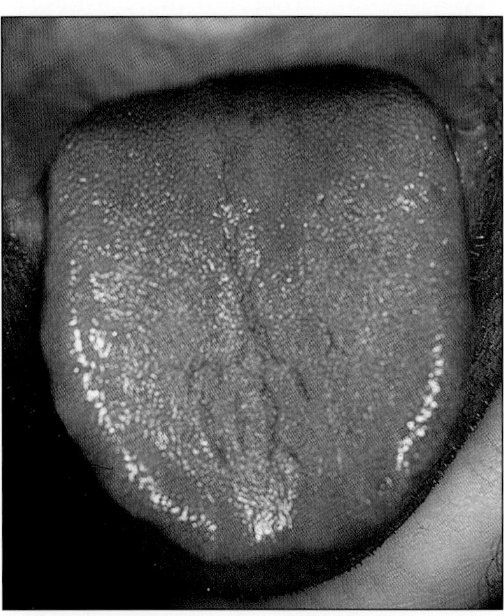

Symptoms

Dry cough
Pain in the chest
Stomach pain
Difficulty sleeping
Tendency to develop high fevers
Irritability

Western diagnosis

Acne vulgaris

Background to disease

Abuse of nicotine, black tea, and cannabis
Irregular lifestyle
Frequent viral and bacterial infections with high fevers

Tongue description	**Chinese diagnosis**
Pale red, pale edges	Spleen qi deficiency with blood deficiency
Deep horizontal cracks in the center and anterior third	Stomach and Lung yin deficiency
Slight swelling in the anterior third	Retention of phlegm in the Lungs
Red in the anterior third	Heat in the upper burner
Dry	Deficiency of fluids

Symptoms

Chronic cough with profuse, white, and slightly yellow mucus
Nasal congestion
Dry throat
Exhaustion
Mood swings

Western diagnosis

Chronic sinusitis
Chronic bronchitis

Background to disease

Repressed emotions
Excessive consumption of spicy foods

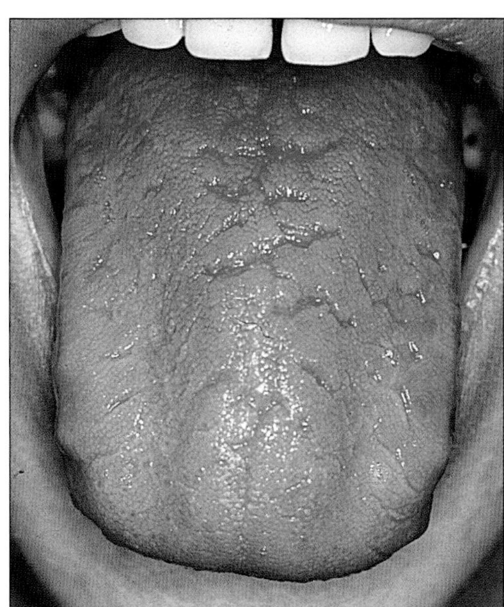

Fig. 5.2.2
Female
28 years old

Tongue description	**Chinese diagnosis**
Red	Kidney yin deficiency
Vertical cracks on the anterior third	Lung yin deficiency
Slightly reddish, cracked center	Stomach yin deficiency
Curled, reddish edges	Liver qi stagnation with developing heat
Yellow, thin coating at the root	Normal

Symptoms

Dry cough, shortness of breath
Hoarseness
Burning of the tongue
Insomnia
Night sweats
Pressure below the ribs

Western diagnosis

Chronic bronchitis

Background to disease

Mental taxation
Lack of sleep
Smoking for 25 years

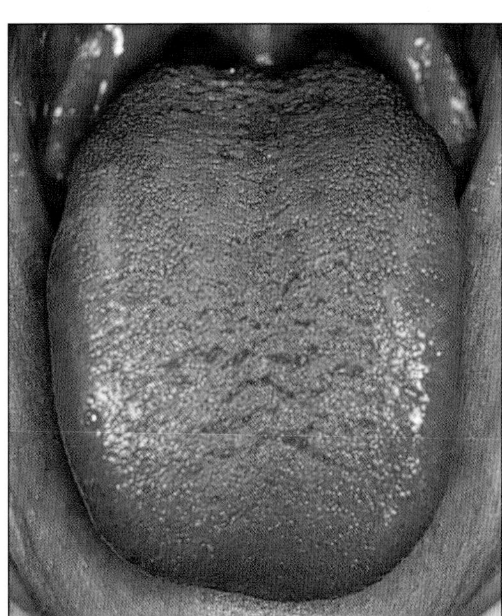

Fig. 5.2.3
Female
43 years old

Tongue description	**Chinese diagnosis**
Deep red	Kidney yin deficiency with lack of fluids
Contracted, red, dry, peeled in anterior third	Lung yin deficiency

Fig. 5.2.4
Male
71 years old

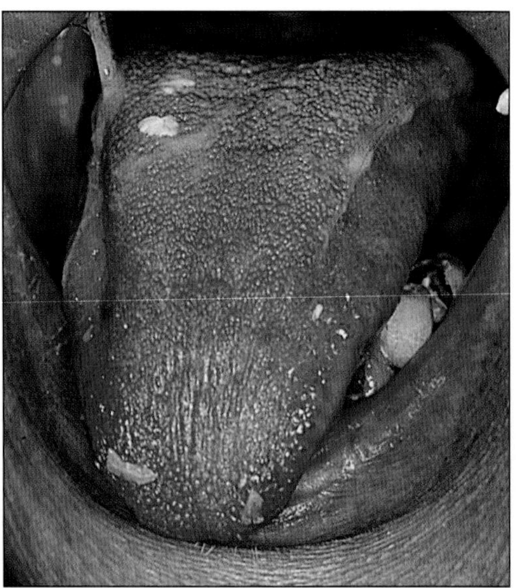

Symptoms

Cough with blood-tinged sputum
Pain in the chest
Dry throat and mouth
Night sweats
Exhaustion

Western diagnosis

Bronchial cancer

Background to disease

Smoking for 50 years

About this case history

The following is a good example of a person suffering from different diseases of the respiratory tract since childhood. The resulting pathomechanisms among the Lungs, Spleen, and Heart are discussed.

CASE HISTORY After contracting pneumonia at the age of four, the patient experienced years of breathing difficulty and asthma. The symptoms diminished with the onset of puberty and were followed by ten years without complaints. Then, a severe cold initiated severe asthma attacks that hospitalized the patient and resulted in the taking of various medications.[8] Physical exertion, emotional stress, and cold, windy weather triggered breathlessness, difficulty inhaling, and tightness in the chest. Six months before coming to the clinic, the patient developed allergic rhinitis, which aggravated her breathing problems. She suffered from a runny nose and occasional sneezing fits, and from recurring colds and infections.

The patient had troublesome premenstrual problems. About ten days prior to menstruation, her breasts became distended. Her menstruation, however, was regular and problem-free. She appeared tense. She described herself as a perfectionist, which put pressure on her internally. Her appetite and digestion were normal, although she complained of thirst and dryness of the mouth; she drank very little, however. She slept well but had night sweats. Her pulse was floating and slippery. The right, distal pulse was remarkably sinking and frail.

Analysis. The patient had asthma. Her acute symptoms must be seen in relation to her childhood illness, which laid the foundation for a weakened constitution based on underlying Lung and Spleen qi deficiency. Her childhood bout with pneumonia, and the ensuing asthma, weakened her exterior, resulting in recurrent colds and infections. This further weakened her Lung qi, as reflected in the sinking and frail right distal pulse.

The tongue body also reflects her weakened constitution. The tongue surface presents with many cracks, especially on the anterior third. The cracks are deep and wide, and signal an injury to the Lung yin. The nature of the cracks highlights a disease process that, in the past, injured

Tongue description	Chinese diagnosis
Pale red with deep cracks on the sides	Spleen qi deficiency
Wide	Accumulation of dampness
Deep, wide cracks on the anterior third	Lung yin deficiency
Curled-up edges	Liver qi stagnation
Reddish, curled-under tip	Heat in the Heart
Slightly contracted root	Onset of Kidney essence deficiency
White, slippery coating	Externally-contracted cold
Peeled coating at the root	No diagnostic significance

Symptoms

Tightness of chest, difficulty breathing
Panting and wheezing
Runny nose, sneezing fits
Thirst, dryness of mouth
Night sweats
Distended breasts and irritability prior to menstruation

Western diagnosis

Allergic rhinitis, bronchial asthma, premenstrual syndrome

Background to disease

Pneumonia in childhood
Overwork
Emotional problems

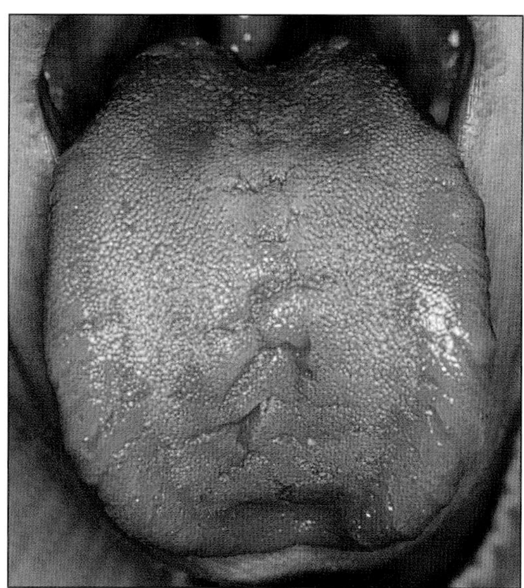

Fig. 5.2.5
Female
36 years old

the yin and set the stage for an ongoing pattern of deficiency. Cracks on the sides of the tongue generally indicate severe Spleen qi deficiency. In this case the cracks appear predominantly on the anterior third of the tongue and may denote Lung yin deficiency.

The patient was free of symptoms for several years before a severe cold—an external pathogenic factor—impaired her constitutionally weak Lung qi. This resulted in renewed asthma attacks and bouts of breathlessness. Medical treatment at a hospital alleviated the breathing problems, but the underlying causes of the disease remained.

The wheezing and panting, difficulty inhaling, and tightness of the chest are triggered by the following factors:

- *Physical exertion.* This is possibly indicative of one of two patterns: Lung-Kidney disharmony, or weak or obstructed Lungs. The Lungs cause the qi to descend and control exhalation. The Kidneys receive the qi. When these functions are normal, respiration is regulated and harmonized. The patient's difficulty inhaling on physical exertion and related breathing problems signal a disharmony of the Lungs and Kidneys. The Kidney qi is too weak to receive the qi from the Lungs, so it 'bounces back' to the chest. In theory, the inability of the Kidney qi to receive and grasp the qi can be attributed to an underlying deficiency of Kidney yang, especially when the breathlessness is triggered by exercise. In this case, however, there are no signs pointing to such a deficiency: the tongue is neither swollen nor particularly wet, and the pulse is neither frail nor sinking. The patient does not feel especially tired, nor does she easily feel the cold. Only the slightly contracted root of the tongue signals the onset of weakness in the Kidney essence,

Pathomechanism

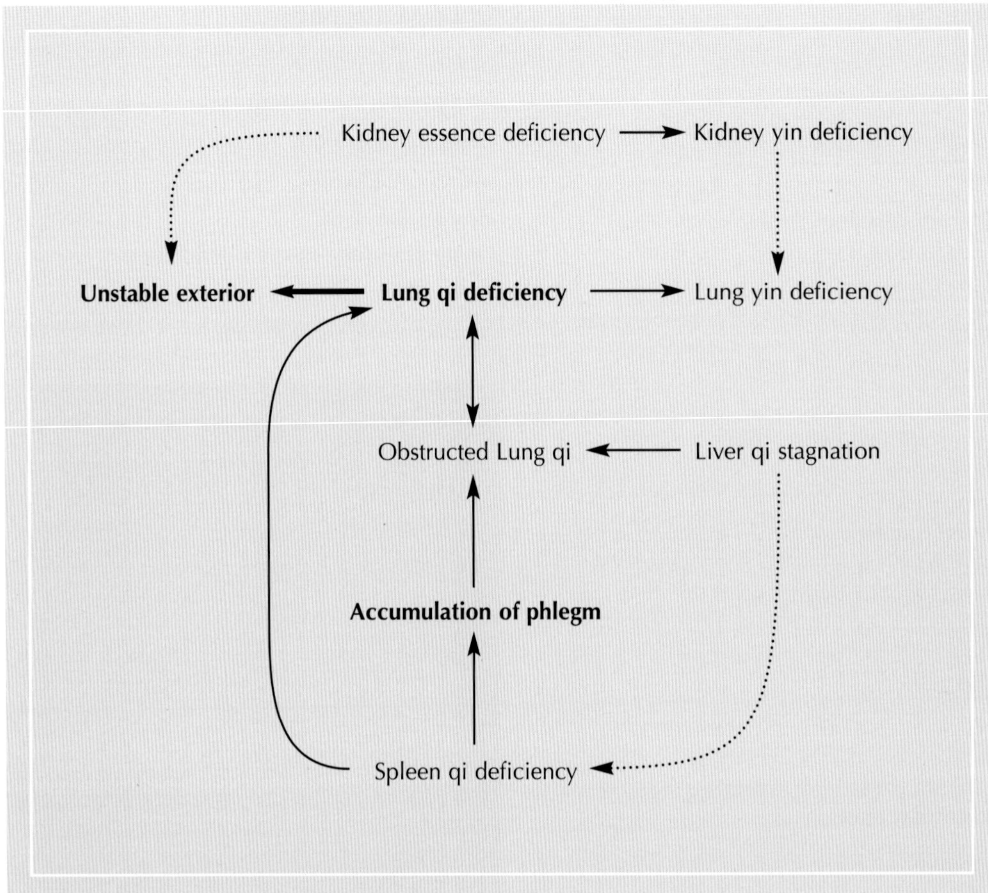

possibly due to the long history of the illness and the patient's frequent colds.

This suggests that the breathlessness, triggered by exercise, is caused by weak and obstructed Lung qi. The Lungs send qi and fluids down to the Bladder.[9] If the Lung qi is weak, the qi and fluids cannot reach the Kidneys, resulting in an accumulation of fluids in the Lungs that congeal into phlegm. A condition of fullness in the Lungs ensues, which causes coughing, wheezing, panting, and tightness of the chest.

- *Cold, windy weather*. The patient's aversion to wind and cold highlights the fact that her protective qi has been affected by the underlying Lung qi deficiency. In a healthy person, the protective qi warms and stabilizes the exterior and protects the body from the penetration of external pathogenic factors. Here, because of the weakness of the protective qi, the exterior is unstable and allows frequent penetration, which, in turn, compounds the congestion and weakness of the Lung qi.

For the first time in her life, early sprouting plants give the patient a runny nose and make her sneeze. Shortly before the onset of these symptoms, she was exhausted from working too hard. These acute symptoms, caused by externally-contracted wind-cold, impair the Lung function of descending and dispersing. The resulting accumulation of phlegm constrains the Lung qi even more, resulting in breathlessness.

Wind attacks the nose and sets off sneezing fits. The Lungs lose their control over the nose as a result of the penetration by wind-cold. This leads to constant nasal discharge. The external wind-cold is manifested in the quality of the nasal secretion (typically clear and watery), in the white and slippery tongue coating, and in the floating pulse. The patient now suffers from allergic rhinitis because of the weakened quality of the protective qi. The strength of the protective qi depends on the integrity of the Lungs and Kidneys, and the origin of the protective qi is located in the lower burner.[10]

- *Emotional stress.* This has led to Liver qi constraint. Because she is a perfectionist, the patient feels tense and under pressure. If she cannot fulfill all her expectations, she becomes frustrated. This behavior has contributed to constraint of Liver qi, as reflected in the curled edges of the tongue. Stress sets off breathlessness and wheezing because the constrained Liver qi rebels upward to the chest and hinders the Lung qi from descending. This mechanism is clarified by studying the course of the Liver channel: A branch of the primary channel crosses the diaphragm and spreads in the Lungs. (The rebellious movement of constrained Liver qi is also responsible for the distended breasts prior to menstruation and her irritability during her menses.)

Although the patient expectorated very little phlegm, Chinese medicine regards it as a causative factor in most forms of asthma. The lack of obvious phlegm is not unusual in patients who are treated with Western biomedicine. Despite this, phlegm is often present, but is lodged deeply in the Lungs; it only moves if it is activated by externally-contracted pathogenic factors. The tongue does not reflect any sign of this phlegm, but the slippery quality of the pulse is an indication of this disease pattern.

Night sweats are often the first sign of Kidney yin deficiency, which favors the development of heat from deficiency. This deficiency is responsible for the dryness of the mouth and thirst without the desire to drink. The tip of the tongue is reddish, which is interpreted as heat developing in the Heart, probably as a result of the use of bronchodilators.[11]

Treatment strategy. Release the exterior wind-cold, induce the Lung qi to descend, regulate the Lungs and Kidneys, transform the phlegm, and stabilize the exterior.

The patient wanted to be treated with acupuncture. The goal of the first treatment was to relieve the acute symptoms. A draining technique was used at the following points:

- BL-12 *(fēng mén)* and BL-13 *(fèi shū)* expel exterior wind and regulate the Lung's descending and dispersing functions.
- LU-7 *(liè quē)* induces the Lung qi to descend and releases the exterior.
- TB-5 *(wài guān)* releases the exterior and expels wind.

A tonifying needling technique was used at KI-3 *(tài xī)* and KI-7 *(fù liū)* to strengthen the Kidneys. After ten acupuncture treatments, the sneezing fits and runny nose had disappeared, but the tight chest and breathlessness had not improved very much. The patient is continuing with the treatment.

5.3 Special Tongue Signs

Swelling in the anterior third of the tongue is indicative of retention of phlegm in the Lungs. Very often, this tongue sign will appear in conjunction with a pale tongue body. The damp-phlegm in such cases is associated with underlying Spleen qi deficiency. Fluids accumulate and form phlegm if the Spleen qi is too weak to transform and transport solids and liquids. The phlegm is retained in the Lungs where it interferes with the qi mechanism and leads to coughing with copious white and easily-expectorated sputum. This may show up on the tongue as a white, slippery coating. The swelling in the anterior third of the tongue reflects the chronic nature of this pathology.

Tongue description	**Chinese diagnosis**
Pale red	Slight Spleen qi deficiency
Swollen in the anterior third	Retention of damp-phlegm in the Lungs
Red points on the anterior third	Acute, externally-contracted wind-heat
Yellow, slippery coating at the root	Retention of damp-heat in the lower burner

Fig. 5.3.1
Female
48 years old

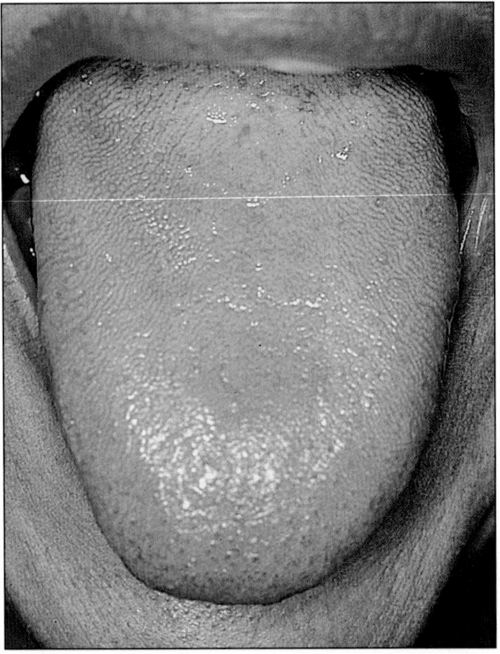

Symptoms

Sore throat
Dry cough
Joint pain
Weight gain
Inability to sleep through the night

Western diagnosis

Acute cold
Ovarian cancer
Hypothyroidism

Background to disease

Condition followed chemotherapy

Tongue description	**Chinese diagnosis**
Pale	Spleen qi deficiency
Swollen in the anterior third	Retention of phlegm in the Lungs
White, wet coating	Acute, externally-contracted wind-cold

Fig. 5.3.2
Female
36 years old

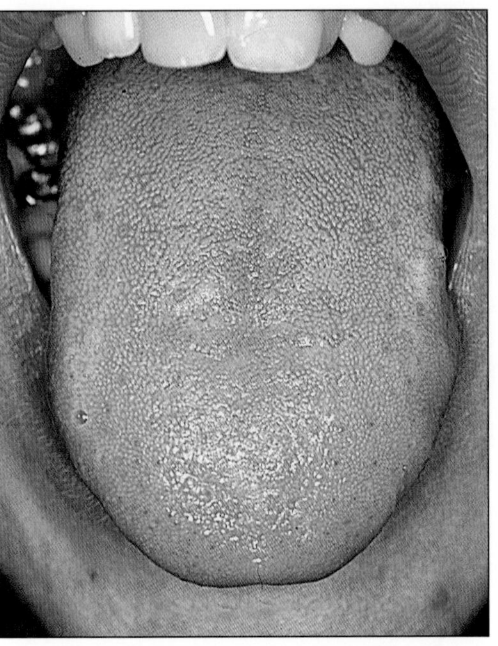

Symptoms

Cough with profuse white mucus
Tendency toward chronic bronchitis
Catches colds easily
Fatigue
Profuse menstrual bleeding

Western diagnosis

Iron deficiency anemia
Acute cold, chronic bronchitis

Background to disease

Sadness and grief after the death of mother
Repeated use of antibiotics

5.4 Tongue Signs Associated with Constitutional Weakness of the Lungs

Two vertical, parallel cracks in the anterior third of the tongue are indicative of an inherited disposition toward weakness of the Lungs. If a parent or grandparent had contracted or died of tuberculosis, this tongue sign may appear one or two generations later. In my experience these cracks suggest the frequent appearance of chronic illness of the respiratory tract, for example, bronchial asthma. They point to a tendency toward both Lung qi and yin deficiency. In these cases, the diagnosis of the tongue provides important information about the constitution of the patient. When such cracks are evident, the practitioner must inquire about the family history. A positive answer indicates a constitutional weakness of the Lungs, which must be taken into consideration when determining the treatment plan as discussed. In the case history at the end of this chapter.

Tongue description	**Chinese diagnosis**
Pale red, slightly wet	Spleen qi deficiency
Two parallel, oblique cracks in the anterior third	Constitutional Lung yin and qi deficiency

Symptoms

Palpitations with or without exertion
Tendency to catch colds
Painful knees
Fatigue

Western diagnosis

Cardiac arrhythmia
Reiter's disease

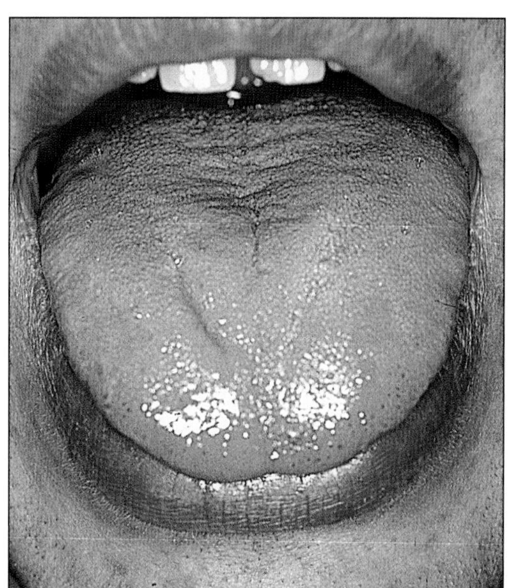

Fig. 5.4.1
Male
37 years old

Tongue description	Chinese diagnosis
Pale red with cracks on the side	Spleen qi deficiency
Slightly bluish	Blood stasis
Slightly swollen	Accumulation of dampness
Slight reddening on the anterior third	Development of heat in the upper burner
Two oblique cracks on the anterior third	Constitutional weakness of the Lungs
Slight depression at the root	Onset of Kidney essence deficiency

Fig. 5.4.2
Female
36 years old

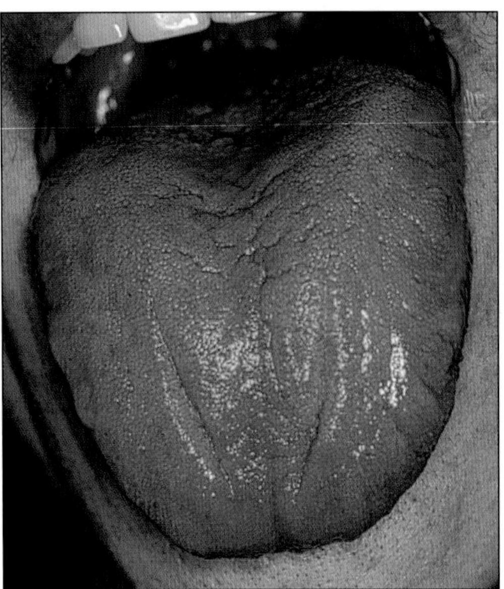

Symptoms

Retrosternal pain
Breathlessness on exertion, shortness of breath
Strong sweating on exertion
Exhaustion
Premenstrual irritability
Menstrual pains

Western diagnosis

Extrasystolic heartbeats

Background to disease

Mental stress
Lack of sleep
Family history of chronic respiratory illness

CASE HISTORY This 36-year-old taxi driver was feeling desperate because of her ill health. Her physical strength was so limited that she could not work properly: She could only manage to drive three nights a week. After endless conventional exams, the only finding was that of extrasystolic heartbeats. However, the patient's symptoms could not be explained by this finding. Physical movement caused extreme breathlessness with retrosternal pain and a feeling of tightness in the chest. She also sweated intensely on the slightest physical exertion. A nitroglycerine spray brought quick relief, but the attacks greatly weakened her. She was constantly exhausted, cried easily, and felt emotionally unstable. She could not remember a specific time when the symptoms began (about 20 years before), and she could not find a cause for the attacks.

Her menstruation was extremely painful during the first 48 hours, although the bleeding was normal. She suffered from quite noticeable hair growth on her face, especially on the chin. Her appetite, thirst, and digestion were normal. Her pulse was sinking and frail.

Analysis. The two oblique cracks in the anterior third of the tongue body signal a constitutional or hereditary weakness associated with the Lungs. These particular cracks reflect an underlying weak constitution associated with the Lungs. The patient's mother and sister both suffered from bronchial asthma and her father had died of coronary heart disease.

For 20 years the patient had suffered from retrosternal pain as well as a feeling of pressure in the chest, shortness of breath, and extrasystolic heartbeats. All of these symptoms were aggravated by physical exertion. The constitutionally-related Lung qi deficiency is responsible for the shortness of breath and breathlessness. This occurs on exertion of any kind and disappears with rest.

Sweating upon the slightest exertion is caused by a weakness of Lung and Heart qi. The

Pathomechanism

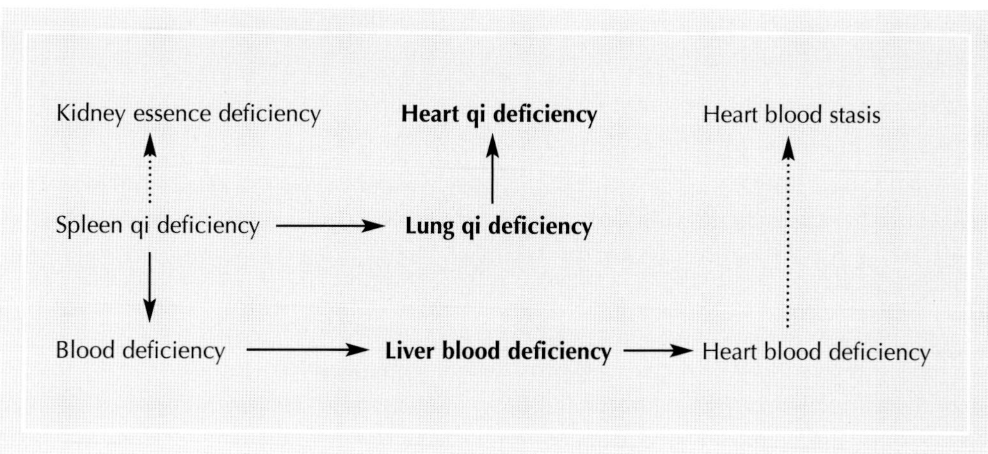

Lungs control the pores and the skin[12] and govern all the qi in the body. Sweat is the fluid of the Heart.[13] Due to the weakness of both yin organs, the exterior is not consolidated and the fluids are allowed to leak out in the form of sweat. When even the slightest physical exertion triggers excessive sweating, deficiency of Heart and Lung qi is implied.

In addition, because of the deficient circulation of qi in the upper burner, the Heart blood is not moving appropriately and blood stasis ensues. When the patient exerts herself, the flow of Heart blood slackens due to the increased demand placed on the Heart and Lung qi, manifesting in retrosternal pains. These pains disappear immediately when the patient uses her nitroglycerine spray. This substance has a dilatory effect on the coronary vessels, and in this sense, nitroglycerine enhances the movement of Heart blood.

The deficient circulation of qi in the upper burner is also responsible for the irregular heartbeat. The Heart engenders the pulse and controls the heartbeat. In order to perform this task, the Heart needs an adequate supply of qi and blood. The patient's irregular heartbeat is the result of Lung qi deficiency as well as Heart qi and blood deficiency.

The patient's desperation, sadness, and obsessive thought about the state of her health have contributed to the stagnation of qi in the upper burner.[14] The slightly reddish anterior third of the tongue signals the development of heat in the upper burner, which readily appears in a pattern of concurrent constraint of qi and blood.

The long-standing qi deficiency in the upper burner, in combination with Spleen qi deficiency, has resulted in the development of Heart blood deficiency. This deficiency can be seen in the slightly indented tip of the tongue. As mentioned earlier, the patient's emotions, as well as the described pathomechanisms, are responsible for the Heart blood deficiency, which in turn contributes to her mental instability.

The Heart has a close connection to the uterus via the vessels of the gestation membranes *(bāo mài)*. If the Heart blood is weak, the Heart qi is unable to descend to the uterus.[15] In this case, the Heart blood deficiency as well as the stasis of blood in the Heart produces stagnation of qi and blood in the Penetrating vessel, which results in extreme menstrual pain.

The retrosternal pain and feeling of pressure are further indications of an obstruction of the Penetrating vessel, since its blockage may result in a counterflow (rebellion) of qi. In my experience, strong hair growth on the face indicates a condition of excess caused by blood stasis and is indicative of an imbalance in the Penetrating vessel. Because women lose blood on a regular basis through menstruation, the Penetrating vessel lacks sufficient blood to carry to the chin and lips. Therefore, women do not have much facial hair.[16]

The patient's constant tiredness is caused by the deficiency of the Lung and Spleen qi. The cracks on the sides of the tongue, the slight teeth marks, and the deep, weak pulse are all indications of this deficiency. The postnatal essence in this patient is not strong and does not sufficiently nourish the Kidney essence. The slight depression at the root of the tongue reflects the onset of this deficiency.

Treatment strategy. Strengthen the Heart and Lung qi, nourish and regulate the Heart blood, regulate the heartbeat, and enrich the Kidney essence.

The first prescription was for Generate the Pulse Powder *(shēng mài sǎn),* modified by the addition of Salviae miltiorrhizae Radix *(dān shēn)* and Fructus Trichosanthes *(guā lóu).* After taking this decoction for two weeks, she felt much stronger, but the extrasystolic heartbeats had increased.

This reaction did not make sense, so I deduced that it was because the prescription did not tonify the blood. A modified version of Honey-Fried Licorice Decoction *(zhì gān cǎo tāng)* reduced the extrasystolic heartbeats but unfortunately also reduced the patient's energy. Because this prescription had also failed, the patient became very angry during the next consultation. When her anger subsided, she cried.

Although the tongue did not show any signs of Liver blood deficiency, her reaction clarified the diagnosis: I had not sufficiently considered the disharmony of the Liver. The general lack of qi and blood, as well as the emotional state of the patient, had impaired the circulation of Liver qi and contributed to an insufficient supply of Liver blood. A deficiency of Liver blood results in a deficient rooting of the ethereal soul *(hún).* Closer questioning of the patient revealed that she had no goals and her life had become meaningless. She thought this was due to her chronic ill-health.

After this, I decided to soften the Liver in order to treat the episodic pains and to calm the spirit. Although the prescription Peony and Licorice Decoction *(sháo yào gān cǎo tāng)* is used for spasmodic and episodic abdominal pain, I prescribed it here because of its ability to ease spasmodic types of pain, which here were caused by Liver blood and yin deficiency. The herb Polygalae Radix *(yuǎn zhì)* was added to the prescription. After taking this decoction for two weeks, the patient had no further symptoms. And after another month with the same prescription, the extrasystolic heartbeats had not reappeared. The patient felt much more content and stopped taking nitroglycerine. Six months later she still felt very well and had gone back to school.

Endnotes

1 Anonymous. *Su wen* [Basic Questions], edited by He W-B et al. Beijing: China Medicine Science and Technology Press, 1996: 9:54.

2 Maciocia G. *Tongue Diagnosis in Chinese Medicine*, rev. ed. Seattle: Eastland Press, 1995: 72.

3 *Tongue Diagnosis in Chinese Medicine*, 72.

4 Zhu D-X. *The Heart and Essence of Dan Xi's Methods of Treatment,* translated by Yang S-Z. Boulder, CO: Blue Poppy Press, 1993: 18:75.

5 Li D-Y. *Treatise on Spleen and Stomach: A Translation of the Pi Wei Lun,* translated by Yang S-Z. Boulder, CO: Blue Poppy Press, 1993.

6 *Tongue Diagnosis in Chinese Medicine*, 51.

7 The following passage appears in *Compendium of Charts and Books Past and Present: Complete Collection of the Medical Section (Gu jin tu shu ji cheng: Yi bu quan lu)*. Beijing: Peoples Medical Publishing House, 1991; 5:81: "The tongue looks red and shows a crack that resembles the character for man (*rén*), which means that the ministerial fire is blazing and toxic heat burns. It is appropriate to administer Cool the Diaphragm Powder *(liáng gé sǎn)*." The patient here shows this tongue sign. It is interesting to note that within a year after the photo was taken, he developed acute porphyria cutanea tarda (a hepatic disorder). Ten years later he is well, but sill smoking. His tongue has taken on quite a red coloring.

8 When she first came for treatment the patient was taking theophylline, corticosteroids, and beta-2-sympathomimetics (adrenergic agents).

9 *Basic Questions*, 21:133.

10 Anonymous. *Huang di nei jing ling shu yi shi* [Translation and Explanation of the Yellow Emperor's Inner Classic: Divine Pivot], edited by Nanjing College of Traditional Chinese Medicine, Traditional Chinese Medicine Department. Shanghai: Shanghai Science and Technology Press, 1997: 18:263.

11 Maciocia G. *The Practice of Chinese Medicine*. London: Churchill Livingstone, 1994: 140.

12 *Basic Questions*, 23:147.

13 Ibid.

14 Ibid., 39:233. The text here describes how sorrow and sadness can lead to an expansion of the Lungs that presses upward and causes stagnation in the upper burner. Later in the chapter, the text describes how narrowly-focused thoughts that revolve around one thing can also contribute to the stagnation of qi.

15 Maciocia G. *Obstetrics and Gynecology in Chinese Medicine*. London: Churchill Livingstone, 1998: 40.

16 *Divine Pivot*, 65:393-94.

CHAPTER 6

Tongue Signs Associated with Heart Disharmonies

The Heart has a special position among all the organs: "The Heart is the ruler, and from it issues the spirit and mind."[1] The Heart allows a person to consciously perceive and cope with life's experiences and to develop a consciousness about the meaning and path of one's life.

The Heart houses the spirit.[2] From birth to death, the spirit influences our perceptions about our lives and our state of mental and physical health. In a healthy person, the spirit resides peacefully in the Heart and can be recognized by a radiant shine in the eyes. On a nonphysical level the spirit manifests in several ways, for example, the ability to meet new situations freely and appropriately, to utilize memory, to think clearly, and to exercise control over the emotions. To accomplish these functions, the spirit needs a place to reside, which is provided by the Heart. But if the spirit lives in a disquieted, neglected residence, disharmony between the spirit and the Heart will ensue. This can cause physical as well as mental symptoms.

The spirit lies beyond yin and yang in that it cannot be measured by either yin or yang. As a result, the condition of the spirit is not directly visible on the tongue. However, energetic conditions that are responsible for the appropriate anchoring of the spirit are reflected in the color and shape of the tongue body. Therefore, the 'spirit of the tongue' refers to the appearance of the tongue. If the tongue possesses spirit, it will be moist and fresh looking, with a pale red color. By contrast, a tongue without spirit will be dry and parched, and have a dull color.

6.1 Tongue Signs Associated with Deficiency

6.1.1 Tongue Signs Associated with Heart Qi/Yang Deficiency

All disease patterns originating from a disturbance of the Heart can manifest in emotional, spiritual, and/or physical symptoms. However, in cases of Heart qi and yang deficiency, as well as Heart blood stasis, the physical symptoms are uppermost. These patterns are characterized, for example, by palpitations or shortness of breath on exertion, or retrosternal pains, and are also often responsible for noticeable heart diseases. Heart qi deficiency may be triggered by a serious emotional shock or by deep sadness. Individuals with constitutional Heart qi deficiency tend to be anxious or easily startled. They often lack energy and complain about a lack of stamina.

Tongue signs of Heart qi deficiency: pale or pale red. As mentioned earlier, the paleness of the tongue body as such is not indicative of this pattern. The degree of paleness in conjunction with other clinical signs and symptoms can help to evaluate the qi deficiency (see Ch. 2).

Tongue signs of Heart yang deficiency: very pale, swollen, and wet. In the case of Heart yang deficiency, in addition to Heart qi deficiency, the extremities may feel ice-cold, with marked shortness of breath on exertion. On a mental/emotional level this is reflected in a lack of zest or drive or by introversion.

6.1.2 Tongue Signs Associated with Heart Blood Deficiency

Blood deficiency in the body will reduce the supply of blood to the tongue, which will thereupon become pale and dry. There are three visible manifestations of this pathology on the tongue:

1. The tip of a normal tongue is red or shows many red, small, and fine points while the tongue body is pale or pale red. A slight reddening of the tip is likewise normal and important as it reflects good communication between the gate of vitality *(mìng mén)* and the Heart. The physiological fire at the gate of vitality causes this slight redness in the tip of the tongue.

2. A pale or pale red tongue with a curled-down tip indicates heat from deficiency of the Heart (Fig. 6.1.2.3). When accompanied by a pale tongue body, there will be a tendency toward depressive moods.

3. In my opinion, pale tongues that show contracted or indented tips also reflect Heart blood deficiency. I could not find any reference to this tongue shape in the literature. This sign might be said to reflect a lack of 'substance' with which to fill out the tip of the tongue, thus depriving it of its normal shape. By contrast, the long and very pointed tongue indicates a completely different pathology. Here it is heat that injures the blood, yin, and fluids, depriving the tip of its 'substance.' The presence of heat or fire in the Heart is much stronger and more vigorous than in the situations described above, and results in an extreme protuberance of the tongue, quite the opposite of what is observed with pale and dry tongues.

Heart blood deficiency is frequently seen in the clinic. It may be initiated by underlying Spleen qi deficiency, by protracted fear and worry, or by a loss of blood. The manifestations of weakened Spleen qi and Heart blood are poor memory, difficulty concentrating, and lack of clear thinking. The Heart blood serves the important function of nourishing and anchoring the spirit. Difficulty falling asleep and/or dream-disturbed sleep signals an insufficient anchoring of the spirit. As with constitutional Heart qi deficiency, an undernourished spirit tends to be anxious or easily startled (Fig. 6.1.2.5).

Over the long term, Heart blood deficiency may lead to heat from deficiency of the Heart. Because blood pertains to yin, over time Heart blood deficiency can also affect the Heart yin. Both processes can be seen when the tongue tip is red and the tongue body is pale (Heart blood deficiency with flaring heat from deficiency) or there is a pathological change in the shape of the tip (Fig. 6.1.3.2).

Tongue signs of Heart blood deficiency

- pale or pale red tongue body with an indentation at the tip (Fig. 6.1.2.1)
- pale or pale red tongue body with an indentation at the tip that has reddened: Heart blood deficiency with heat from deficiency
- pale or pale red tongue body with a red tip: Heart blood deficiency with heat from deficiency
- pale or pale red tongue body with a red tip and a crack just at the tip: Heart blood and Heart yin deficiency with heat from deficiency (Fig. 6.1.2.4)

Tongue description	**Chinese diagnosis**
Pale, swollen, slight teeth marks	Spleen qi deficiency (accumulation of dampness and deficiency of blood)
Indentation of the tip	Heart blood deficiency
White, thin coating	Normal

Symptoms

Headaches for past 20 years, especially during menstruation
Nausea in the mornings
Lack of concentration
Fatigue

Western diagnosis

Hypothyroidism

Background to disease

Family history of headaches
Long-standing emotional problems
Excessive anxiety

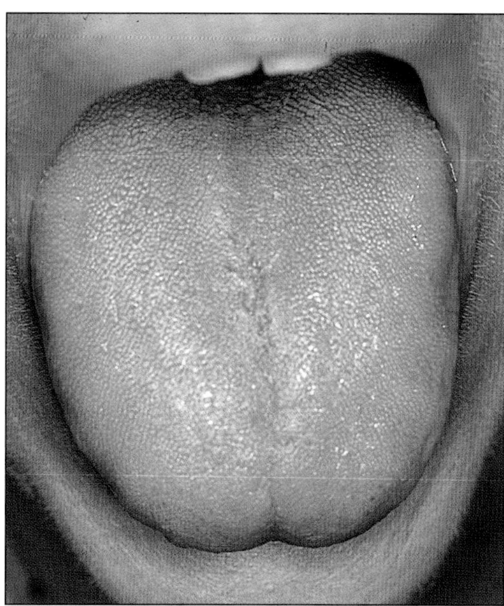

Fig. 6.1.2.1
Female
38 years old

Tongue description ------------------------ **Chinese diagnosis**

Tongue description	Chinese diagnosis
Pale red, soft	Spleen qi deficiency
Indentation of the tip	Heart blood deficiency
Swollen in the anterior third	Possible Heart qi deficiency
Yellow, thin coating with red points at the root	Heat in the lower burner

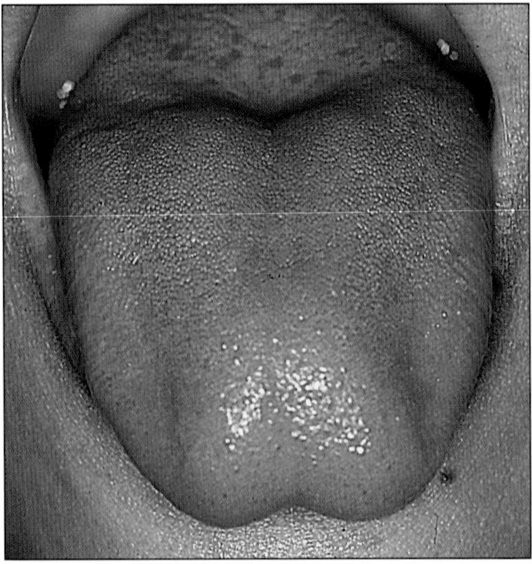

Fig. 6.1.2.2
Female
28 years old

Symptoms

Long-lasting, profuse menstrual bleeding
Lower abdominal pain during menstruation

Western diagnosis

Menorrhagia
Infertility

Background to disease

Long-standing emotional problems

Tongue description ------------------------ **Chinese diagnosis**

Tongue description	Chinese diagnosis
Pale, slightly swollen	Spleen qi deficiency (accumulation of dampness)
Curled-down tip with red points	Heat from deficiency of the Heart

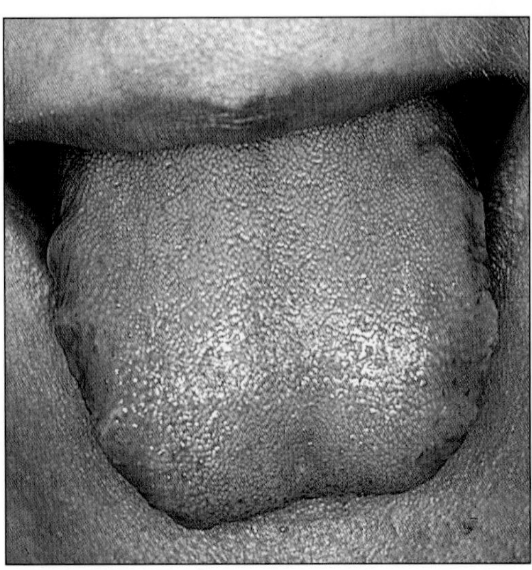

Fig. 6.1.2.3
Female
40 years old

Symptoms

Insomnia, exhaustion
Feeling hot at night
Anger and depressive moods
Cough
Shortness of breath

Western diagnosis

None

Background to disease

Unwanted divorce
Overwork
Lack of rest after the birth of her first child

Tongue description	**Chinese diagnosis**
Pale, swollen	Spleen qi deficiency (accumulation of dampness)
Dry	Lack of fluids in the Stomach
Small, deep cracks in the center and anterior third	Onset of Stomach and Lung yin deficiency
Deep crack in the tip of tongue	Heart qi and yin deficiency

Symptoms

Severe exhaustion
Shortness of breath
Inner tension

Western diagnosis

Non-Hodgkin's lymphoma
Right heart insufficiency

Background to disease

Condition after chemotherapy, radiation therapy, and splenectomy

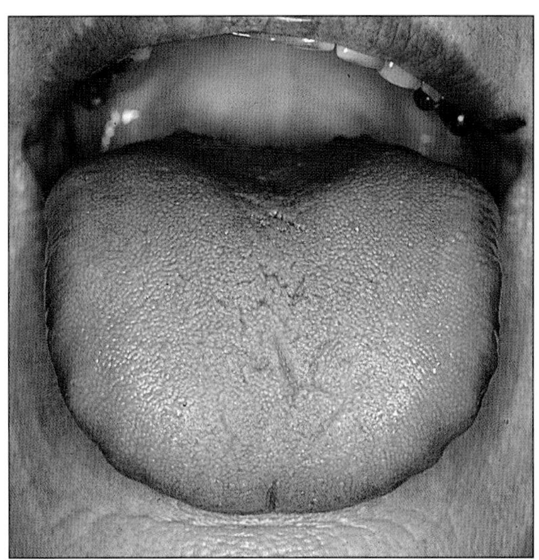

Fig. 6.1.2.4
Female
63 years old

Tongue description	**Chinese diagnosis**
Very pale	Spleen qi and yang deficiency → blood deficiency
Slightly swollen	Accumulation of dampness
Indentation of the tip	Heart blood deficiency
White, thin, and moist coating	Accumulation of dampness
Light yellow, slightly greasy coating on the posterior third	Retention of damp-heat in the lower burner

Symptoms

Incessant feelings of hunger, desire to vomit
Constipation
Poor memory
Anxiety
Mental and physical exhaustion

Western diagnosis

Bulimia nervosa

Background to disease

Unhappy childhood, irregular diet

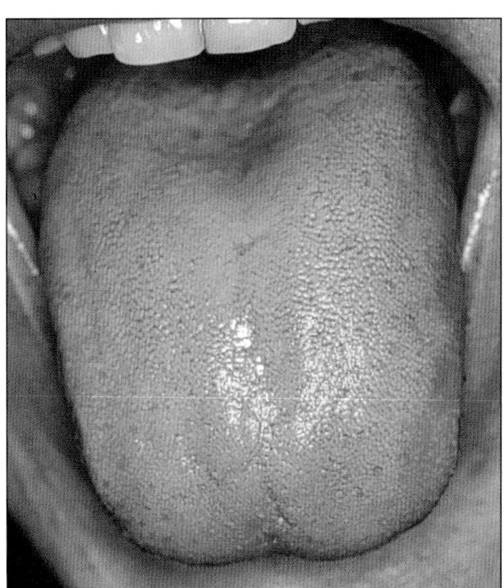

Fig. 6.1.2.5
Female
25 years old

About this case history

The close relationship between the Spleen and Heart is discussed (Fig. 6.1.2.5).

CASE HISTORY From the age of eight this patient had suffered from voracious hunger attacks and incessant eating. During these attacks, she mainly ate chocolate. After eating, she forced herself to vomit, and she occasionally used laxatives. The attacks occurred about once a week and were triggered by critical remarks about her person, arguments with her boyfriend, or weight gain. She was never punctual, was frequently absent from work, and did not work conscientiously. She appeared dull and dreary, and excessively brooding. Her neglected appearance and entire aura smacked of a psychological disorder.

She was always tired and suffered from a lack of drive. Her stools were hard and formed, and, unless she took laxatives, she had only two or three bowel movements a week. Her sleep and menstruation were normal. Her pulse was sinking and rough.

Analysis. A disharmony of the Heart and Spleen lies at the core of this patient's pathomechanism. The pale, swollen tongue body reflects Spleen qi and yang deficiency resulting in accumulation of dampness. The intensity of the pale tongue color is significant as it lacks any sign of vital reddening. This signals not only a pattern of blood deficiency, but also a lack of yang and physiological fire based in the gate of vitality *(mìng mén)*, especially since there is no redness at the tip of the tongue. The indentation at the tip signals Heart blood deficiency caused by underlying Spleen qi deficiency. The tip of the tongue lacks proper nourishment because of the lack of blood; consequently, it has become misshapen.

It is unclear which of the two yin organs is responsible for the ensuing pathology. The illness developed gradually, characterized by fits of voracious eating, including chocolate, followed by vomiting. When the patient starts brooding or feels unwell, she eats chocolate in the belief that it will calm her down. Chapter 63 of the *Divine Pivot* describes the energetic effect of eating sweet foods: "If sweet food reaches the Stomach, and the qi [of the sweetness] is weak, it cannot ascend to the upper burner. It remains in the Stomach together with food. Due to this, [the qi of the Stomach] becomes soft and damp and slows down [its function]."[3] Because of her weight gain, the patient forced herself to vomit. She could not control her behavior. Her eating habits and repeated vomiting injured both the Spleen and Stomach qi.

The following factors contribute to Spleen qi deficiency:

- Excessive brooding injures the Spleen.[4]
- Frequent and excessive consumption of sweets injures both the Spleen and Stomach qi. Taken in small amounts, sweet foods may have a moistening effect. However, if eaten to excess, they contribute to the formation of phlegm, which aggravates the Spleen qi deficiency.

This process is a vicious circle: Spleen qi deficiency leads to an accumulation of dampness, which is reflected in the white, thin, and moist coating. The thickening of the collected fluids results in the formation of phlegm, aggravating the Spleen qi deficiency. In this case, the firmness of the swollen tongue body specifically points toward the presence of phlegm. By contrast, a swollen tongue body that often appears soft denotes an accumulation of dampness (Fig. 2.1.4).

Dampness and phlegm can hinder the ascent of clear yang, and this disease process is partly responsible for the patient's mental exhaustion and inability to concentrate. Her thinking or intention *(yì)*, which is governed by the Spleen,[5] is therefore muddled. In addition, her forgetfulness and lack of concentration can be attributed to the Heart blood deficiency, which is reflected in the rough pulse. Since the blood is deficient, the spirit is not properly nourished; this accounts for the patient's phobias, fearfulness, and forgetfulness. Her disturbed spirit also leads to poor emotional control, as evidenced in her pathological eating habits.

Pathomechanism

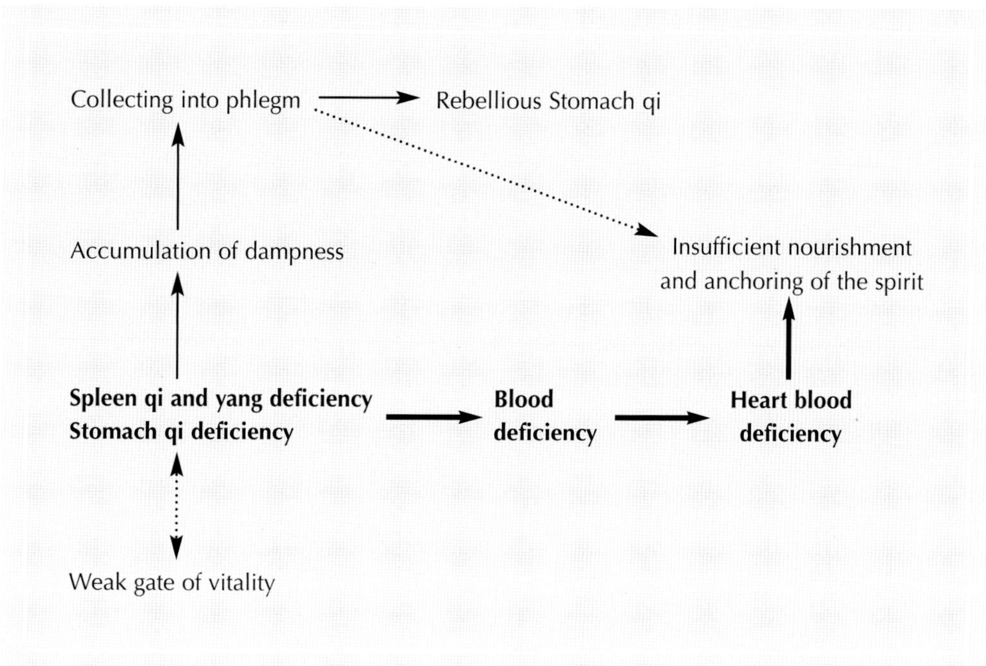

The Spleen needs warmth to transform and transport food. The patient's poor nutrition and frequent vomiting have injured the yang qi of the middle burner, reducing the warmth and strength of the gate of vitality. In a healthy person, the gate of vitality provides warmth to all the inner organs and determines their vitality. The gate of vitality also communicates with the Heart, rising upward and supporting the Heart's function of anchoring the spirit. When the gate of vitality is weak, the individual is easily depressed and there is a noticeable lack of drive. The tip of the tongue will have a slight red color when the gate of vitality is strong and is communicating with the Heart. In this case, however, the slight reddening is missing, signaling that the Heart yang is deprived of warmth and proper nourishment. In other words, the Heart is deficient, which manifests in Heart blood and yang deficiency. Steve Clavey describes it thus: "If Heart yang activity is not supported by yin blood, it will fail to move and fluids will collect into phlegm. It also implies that as the phlegm is the result of deficiency, its treatment will require tonification rather than attack."[6] The patient's inability to manage her time, her unkempt appearance, and dull mental attitude are interpreted as manifestations of a pathology caused by phlegm.

Because of the frequent vomiting, there is rebellious movement (counterflow) of the Stomach qi. The Stomach qi is thus unable to descend, which contributes to the slack bowel movements. The lingering stools may engender development of damp-heat in the Large Intestine, which is perhaps suggested in the light yellow coating at the root of the tongue.

Treatment strategy. Calm the spirit, nourish the Heart blood, strengthen the Spleen and Stomach qi, and transform the phlegm.

The patient was treated with acupuncture. Because she often forgot her appointments there were long intervals between treatments. However, she always felt good after treatment, and her eating binges and vomiting had declined in frequency to about once a month. She also started psychotherapy. Tonifying needling with moxibustion was performed at ST-36 *(zú sān lǐ)* and SP-6 *(sān yīn jiāo)*, and needling with a draining technique was performed at SP-9 *(yīn líng quán)* and PC-5 *(jiān shǐ)*.

6.1.3 Tongue Signs Associated with Heart Yin Deficiency

Heart yin deficiency occurs frequently in older people. Symptoms caused by this deficiency tend to be sleeping disorders, night sweats, increased mental restlessness, palpitations, and dry mouth (especially at night). The diminished strength of Kidney yin, which is less able to nourish the Heart yin, is physiologically normal in old age. The Heart is linked to the element fire and has a close affinity to heat. As the cooling, calming qualities of yin diminish, heat tends to rise faster.

Heart yin deficiency can also develop in young people and is related to long-standing emotional problems, intensive study periods with exams, agitation, stress, hectic lifestyles, drug abuse, or a constitutional weakness of the Heart.

It should be noted that Heart blood and Heart yin deficiency share some common symptoms: palpitations, anxiety, forgetfulness, and dream-disturbed sleep. However, the two can be distinguished by their effect on sleep and differences in tongue signs. In the case of blood deficiency, the patient may find it difficult to fall asleep, but once asleep, she will continue to sleep through the night. In addition, because the blood that reaches the tongue is inadequate, the tongue body color will be pale. By contrast, in the case of Heart yin deficiency, the patient will wake up frequently during the night and be very restless. Also, the tongue body color tends to be red.

The symptoms of heat or fire from deficiency of the Heart (irritability, palpitations with anxiety, insomnia, restlessness, and a dry mouth and throat) are much more pronounced in Heart yin deficiency than in Heart blood deficiency. In the former case, the tongue body will be red with a strongly discolored red tip, or there may be, in addition to a peeled coating, a long vertical midline crack.

Disharmonies of the tongue are most commonly manifested by a change in the color or shape of the tip of the tongue. It is important to closely inspect this part of the tongue, as it reflects the state of the Heart energies.

Tongue signs of Heart yin deficiency

- red tongue body without coating: Heart yin and Kidney yin deficiency (Fig. 5.2.4)
- red tongue body without coating, tip reddened: Heart yin and Kidney yin deficiency with heat from deficiency (Fig. 3.6.3)
- red, swollen tip: flaring-up of heat from deficiency of the Heart[7] (Fig. 6.2.1)
- red, cracked tip: Heart yin deficiency with heat from deficiency
- long midline crack on a red and peeled tongue: Heart yin and Kidney yin deficiency

Tongue description	**Chinese diagnosis**
Pale red, thinning out toward the tip	Heart blood deficiency with heat from deficiency
Long	Constitutional weakness of the Heart
Contracted, flattened, reddened tip	Onset of Heart yin deficiency

Symptoms

Inability to fall asleep and to sleep through the night
Sexual dreams
Occasional night sweats
Inability to form relationships

Western diagnosis

None

Background to disease

Excessive masturbation

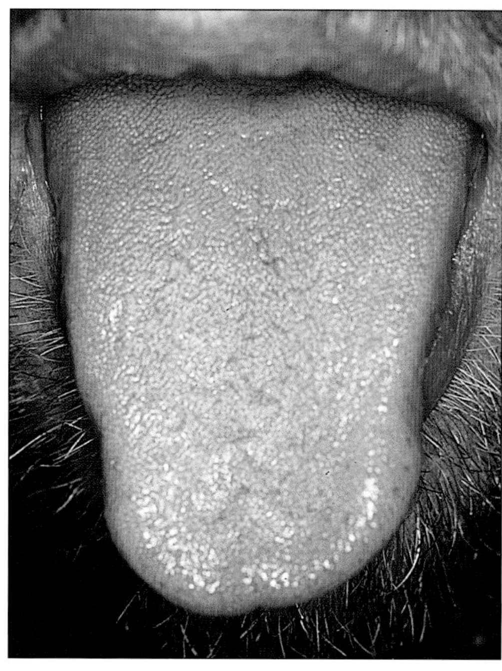

Fig. 6.1.3.1
Male
47 years old

Tongue description	**Chinese diagnosis**
Reddish	Heat from deficiency
Pale edges	Liver blood deficiency
Red, very pointed and contracted tip	Heart blood and yin deficiency with heat in the Heart
Whitish, dry coating	Slight dryness in the Stomach

Symptoms

Palpitations
Insomnia for 10 years
Anxiety on awakening
Painful and swollen wrist and ankle joints
Backache

Western diagnosis

Chronic polyarthritis

Background to disease

Long-standing problems with relationships
Severe mental demands at work

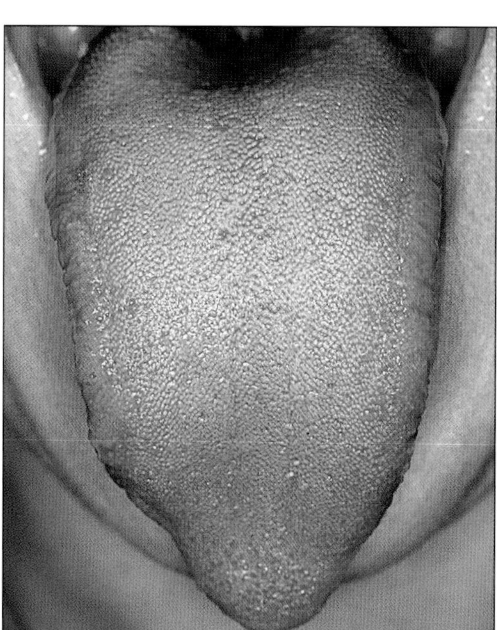

Fig. 6.1.3.2
Female
46 years old

6.1.4 The Tip of the Tongue

Before moving on to the discussion of patterns of excess associated with the Heart, we should consider the possible changes at the tip of the tongue. This concerns especially the shape and color, which give information about the condition of the Heart blood and yin.

The slight redness at the tip of the tongue is due to a reddening of the papillae filliformes. This is considered normal when it appears with a pale or pale red tongue. It shows that the communication between the Heart and gate of vitality *(mìng mén)* is functioning. The gate of vitality warms the Heart and supports the Heart in housing the spirit.

A red tongue tip that appears during an illness as a result of internal factors (e.g, long-term qi constraint and depression, strong emotional pressures, and consumption of drugs like cocaine and ecstasy) denotes the presence of heat or fire in the Heart. The degree of intensity of the red discoloration of the tongue body has an influence on the diagnostic significance of the red tongue tip. If the tip is very red or dark red, the intensity of the redness of the tongue body color reflects the severity of the pathology. This tongue type will be accompanied by strong palpitations, mouth ulcers, a feeling of heat in the body, restlessness, and insomnia. The presence of Heart fire will also result in increased agitation and diminished mental clarity. In addition to a strong reddening of the tip, in extreme cases the tip may also be slightly swollen. Here, the extreme heat leads to clumping of fluids that have transformed to phlegm-fire in the Heart, which can lead to very serious psychiatric disorders (Fig. 6.2.5).

The symptoms associated with heat from Heart yin deficiency tend to be less severe than those associated with Heart fire. In this case, the tongue tip will be red, but the tongue body will often be red with a peeled coating, as Heart yin deficiency is closely linked with Kidney yin deficiency.

Long-standing Heart blood deficiency can also lead to Heart yin deficiency, which in turn will give rise to heat from deficiency of the Heart. This may be reflected in a less red tongue body, but the tip will still look very red, or will occasionally be turned upwards (Fig. 6.2.1).

Heat in the Heart is generally caused by too much stress and a hectic lifestyle, especially if combined with an unfulfilled emotional life. Constant, long-term grief and worry will slowly lead to the formation of heat in the Heart, which will impair its function of storing the spirit; this manifests in a reddening at the tip of the tongue.

In general, it is important to judge the redness of the tongue tip in relation to the intensity of the redness of the tongue body. Heart fire will have more serious consequences in an individual with a red tongue than with a pale tongue.

Tongue signs

- pale tongue body with a red tongue tip: Heart blood deficiency with heat from deficiency of the Heart (Fig. 6.1.4.1).
- red tongue tip: presence of heat or fire in the Heart (Fig. 6.2.7)
- red tongue tip turned upwards: heat in the Heart (Fig. 6.1.4.2)
- red tongue tip with red tongue body and peeled coating: Heart yin and Kidney yin deficiency with heat from deficiency
- strong reddening of the tip and swelling of the tip: flaring up of heat or fire in the Heart (Fig. 6.2.5)

It is also important to distinguish between a red tongue tip caused by heat in the Heart and red points at the tip of the tongue caused by an externally-contracted wind-heat disease, for example, an acute infection like tonsillitis or bronchitis. More often than not, these points often appear fresher, bigger, and coarser than the points that result from heat in the Heart.[8] In addition, the points associated with externally-contracted wind-heat are located not only at the tip of the tongue, but also in the anterior third, which denotes that the heat resides in the superficial layers of the body, specifically the Lungs.

A dark red tongue with a very red tip may be caused by toxic heat entering the nutritive and blood levels. To differentiate between these red points and those described above is not difficult, as the acute symptoms of toxic heat include high fever, skin rashes, sudden nose bleeds, blood in the urine, restlessness, and even loss of consciousness and coma. (In Ch. 9, red points that are indicative of externally-contracted wind-heat and toxic heat are discussed at greater length.)

Another diagnostic meaning of red tongue points was suggested in the following study: 500 patients were examined in a Guiyang hospital[9] to study the appearance of red points at the tip of the tongue. Here, however, it was found that they were an expression of Liver qi constraint. The investigation showed a direct correlation between the red points and the inability of some patients to freely express their emotions. This is not entirely surprising, as long-standing Liver qi constraint will eventually lead to heat formation, which in turn will agitate the Heart.

Another clinical investigation in China[10] showed a connection between red points at the tip of the tongue and menstruation. It was observed that three to seven days before the onset of the period the tongue papillae would swell up, fill with blood, and turn red. In fact, the tongue papillae became even redder with the actual start of menstruation, then became smaller and lost their intense color three to seven days after menstruation. According to this investigation, the appearance of the red points at the tip shortly before menstruation has no diagnostic significance.

In the case of long-standing heat in the Heart, besides the reddening of the tip of the tongue, a pathological change of the tongue shape may also occur. There seem to be two mechanisms responsible for this change in shape:

1. Heat evaporates the fluids. The blood that is formed by the Heart is thinned by the body fluids *(jīn yè)*; the blood thereby remains liquid and contributes to giving the tongue, especially the tip, its soft, elastic, and slightly rounded form. However, if there is constant heat, the tip of the tongue will no longer receive adequate nourishment from the blood and fluids. The slightly rounded shape of the tip will then disappear and instead become very pointed.

2. Heat vigorously moves the remaining fluids. This process pushes the tip to the outside and results in a pathological tongue shape. (The same process is observed in the case of long tongues.) The heat moves the blood so vigorously that, besides the reddening of the tongue, the tip may also take on an unusual shape. This is reflected in the photographs of the following section.

Patients with these tongue signs are often psychologically unbalanced or ill. If there are no signs or symptoms of a disturbance of the spirit, the patient may show a tendency to easily lose his mental balance.

Tongue description	Chinese diagnosis
Pale red	Normal
Long, narrow	Constitutional weakness of the Heart, onset of fluid deficiency
Red, flattened tip with red points	Heart blood deficiency with heat in the Heart

Fig. 6.1.4.1
Female
34 years old

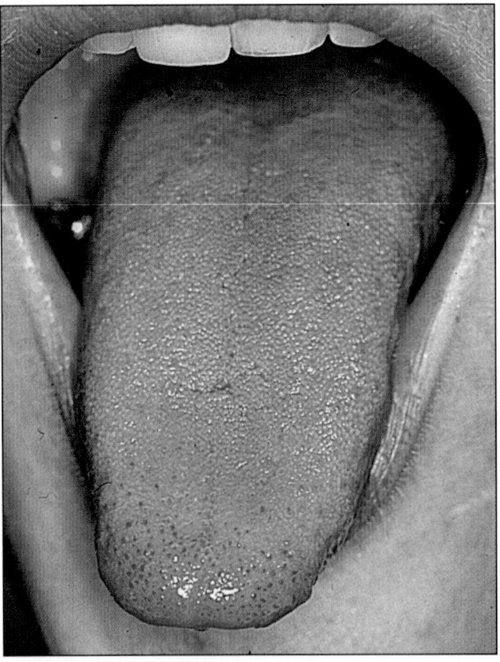

Symptoms

Night sweats
Severe sweating on the chest
Severe itchiness
Formation of pustules on the skin
Strong menstrual pains

Western diagnosis

Lichen sclerosus et atrophicus (a chronic skin disease) for the past 18 years

Background to disease

Unclear

Tongue description	Chinese diagnosis
Pale red, slightly bluish	Slight stasis of blood
Curled-up, flattened, red tip with red points	Heart blood deficiency with heat in the Heart
White, thin, dry coating	Externally-contracted wind-cold

Fig. 6.1.4.2
Female
44 years old

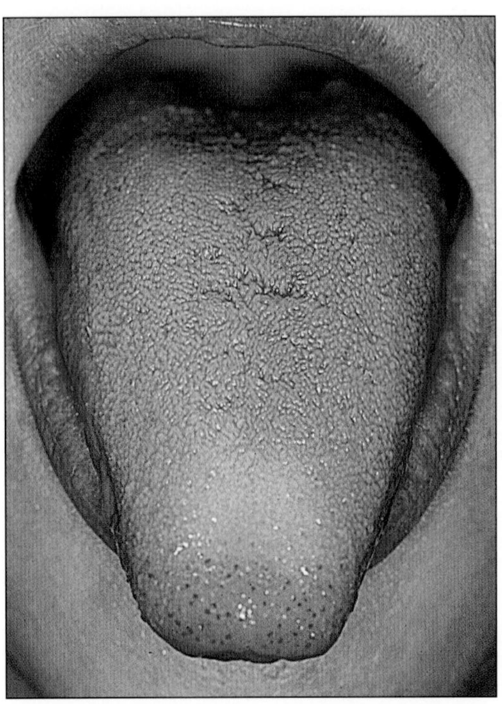

Symptoms

Scratchy throat
Backache
Feeling of tension
Nervousness
Severe stage fright

Western diagnosis

Psoriasis

Background to disease

Divorce
Overwork

Tongue description	Chinese diagnosis
Pale red	Normal
Slight indentations and slightly reddish edges	Developing heat in the Liver
Long, thin, vertical midline crack	Constitutional disharmony of the Heart
Pointed, swollen tip	Heat in the Heart
Pale tip	Onset of blood stasis
Light yellow, slightly greasy coating	Retention of damp-heat

Symptoms

Palpitations
Insomnia
Vertigo
Irritability, bouts of anger
Bitter taste

Western diagnosis

High blood pressure

Background to disease

Dissatisfaction with her living conditions
Excessive consumption of greasy foods

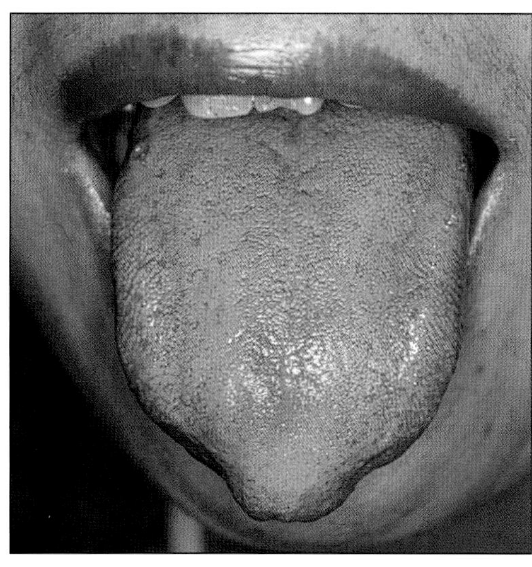

Fig. 6.1.4.3
Female
41 years old

Tongue description	Chinese diagnosis
Reddish, long tongue body	Constitutional heat in the Heart
Pale edges	Liver blood deficiency
Red, very pointed tip with dark red points	Heart fire
White, thin, dry coating with rootless coating at the root	Onset of deficiency of fluids and Stomach yin

Symptoms

No desire to sleep
Restlessness
Increased drive
No appetite
Strong thirst

Western diagnosis

Bipolar disorder

Background to disease

Family history of bipolar disorder

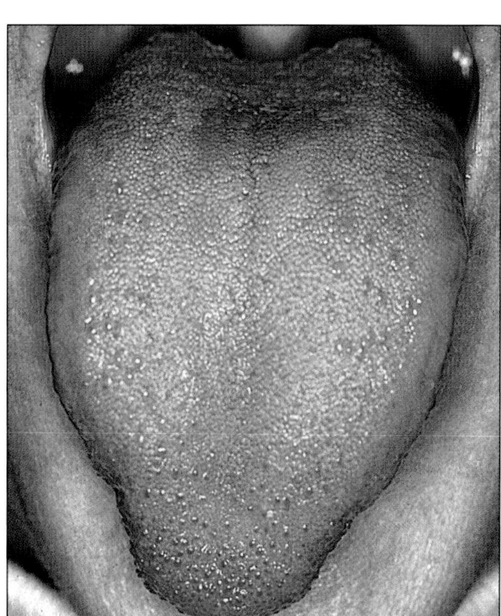

Fig. 6.1.4.4
Female
35 years old

Tongue description	**Chinese diagnosis**
Pale red	Normal
Pale edges	Liver blood deficiency
Many small cracks	Stomach yin deficiency
Red tip with protrusion	Heat in the Heart
Depression at the root of the tongue	Essence deficiency

Fig. 6.1.4.5
Female
52 years old

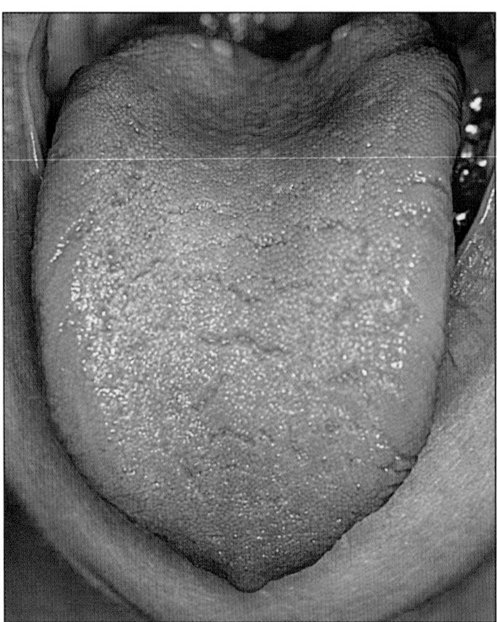

Symptoms

Twitching of facial muscles
Sudden attacks of fright
Insomnia

Western diagnosis

Compulsive neurosis

Background to disease

Condition began after hysterectomy

About these case histories

In the first case, long-standing emotional problems engendered heat in the Heart, which here gave rise to recurrent bladder infections. Here the tongue is very helpful to obtain the right differential diagnosis.

In the second case, depression as the result of long-standing unhappiness produced not only insomnia but also body pains. The relationship to the Heart is presented, which is emphasized by the unusual tongue shape.

CASE HISTORY The separation from her husband was very difficult for the patient. Although the couple did not live together, they still kept in frequent contact. Their meetings were characterized by quarreling and sadness, but they always ended with sexual intercourse. Usually on the morning after, the patient felt a strong burning sensation or pain when urinating. The urine was dark yellow. If she drank copious amounts of fluids, the symptoms would often disappear after 24 hours. She developed a fever, pain in her sides, and a strong thirst that was not alleviated by drinking. For the past 12 months she had taken a course of antibiotics, as pyelonephritis was suspected.

From the age of 18, the patient suffered from severe insomnia. She had difficulty falling asleep and sleeping through the night. She felt that she only slept deeply for a few hours each night. Thus she was constantly tired, which she believed accounted for her increasing irritability and restlessness. Her appetite and digestion were normal. Her pulse was rapid and slightly thin.

Analysis. The present condition of this patient revolves around heat and fire in the Heart that has caused excess in the Heart channel, which has been transferred to the Small Intestine.

Tongue description	**Chinese diagnosis**
Reddish	Internal heat
Short, small tongue body	Possible protracted heat in the Liver[11]
Red points along the edges and at the tip	Heat in the Liver and Heart
Whitish, *dry*, thin coating	Onset of injury to body fluids

Symptoms

Painful urination
Cramp-like sensation in the bladder
Insomnia
Irritability and restlessness
Thirst

Western diagnosis

Recurrent cystitis

Background to disease

Long-standing emotional problems

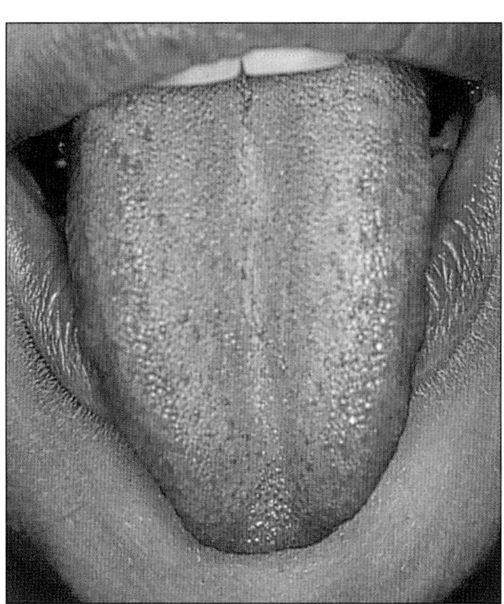

Fig. 6.1.4.6
Female
29 years old

The function of the Small Intestine is to separate the pure from the most impure fluids in order to send them for excretion to the Bladder and Large Intestine. This function of filtering the fluids is disrupted by the heat in this channel, which manifests as a burning sensation during urination. The heat causes the fluids to congeal, resulting in the dark yellow urine. The heat in the Heart channel, reflected in the red tip of the tongue and the red points in this area, is responsible for her strong thirst. The whitish, dry coating is surprising, but its dryness indicates the onset of injury to the fluids as a result of the internal heat. The rapid pulse can be attributed to developing heat.

The patient's long-standing emotional problems have caused Liver qi stagnation that engendered Liver heat, which in turn agitated the spirit. Liver heat and fire is readily transferred to the Heart. This pathological development is shown in the red tongue edges and the spots that cover the entire length of the tongue edges. The red spots are a very important sign because they implicate the underlying disharmony of the Liver as the source of the heat, rather than an invasion by an external pathogenic factor.

Arguments with her partner precede the onset of the bladder disorder. The conflict is harmonized for only a short period of time by the ensuing sexual intercourse. Her anger intensifies the Liver qi stagnation and its transformation into fire. The ensuing sexual desire awakens the ministerial fire which, on the one hand, "opens the womb,"[12] and on the other hand, agitates the spirit. These events intensify the heat in the Heart and indirectly cause her urinary problems.

The findings on the tongue are very helpful in evaluating the origin of the bladder disorder. In clinical practice, bladder disorders are frequently caused by the retention of damp-heat in the Liver and Gallbladder or in the Bladder. In both patterns, the tongue coating, which is often localized on the posterior third, is yellow and thick. The presence of many red spots or raised papillae in this area signifies an acute infection (Figs. 9.2.3 and 9.2.4).

The long-standing sleeping problems, as well as the restlessness of the patient, result from blazing Heart fire that disturbs the sprit. Problems with falling asleep are often caused by Heart

Pathomechanism

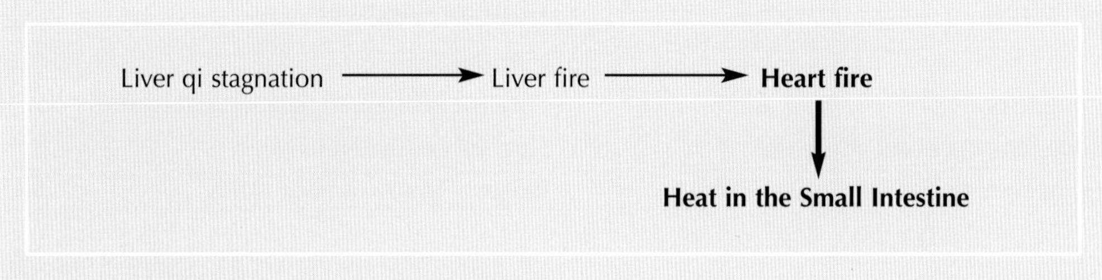

blood deficiency, which fails to provide a satisfactory 'residence' for the spirit. Failure to sleep through the night usually occurs when the yin is too weak to anchor the spirit. There are only a few signs of deficiency here; the thin pulse possibly signals blood deficiency.

The short and relatively small tongue body suggests a constitutional weakness of the blood or yin, which implies a tendency to develop heat. This may have contributed to the patient's poor sleep quality over the years. It cannot be determined whether the internal heat, which is reflected in the red tongue body, has developed because of an underlying constitutional weakness or because of the emotional state of the patient.

Treatment strategy. Clear the Heart, calm the spirit, and regulate the Liver qi.

The first acupuncture treatment consisted of draining HT-7 *(shén mén)*, PC-7 *(dà líng)*, and LU-9 *(tài yuǎn)*. Following this treatment, the patient slept well for a few nights. This point combination is used in cases of restlessness and apprehensiveness when the pulse is strong or full. The use of this combination contributes to calming the spirit and regulating the circulation of qi and blood in the upper burner. These are source points and are suitable for disorders of the yin organs.[13] They correspond to the earth phase and can be used to reduce excess in the fire phase.

After another argument with her ex-husband, her sleeping problems returned, and the patient immediately experienced a cramp-like sensation in her bladder. The formula Guide Out the Red Powder *(dǎo chì sǎn)* was prescribed for three days. The bladder pain disappeared instantly and only returned once in the space of 12 months; it was again successfully treated with the same prescription. During this time, the patient came for occasional acupuncture treatments. She started practicing tai qi, which made her more emotionally stable. She improved enormously, and her sleeping was much better unless she became agitated. Two years later, she was still sleeping well and had not suffered another bladder attack. Later on, after living with her husband again, she became pregnant and gave birth to a child that suffered from Down Syndrome.

CASE HISTORY The patient gave the impression of being very controlled and tense. She was unhappy about her long-standing insomnia, as she could not fall asleep or sleep through the night. It had become worse over the previous five years and her psychiatrist had therefore prescribed neuroleptic drugs at or below the neuroleptic threshhold. With their help, she was able to sleep for about five hours nightly.

The sleeping problems started when she discovered that her husband had been having an affair. When he left her, she shied away from any close contact with people.

Her muscles were very tense, especially in the neck and shoulder region. In addition, she complained of constant body pains, mainly in the extremities and lower back. She had taken painkillers for years. Otherwise she had no complaints. Her digestion was normal. Her dry and lined skin was very noticeable. Large uterine fibroids had caused severe menstrual bleeding. Therefore, seven years ago, she had a hysterectomy. Her pulse was tight and thin.

Tongue description	**Chinese diagnosis**
Pale, slightly dull	Blood deficiency and onset of blood stasis
Long	Constitutional disharmony of the Heart
Pointed tip with a long, thin crack	Heart yin deficiency
Small cracks in the center	Injury to fluids
Whitish, greasy, thin coating	Retention of dampness

Symptoms

Disturbed sleep
Body pains
Tight muscles in the neck and shoulder region
Inner tension
Mood swings

Western diagnosis

Insomnia
Depression

Background to disease

Unwanted divorce after 20 years of marriage
Excessive brooding

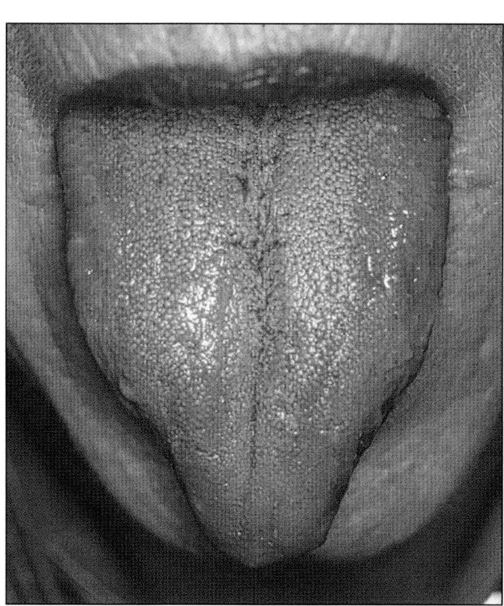

Fig. 6.1.4.7
Female
54 years old

Analysis. The tongue body is firm, and its anterior third appears to be disconnected from the rest of the tongue body, suggesting a disharmony of the Heart. In addition, the tongue is long, an indication of a constitutional imbalance of the Heart.

Depending on one's constitution and disposition, long-standing emotional problems can dramatically affect the Liver and Heart. Both yin organs are sensitive to mental and emotional suffering. A long and red or reddish tongue body reflects a predisposition toward an agitated spirit.

A study of the tongue of this patient reveals the injury to her Heart yin and blood. The yin and blood give the tongue body its normal volume. The anterior third of the tongue is extremely contracted, which suggests an inadequate supply of yin and blood to the Heart. The thin crack in the anterior third underlines the development of yin deficiency.

The formation of this extraordinary tongue shape suggests the following disease process: The patient's traumas caused the development of heat in the Heart, which in turn injured the yin and blood. As a rule, heat in the Heart will be reflected in a red tip on the tongue, which is not present in this case. This fact reinforces the underlying pattern of deficiency. It is possible, however, that the intake of neuroleptic drugs is partly suppressing the heat in the Heart, especially because the patient cannot sleep without them. The shape of the tongue tip signals a long-standing and serious disturbance of the spirit. The deep emotional injury 'broke the heart' of the patient, which, in turn, weakened her Heart yin and blood. This is partly responsible for her inability or lack of desire to allow intimacy back into her life. In addition, the dryness of her facial skin, resulting in so many lines, is another sign of insufficient moistening and nourishment by the blood. The vitality of the Heart manifests in the complexion; in this case, her skin is further confirmation of blood and yin deficiency.

Emotionally, the patient was 'blocked.' She gave the impression of being armor-plated. Physically, she also appeared to be stiff, as her musculature was very hard. When asked why she

Pathomechanism

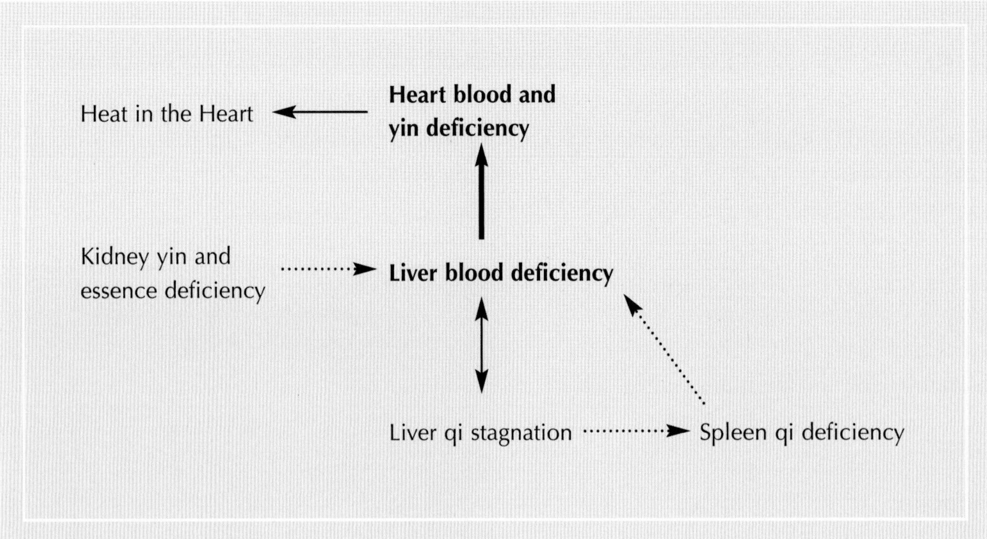

protected herself so much, she burst into tears and wept uncontrollably. Her response indicated that her spirit had lost its ability to react appropriately. The question had activated her memory, and, because the memory is governed by the Heart, it brought her deep desperation and sadness to the surface. The patient revealed that she had not cried for years, and that she had only now realized that she had not got over the breakup with her husband. These unresolved emotions contributed to the development of Liver qi stagnation. Chapter 8 of the *Divine Pivot* observes: "If sadness affects the Liver and injures the ethereal soul, the yin retracts, the muscles become tense, and the ribs do not expand anymore."[14] This would suggest an emotional origin to the patient's pain. Usually, body pains are a sign of obstruction, but this was not so in this case. The pains were not caused by externally-contracted pathogenic factors.

The pale, dull color of the tongue indicates blood deficiency as well as slight stagnation in the flow of blood. As is often the case with Liver blood deficiency, the sinews and tendons were not sufficiently nourished or moistened, and were therefore tense. The blood deficiency, reflected in the thin pulse, aggravated the constraint of Liver qi. Thus the constrained circulation of Liver qi, insufficient nourishment from the blood, and onset of blood stagnation combined to impair the flow of qi and blood; each of these factors is responsible in part for the pain and the hard and tense musculature. The patient's tight pulse, common with painful disorders, confirms this diagnosis.

There are a few possible explanations for the blood deficiency:

- *Excessive menstrual bleeding*. Seven years before, the patient underwent a hysterectomy because of severe bleeding caused by uterine fibroids. The menstrual bleeding lasted for several months and exhausted her. Her essence and blood were seriously weakened. However, the current blood deficiency cannot be linked to the blood loss from that time because the patient is no longer menstruating and is eating well.
- *Liver acting on the Spleen*. Although the symptoms do not indicate the participation of the Spleen in the disease process, a malfunction of this organ must be considered because of its essential role in the production of blood. If the Spleen does not provide enough extracted essence from food, a pattern of blood deficiency may ensue. This implies that the Liver has 'overacted' on the Spleen, impairing the production of blood.
- *Deficiency of Kidney yin and essence*. A pattern of blood deficiency can also arise from deficiency of Kidney yin and essence. Here, however, the tongue and pulse do not confirm this pattern. Yet because of her age and history, this possibility must be considered. It is reflected in the treatment strategy.

The tongue coating is whitish and greasy and mainly covers the center of the tongue, indicating an accumulation of dampness in the middle burner. This, however, is not causing any problems. The small, thin cracks that appear in the center of the tongue are disregarded in this diagnosis, as there are no symptoms reflecting Stomach disharmony. It is possible that taking painkillers for so long has injured the Stomach fluids, and may have led to the formation of the cracks. Years ago, when the patient started taking the painkillers, she initially suffered from heartburn; however, this does not trouble her anymore.

Treatment strategy. Enrich the Heart blood and yin, regulate the Liver qi, improve the circulation of qi and blood in the channels, and nourish the Kidney yin and essence.

Acupuncture was chosen in the treatment of this patient. Here are three point combinations that were used:

HT-5 *(tōng lǐ)*, LR-8 *(qū quán)*, KI-3 *(tài xī)*, BL-23 *(shèn shū)*, and N-HN-54 *(ān mián)*

PC-6 *(nèi guān)*, LR-3 *(tài chōng)*, GB-41 *(zú lín qì)*, and N-HN-54 *(ān mián)*

HT-6 *(yīn xī)*, KI-6 *(zhào hǎi)* SP-6 *(sān yīn jiāo)*, BL-11 *(dà zhù)*, and N-HN-54 *(ān mián)*

In addition, spontaneously painful points were regularly treated. Following these treatments, the patient felt much more relaxed, but the pain had not improved. After five acupuncture treatments, the patient chose not to continue. Instead, she decided on a course of osteopathy, which she discontinued after seven sessions. Her condition had not improved.

6.2 Tongue Signs of Excess Associated with the Heart

1. *Blazing Heart fire.* This pattern often arises as a result of Liver fire affecting the Heart. A frequent cause of this pathology is the stagnation of Liver qi that transforms into fire. Serious emotional injury plays an important role in the development of this pattern, but overconsumption of fatty, fried foods as well as abuse of caffeine and alcohol can also contribute to its development. Abuse of hallucinogenic drugs may also initiate a pattern of Heart fire. The patient with Heart fire may experience distinct feelings of heat and thirst, restlessness, and impulsiveness. The patient may also display mouth and tongue ulcers as well as blood in the urine.

   Tongue signs

   - marked red tip, red tongue body with yellow coating (Fig. 6.2.7)
   - long, red tongue body, tip reddened (Fig. 6.2.3)

2. *Phlegm misting the Heart.* Phlegm often originates in the Spleen, and phlegm misting the Heart frequently arises from underlying Spleen qi deficiency. When phlegm and fire merge and 'block the pores of the Heart,' the functioning of the Heart and spirit will be severely impaired. Consequently, the spirit cannot return to its residence, and hallucinations as well as manic, confused, or even comatose states may result

   Tongue signs: no special tongue signs, but possible thick, greasy coating

3. *Phlegm-fire agitating the Heart.* The fluids are easily injured by the intensity of the Heart fire and consequently thicken and form phlegm. The intensity of the symptoms depends on whether phlegm or fire dominates the pattern. If phlegm is the dominant element in the disease process, the confusion and lack of clear thinking will be more noticeable; inner restlessness will be more pronounced where Heart fire is the dominant pathology.

Tongue signs

- red, swollen tongue body, with dry, thick greasy, yellow coating (Fig. 6.2.6)
- red, swollen tongue body, with dry, thick greasy, yellow coating covering the entire tongue body
- red tongue with deep midline crack and dry, sticky, yellow coating (Fig. 4.1.5.3)
- red, long tongue body, with greasy, yellow coating (Fig. 6.3.3)

Tongue description	**Chinese diagnosis**
Red, very narrow, contracted	Severe exhaustion of Kidney yin and essence
Long, firm tongue body	Lack of body fluids
Slightly deviated	Onset of internal wind
Red tip	Heat in the Heart
Midline crack over the entire tongue body	Constitutional weakness of the Heart
Old, yellow coating	Injury to body fluids due to heat from excess

Fig. 6.2.1
Female
38 years old

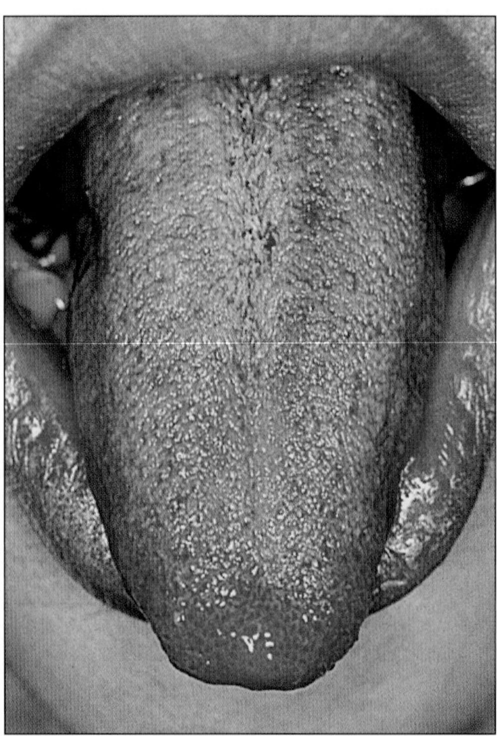

Symptoms

Atrophy and pain of facial muscles
Complete loss of all body and head hair
Facial eczema
Exhaustion
Insomnia
Unwanted weight loss

Western diagnosis

Atypical, progressive collagen-vascular disease

Background to disease

Weak constitution
Nocturnal work for many years
Chronic lack of sleep
Irregular eating habits
Tea and coffee abuse
Overwork
Excessive use of willpower

Tongue description	**Chinese diagnosis**
Reddish, slightly swollen	Slight Spleen qi deficiency (accumulation of dampness)
Long, vertical crack in the center with yellow, thin, greasy coating	Constitutional heat in the Heart with phlegm-fire in the Stomach
Red tip	Heat in the Heart
White, greasy coating	Accumulation of dampness

Symptoms

Panic attacks with fainting spells
Palpitations
Severe feelings of fear
Diarrhea with emotional pressure

Western diagnosis

None

Background to disease

Long unhappy marriage
Overwork
Excessive consumption of chocolate

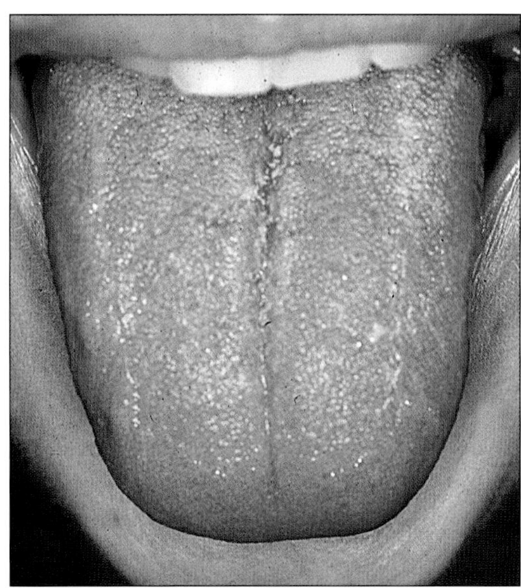

Fig. 6.2.2
Female
35 years old

Tongue description	**Chinese diagnosis**
Slightly pale	Spleen qi deficiency
Long tongue body	Constitutional disharmony of the Heart
Pointed with red tip	Heat in the Heart
Whitish, greasy coating	Accumulation of dampness

Symptoms

Pain and sensation of distention on the left side of the face
Unclear speech due to the pain
Insomnia
Restlessness, tension
Panic feelings
Mentally unclear

Western diagnosis

None

Background to disease

Tooth extraction 10 months prior

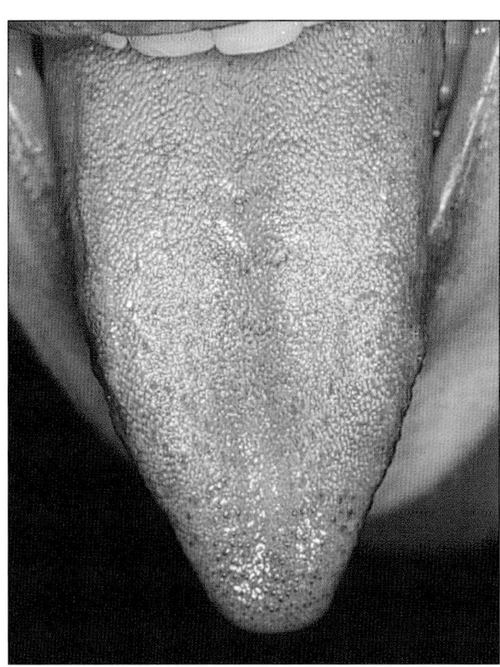

Fig. 6.2.3
Female
29 years old

Tongue description	Chinese diagnosis
Reddish and cracked	Onset of Kidney yin deficiency
Long tongue body	Constitutional disharmony of the Heart
Red and pointed tip	Heat in the Heart with underlying Heart yin deficiency
Slightly indented and red edges	Liver qi stagnation with developing heat
Light yellow, thin, and dry coating	Slight injury to the fluids

Fig. 6.2.4
Male
32 years old

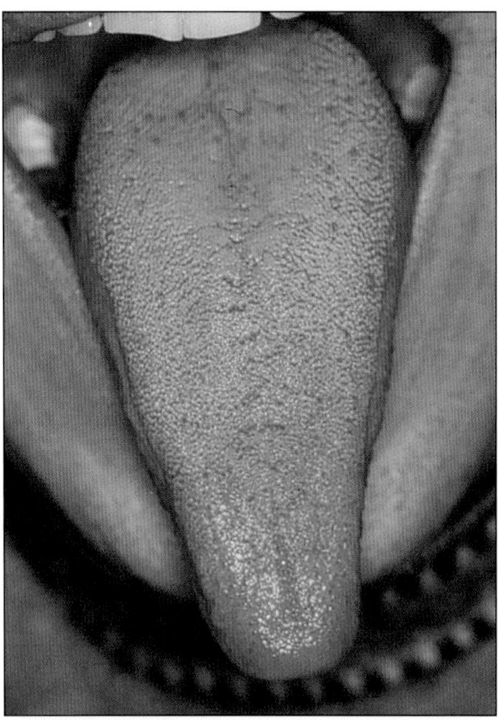

Symptoms

Restlessness
Apprehensiveness, depressive states, irritability
Nightmares
Occasional night sweats

Western diagnosis

None

Background to disease

Long-standing emotional problems

Tongue description	Chinese diagnosis
Red with red sides	Kidney yin deficiency with ascendant Liver yang
Long	Constitutional heat in the Heart
Red, very pointed tip	Heart fire
White, dry coating	Lack of fluids in the Stomach

Fig. 6.2.5
Female
70 years old

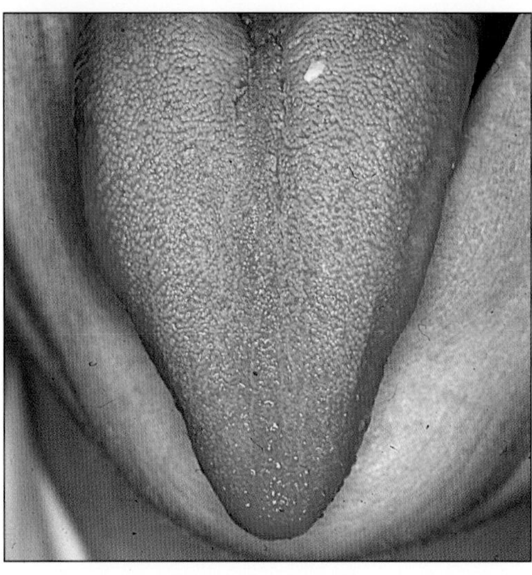

Symptoms

Inability to open her eyes
Severe frontal headaches
Irritability
Depression
Inability to sleep through the night

Western diagnosis

Compulsive neurosis

Background to disease

Shell-shocked as a teenager in World War II

Tongue description

Reddish

Swollen

Deep crack reaching from the anterior third to the tip

Brownish yellow, old, peeled coating

Chinese diagnosis

Developing heat

Retention of phlegm

Possible underlying Heart yin deficiency

Phlegm-heat in the Stomach and Heart with injury to the fluids

Symptoms

Hallucinations, delusions
Restlessness
Irritability
Panic attacks
Disturbed sleep
Dryness of the mouth

Western diagnosis

Schizophrenia

Background to disease

Abuse of 'ecstasy' drug, the stress of examinations

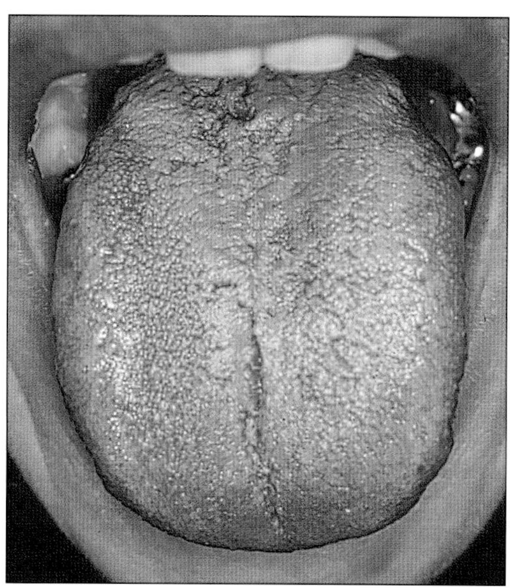

Fig. 6.2.6
Female
29 years old

Tongue description

Pale red

Narrow, firm tongue body

Very red tip

White coating at the sides, with a yellow, thick coating in the middle

Chinese diagnosis

Normal

Injury to the fluids

Heart fire

Phlegm-heat in the Stomach

Symptoms

Teleangiectasia
Fear of going outside, fearfulness
Irritability, mood swings
Bouts of voracious hunger
Thirst

Western diagnosis

Agoraphobia

Background to disease

Unwanted abortion three months prior

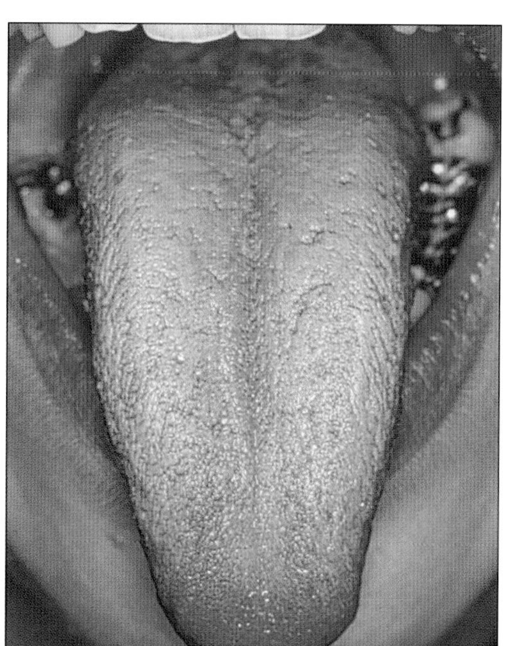

Fig. 6.2.7
Female
27 years old

About this case history

The thick coating covering almost all of the tongue body is a typical sign when phlegm-heat is harrassing the Heart. It usually causes serious mental problems, as with the following patient who suffered from agoraphobia.

CASE HISTORY The patient's long-standing relationship broke up under the strain of an unwanted abortion. She wanted the child, but her partner did not. She agreed, reluctantly, to have the abortion. Physically, she recovered quickly, but emotionally, she felt completely changed, suffering from strong mood swings and irritability. She developed a fear of places and gatherings of people. She also stopped contacting people, preferring to stay in her flat. She attributed this behavior to what she saw as a strong reddening of the right half of her face after the abortion. She believed that everybody was staring at her. The redness of her face, however, was not apparent to anybody else; a few superficial capillaries were noticeable next to the right nostril and cheek.[15] The patient felt constantly hungry, with voracious bouts of appetite, and ate mainly fast foods and sweets. She was very thirsty. Her menstruation was regular and problem free. Her pulse was slippery and rapid.

Analysis. This is a pattern of excess in which an accumulation of phlegm and fire has affected the Stomach and Heart, as evidenced in both the yellow, greasy, thick coating of the tongue and the rapid and slippery pulse. The very red tip of the tongue signals the presence of Heart fire. Phlegm and fire disturb the Heart and agitate the spirit, resulting in the patient's depression and her disturbed perception of reality. She is so agitated that she believes that the right half of her face is significantly red and that everybody is staring at her. Therefore, she only feels secure behind closed doors and no longer participates in life.

Incessant hunger, voracious bouts of appetite, and a strong thirst are indications of Stomach fire; it is also responsible for her uncontrollable eating habits. The fatty nature of fast foods and the overconsumption of sweets have combined to form phlegm-fire in the Stomach, again, as evidenced in the greasy, thick tongue coating. The coating grows more and more yellow toward the center of the tongue, which signals the development of heat in the Stomach. Phlegm-fire can harass the spirit, which contributes here to the severe mental dysfunction of the patient,

Pathomechanism

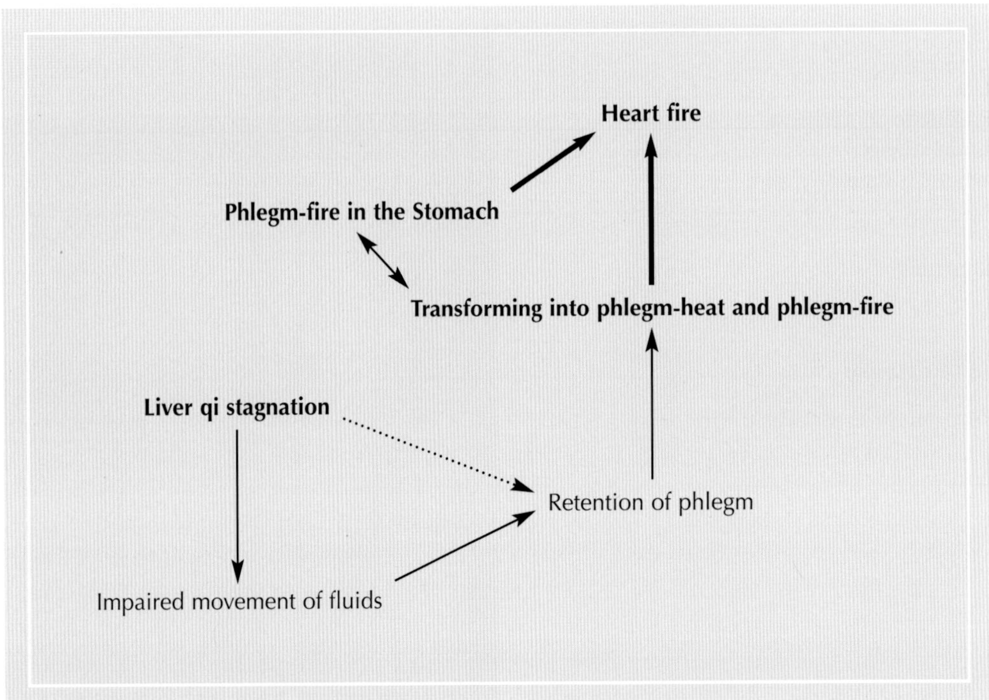

resulting in agoraphobia. The presence of a yellow, greasy, and thick coating in the center of the tongue, and the red tip, are important indicators of this pathomechanism.

The patient dated the onset of her symptoms to her abortion. The period prior to the abortion was characterized by severe quarrels and separation from her partner. These events caused the constraint of Liver qi and increased her irritability. In addition, Liver qi stagnation contributed to the impeded movement of body fluids. As a result, the fluids collected and transformed into phlegm-fire in the Stomach, which was aggravated by the consumption of fried and sweet foods.

The narrow, firm tongue body denotes long-standing heat with resulting injury to the fluids. The fluids are part of the yin and give the tongue body its soft, elastic texture. Phlegm-fire and the subsequent injury to the fluids and yin, as well as the Liver qi stagnation, are the basis of the patient's mental problems. It cannot be determined whether it was the operation itself or the ensuing emotional state of the patient that set off the disturbance in the Heart. Surgery of the uterus can cause a pattern of blood stasis in the Penetrating vessel, impairing the circulation of Heart qi and blood. However, this does not seem to be the case here, as the patient's menstruation did not change after the abortion. What is known is that, following the abortion, she was very angry. Anger and feelings of guilt weighed heavily on her. These strong emotions may have caused the development of Heart fire and possibly Liver fire. Both can result in irritability and inner agitation.

Treatment strategy. Clear the Heart fire, drain the Stomach fire, transform the phlegm, and calm the spirit.

A draining technique was applied at PC-8 *(láo gōng)*, PC-5 *(jiān shǐ)*, and ST-40 *(fēng lóng)* to transform the phlegm and calm the spirit. Other points that were often used include ST-44 *(nèi tíng)* and HT-3 *(shào hǎi)* to eliminate heat from the Stomach and to calm the spirit; LR-2 *(xíng jiān)* to clear the Liver fire; and GV-24 *(shén tíng)* to calm the spirit. After five acupuncture sessions, the patient improved. She felt more relaxed and thought that her face looked normal again. The agoraphobia improved, and then disappeared entirely after the patient underwent behavioral therapy.

6.3 Tongue Signs Associated with Constitutional Disharmony of the Heart

Long Tongues

A long, pale red or pale tongue that is big but within the normal range points to a strong constitution. As a rule, long tongues tend to be narrow or thin. If the tongue is very pointed toward the tip and of a reddish color, it may indicate a constitutional weakness of the Heart.

Tongue signs

- long, reddish or red tongue body or reddish areas on the tongue body surface: presence of internal heat. Heat in the body not only dries the body fluids, it also vigorously moves the qi and blood. This movement of qi and blood causes the tongue to be extended such that it protrudes further from the mouth than normal. The opposite mechanism obtains for short and pale tongues. Cold slows down the flow of qi and blood and its contracting effect manifests in a short, often contracted, tongue body.

  A long, reddish tongue often appears with a firm tongue body. Long-standing heat depletes fluids and yin, which in general causes hardness, firmness, and dryness of the tongue body. On the other hand, an accumulation of yin (dampness) is responsible for a swollen and soft tongue body.

- long tongue with a very red tip or red points on the tip: heat in the Heart. The degree of narrowness of the tongue body reflects the extent of injury to the body fluids and yin.
- long, reddish, and especially a firm tongue: tendency to yin deficiency. Further, since yin deficiency often gives rise to heat from deficiency, which readily affects the Heart, a long tongue may specifically point to an imbalance in the fire phase.

Tongue description	**Chinese diagnosis**
Reddish, *very long*	Constitutional heat in the Heart
Slightly red edges	Heat in the Liver
Yellow, greasy coating in middle and posterior thirds	Retention of damp-heat in the middle and lower burners

Fig. 6.3.1
Female
22 years old

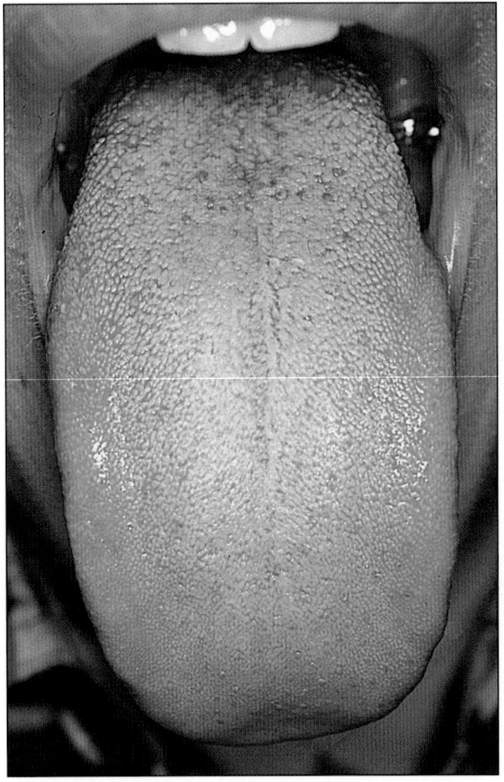

Symptoms

Raised, bleeding skin lesions
Strong itchiness
Soft stools
Inability to fall asleep

Western diagnosis

Lichen simplex (an eczematous dermatitis)

Background to disease

Caffeine abuse
Frustration

Tongue description	Chinese diagnosis
Slightly pale	Slight Spleen qi deficiency (blood deficiency)
Long	Constitutional weakness of the Heart
Vertical crack in the center with rootless coating	Stomach yin deficiency, onset of Kidney yin deficiency

Symptoms

Inability to relax
Inner tension
Headaches with tight neck muscles
Pain and weakness of the lumbar area
Occasional numbness and tingling of the right arm
Insomnia
Fatigue

Western diagnosis

Neck pain
Primary infertility

Background to disease

Overwork
Perfectionist attitude

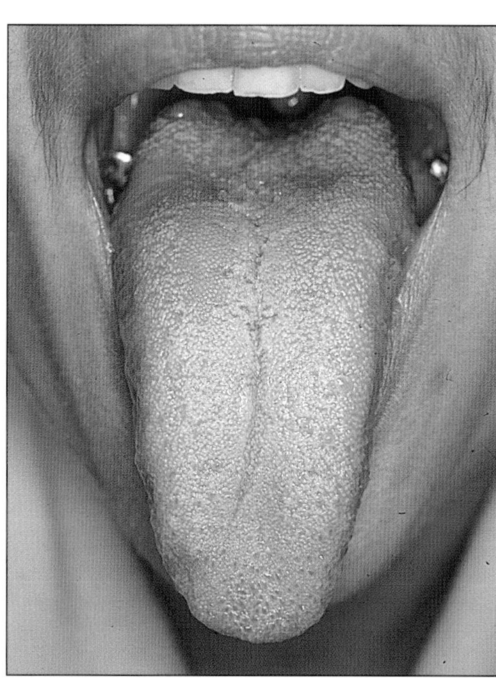

Fig. 6.3.2
Female
32 years old

Tongue description	Chinese diagnosis
Reddish, long, narrow	Heat with injury to the fluids, constitutional heat in the Heart
Slightly yellow, thick, greasy coating	Accumulation of damp-phlegm in the Stomach

Symptoms

Stomach pain with stress
Epigastric fullness
Lack of appetite
Depression
Fatigue

Western diagnosis

Polyps in the stomach

Background to disease

Overwork
Emotional problems due to death of mother and divorce in the same year

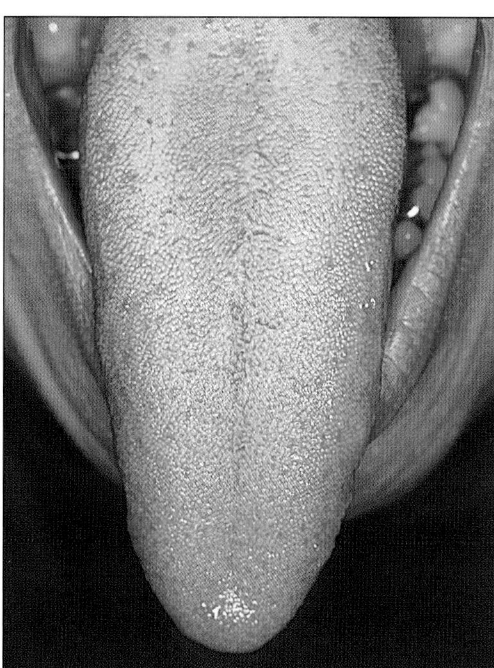

Fig. 6.3.3
Female
42 years old

6.4 Tongues with a Long, Vertical Crack in the Midline

A crack in the midline of the tongue is often seen as an indication of Stomach yin deficiency. The crack appears in the middle third of the tongue and is very often deep and wide. Constitutional weakness of the Heart can also present with a deep midline crack. This crack, however, is much longer than the former. It starts in the posterior third and runs to the tip or just short of the tip. If the tongue body color is pale red or normal, and if the crack is thin, there may be no pathology. The crack may simply indicate that there is possible constitutional weakness of the Heart. If, however, the tongue body is very red and the midline crack is very deep, Heart fire is probably present. In this case there will also be restlessness, irritability, palpitations, and mouth ulcers. If the crack is covered by a yellow, greasy coating, phlegm-fire is agitating the Heart. In this case the patient will exhibit restless agitation, a bad temper, and manic behavior. Finally, a red tongue body with a rootless or peeled coating in conjunction with a long, vertical midline crack indicates deficiency of Heart and Kidney yin.

A constitutional weakness of the Heart does not mean an organic weakness of the Heart. In those with this tongue type there is a tendency toward certain types of mental or emotional discomfort: frequent attacks of melancholy and crying spells, emotional instability, fearfulness since childhood, depression. However, with an appropriate lifestyle, there may be no symptoms at all. Great care must be taken, therefore, when assessing the significance of this crack.

Tongue description	Chinese diagnosis
Reddish, slightly swollen	Spleen qi deficiency (accumulation of dampness)
Long, vertical crack in the center with slightly yellow, thin, greasy coating	Constitutional heat in the Heart with phlegm-heat in the Stomach

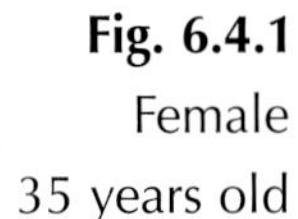

Fig. 6.4.1
Female
35 years old

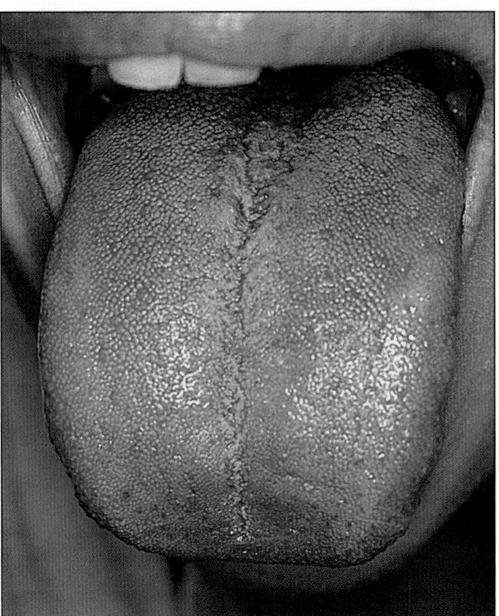

Symptoms

Sudden vertigo
Trembling of the entire body
Numb areas in the extremities
Severe feelings of fear
Tendency to catch colds

Western diagnosis

Chronic fatigue syndrome

Background to disease

Physical and mental demands of competitive sports

Tongue description	Chinese diagnosis
Reddish	Normal
Red edges	Heat in the Liver
Long, vertical crack in the center with a red tip	Heat in the Heart
Yellow, thin, greasy coating	Accumulation of damp-heat

Symptoms

Inability to stay asleep
Hot feet at night
Occasional night sweats
Headaches
Tightness of the neck muscles
Blocked sinuses

Western diagnosis

Uterine fibroids
Allergic rhinitis

Background to disease

Long-standing emotional problems

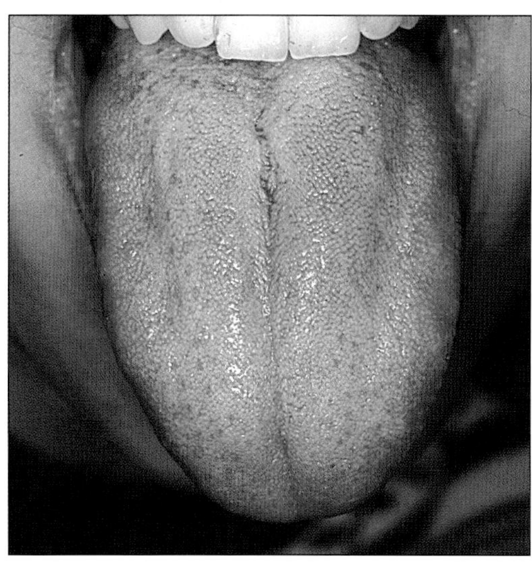

Fig. 6.4.2
Female
38 years old

Tongue description	Chinese diagnosis
Slightly pale and thin	Spleen qi deficiency → blood deficiency
Slight teeth marks	Spleen qi deficiency
Curled edges	Liver qi stagnation
Long, vertical midline crack	Constitutional disharmony of the Heart
Indentation and reddening of the tip	Heart blood deficiency
Red points on the anterior third	Penetration of acute, externally-contracted wind-heat
Whitish, dry, slightly greasy coating	Slight injury to the fluids in the Lung
Light yellow coating in the center	Heat in the Stomach and Large Intestine

Symptoms

Irritability
Mental and physical exhaustion
Restless sleep
Feeling of tightness in the chest
Mood swings
Lack of appetite, constipation
Itching of the eyes and palate
Sneezing fits

Western diagnosis

Allergic rhinitis, depression

Background to disease

Difficult separation from husband
Excessive brooding

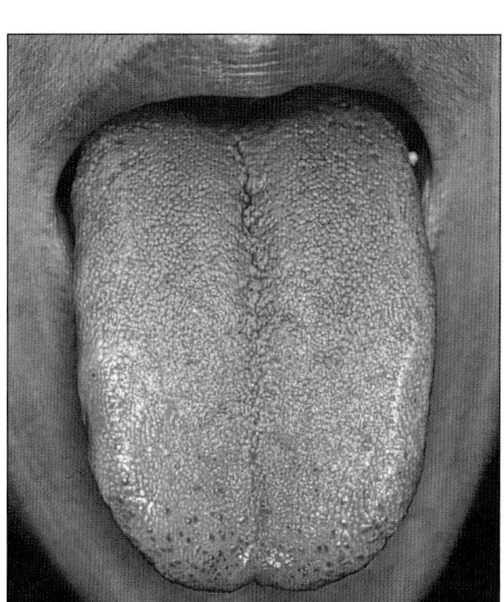

Fig. 6.4.3
Female
44 years old

About this case history

In someone with a constitutional disharmony of the Heart, a difficult or unwanted separation can trigger a range of pathomechanisms that affect the spirit.

CASE HISTORY Quarrels and arguments, followed by separation from her husband, had produced a state of utter mental and physical exhaustion in the patient. She suffered severe mood swings, which ranged from irritability to a lack of interest in life, and frequently felt a tightness or constriction of the chest when she became depressed. She never slept deeply, and consequently never felt refreshed.

The patient was frightened that she would be too weak to go to work or look after her child. After the separation, her son developed alopecia aerata, an inflammatory, patchy loss of hair, which made her feel guilty. She worried about her lack of appetite and the ensuing weight loss. She had a bowel movement every other day, but never felt relieved. The stools were hard and pellet-like. Her urination was normal. Her menstruation was regular, but she bled for only a short time. She also suffered from seasonal hay fever that made her eyes itchy and red, and included sneezing fits and a constant itching of her palate. The symptoms were relieved with antihistamines. Her pulse was floating and frail.

Analysis. The tongue presents with signs that are indicative of both a constitutional disharmony of the Heart the long crack as well as an acquired disharmony of the Heart the indentation at the tip of the tongue. The indentation suggests long-standing Heart blood deficiency, probably as a result of Spleen qi deficiency that led to blood deficiency. The latter is evident in the slightly pale, thin tongue body and the teeth marks. The combination of a constitutional disharmony as well as an acquired disharmony of the Heart has led to the unstable psychological and emotional condition of the patient. The emotional symptoms—a fearful, and often overcritical, attitude toward life—essentially originate from a condition of deficiency, but are complicated by the constraint of Liver qi. The curled edges of the tongue reflect a pattern of Liver qi stagnation that is responsible for the patient's mood swings and irritability.

The acute situation of the patient is characterized by exhaustion, worry, anxiety, and mood swings, all of which worsened after the separation from her husband. Her unsuccessful marriage created feelings of disappointment and frustration. The resulting constraint in the flow of Liver qi affected how she communicated with her husband. He could not live up to her expectations; she constantly criticized him and was unable to see her own part in the breakdown.

Pathomechanism

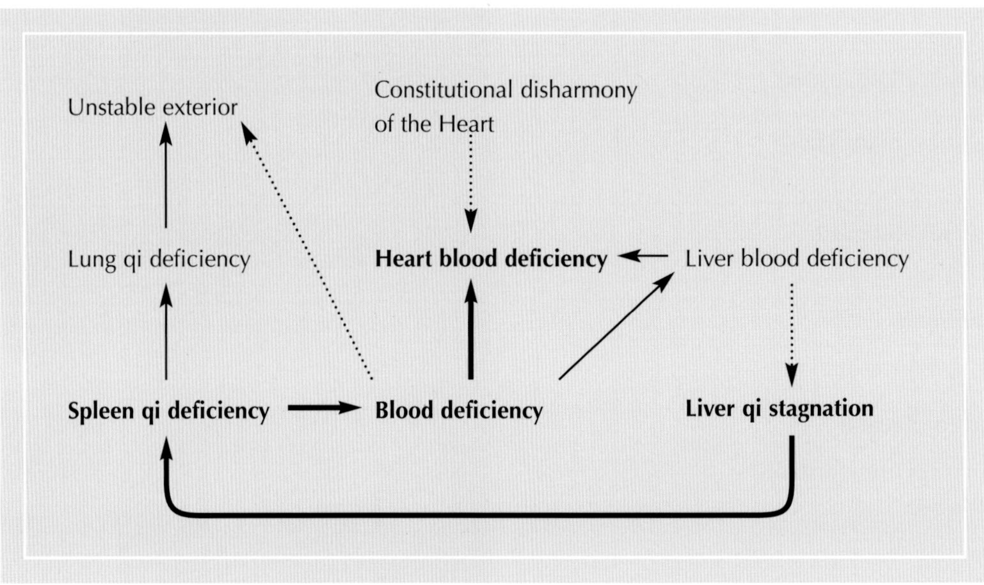

The Liver qi stagnation is also responsible for blocking the movement of qi in the Intestines, which is seen in the hard, pellet-like stools and a feeling of incomplete evacuation of the bowels. Damp-heat in the Intestines, reflected on the tongue by the light yellow, dirty coating on the posterior third, has formed because of the prolonged time that the stool lingers in the Intestines. The stagnation of Liver qi has probably also contributed to the development of Spleen qi deficiency, resulting in physical tiredness and a lack of appetite. The Spleen's function of providing essence, necessary for the production of blood, is impaired. This process is reflected in the thin tongue body, where its slight volume is a sign of blood deficiency.

Both the Liver and Heart depend on an adequate supply of blood. The pattern of Liver and Heart blood deficiency is responsible for the spirit losing its moorings, which is evident in the poor mental state of the patient. At night, the blood returns to the Liver in order to anchor and nourish the ethereal soul. In cases of blood deficiency, the anchoring process cannot occur, resulting in vivid dreams, sleeping problems, or feeling unrefreshed after a night's sleep.

As previously noted, Heart blood deficiency is reflected in the indentation at the tip of the tongue. The patient's unyielding attitude and opinions, and her resistance to accepting or even considering a different style of life, may be an expression of the impaired function of the ethereal soul leading to disharmony of the spirit. Together, their purpose is to examine and regulate one's thoughts and perceptions, tasks that can only be accomplished when they are properly nourished with blood.

The patient constantly worries about her son, work, or weight. Excessive worry knots the qi of the Spleen and Lungs and impairs its circulation. This results in the obstructed flow of qi in the upper burner and causes tightness in the chest when the depressive moods occur.

The red spots on the anterior third of the tongue are a sign of an attack by external pathogenic factors. The itchy eyes and palate result from the invasion of wind-heat. Slight injury to the fluids as a result of the external heat has caused the dry coating. The floating, frail pulse denotes the presence of externally-contracted pathogenic factors with an underlying pattern of qi and blood deficiency.

Treatment strategy. Strengthen the Spleen qi, nourish the blood, regulate the Liver qi, calm the spirit, and release and stabilize the exterior.

The patient responded well to acupuncture. She felt more relaxed and calmer after the following points were needled:

PC-5 *(jiān shǐ)* for depression, when worry and apprehension are in the foreground
LR-3 *(tài chōng)* to nourish the Liver blood and spread the Liver qi
LU-7 *(liè quē)* to regulate the Lung qi and help expel external wind
ST-36 *(zú sān lǐ)* to tonify the qi and blood

After five acupuncture treatments the patient felt much more stable. She reestablished communication with her husband. She is continuing with treatment.

Endnotes

1 Anonymous. *Su wen* [Basic Questions], edited by He W-B et al. Beijing: China Medicine Science and Technology Press, 1996: 8:49.

2 Ibid., 23:147.

3 Anonymous. *Huang di nei jing ling shu yi shi* [Translation and Explanation of the Yellow Emperor's Inner Classic: Divine Pivot], edited by Nanjing College of Traditional Chinese Medicine, Traditional Chinese Medicine Department. Shanghai: Shanghai Science and Technology Press, 1997: 63:373.

4 *Basic Questions*, 5:28

5 Ibid., 23:147.

6 Clavey S. *Fluid Physiology and Pathology in Traditional Chinese Medicine.* Edinburgh: Churchill Livingstone, 1995: 172.

7 Maciocia G. *Tongue Diagnosis in Chinese Medicine,* rev. ed. Seattle: Eastland Press, 1995:70.

8 See Li N-M. *Zhong guo she zhen da quan.*Beijing: Xueyuan Publishing Company, 1994:1197. Investigators in a study undertaken in a TCM hospital in Henan, China felt that red points at the tip of the tongue suggest that the patient has contracted a cold. On the first two days of the cold, the points have a special appearance: they are fresh red, stand together very narrowly, partly 'sprout' in a bunch-like fashion, and do not occupy more than the first third of the anterior part of the tongue. On the third and fourth days of the cold the points slowly became flatter, no longer form a bunch, and the color is not as intense. The area covered by the points becomes bigger, that is, they take up the entire anterior third of the tongue, but not the center. After one week, the points are no longer visible.

9 Ibid.

10 Ibid.

11 Maciocia G. *Tongue Diagnosis in Chinese Medicine.* Seattle: Eastland Press, 1987: 75.

12 Fu Q-Z. *Fu Qing-Zhu's Gynecology,* translated by Yang S-Z and Liu D-W. Boulder, CO: Blue Poppy Press, 1992: 28.

13 *Divine Pivot,* 1:12. The point HT-7 (*shén mén*) is used here but is not mentioned in that text.

14 *Basic Questions,* 44:249.

15 The patient was in no way disfigured. The suggested diagnosis of rosacea could not be confirmed.

C H A P T E R 7

Tongue Signs Associated with Liver Disharmonies

7.1 Tongue Signs Associated with Excess

7.1.1 Restraint of Liver Qi

The Liver ensures the free and smooth flow of qi throughout the body. It also ensures that the qi in the organs moves in the proper direction, thereby preventing the rebellion of qi. Thus, impairment to the frcc flow of qi can involve all the organs and regions of the body.

In many people the pressures of daily life constrain the flow of Liver qi. Frustration, anger, and repressed emotions may all lead to stagnation of qi, which can manifest in such symptoms as hypochondriac pain, a feeling of something caught in the throat, or mood swings. Long-term constrained Liver qi readily leads to Liver heat. In the tongue, this process is reflected in red edges and curled-up sides. The heat represents an intermediate stage between Liver fire and ascending Liver yang.

Liver qi can bind the qi of the middle burner, causing fullness and/or pressure in the chest and abdomen. Inner heat develops when the qi does not flow freely and the constrained qi is not moved. This inhibits the circulation of qi to the extremities, causing cold fingers and toes. In this situation, the remainder of the body is warm and the patient does not experience an aversion to cold.

The intensity of Liver qi constraint varies depending on the particular situation; the associated symptoms are likewise in constant flux. Sometimes patients complain of feeling bloated, wound up, or of having hard, dry, pellet-like stools. On other days they may suffer from soft stools and depressive moods. Quite often the specific tongue signs allow one to evaluate the degree of Liver qi constraint.

Tongue signs

- pale-red tongue body and curled up edges: Liver qi constraint (Fig. 7.1.1.1)

  The presence of Liver qi stagnation can be assumed when the edges of the tongue are curled up; this upward arch is believed to be the result of increased tension on the edges of the tongue. The pathology is probably not very pronounced, which is to say, the disharmony has not affected the fluids or blood when the tongue body color has a pale or pale-red color.

- pale-red tongue body and curled up, red edges: Liver qi constraint with Liver heat

  Over a period of time, if the Liver qi constraint transforms into heat, several outcomes are possible. The heat may harass the Heart and disturb the spirit. This pathomechanism is often reflected on the tongue by curled-up edges and a red tip (Fig. 7.1.1.6). Alternatively, damp-heat is readily engendered by impaired circulation of fluids and a weakened Spleen. The combination of a yellow tongue coating and curled-up edges (Fig. 7.1.1.1) helps identify the pathomechanism and thereby formulate a proper treatment strategy.

- edges of the tongue are markedly curled up, indented, or swollen: long-standing and deep Liver qi constraint (Fig. 7.1.1.2)

  In cases where the edges of the tongue are very curled-up, indented, or swollen, the constraint of Liver qi is likely a primary factor in the development of the illness. Nevertheless, taken by itself, this tongue sign does not give an accurate portrayal of the course of an illness. Rather, it is only meaningful when other signs and symptoms are taken into account; only then can the effect of the Liver qi constraint be determined. Swollen, curled-up edges and indented edges also indicate constraint of Liver qi. The latter appears as a long line, or indentation, along the entire side of the tongue body and gives the impression of being separate from the tongue body (Figs. 7.1.1.2, 7.1.1.4). This sign tends to denote a long-standing constraint of Liver qi that is often connected with old, seemingly irresolvable, emotional problems, for example, sexual abuse during childhood, an unhappy childhood, or repeated problems with relationships. This tongue sign is very important as it reflects the necessity for prolonged treatment in order to resolve the qi constraint. In addition, the chronic nature of this disease pattern can eventually lead to impairment in the functions of the Spleen, Stomach, Large Intestine, or Lungs.

Tongue description	**Chinese diagnosis**
Slightly pale	Slight Spleen qi deficiency
Slightly reddish center	Onset of heat in the Stomach
Curled-up edges	Liver qi stagnation
Slightly reddish tip	Onset of heat from deficiency in the Heart
White, slippery coating, *yellow coating at the root of the tongue*	Accumulation of damp-heat

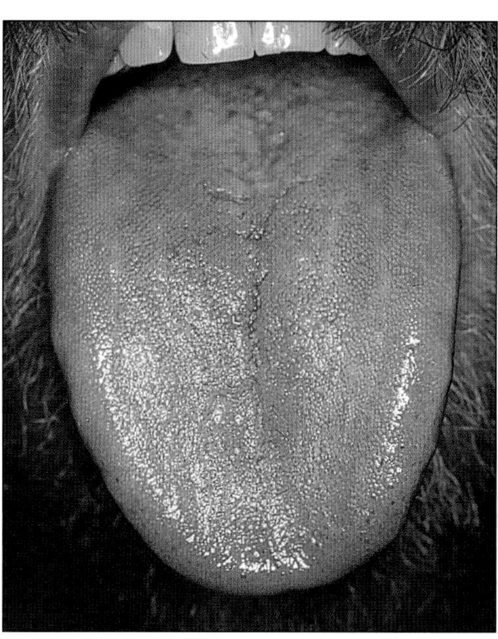

Fig. 7.1.1.1
Male
41 years old

Symptoms

Inability to fall asleep and remain asleep
Occasional night sweats
Stomach pains exacerbated by stress
Bad breath
Occasional diarrhea

Western diagnosis

Insomnia

Background to disease

Separation from partner

Tongue description	**Chinese diagnosis**
Slightly pale tongue body	Slight Spleen qi deficiency
Indented edges	Liver qi stagnation
Slightly pale edges	Slight Liver blood deficiency
Slight indention of the tip	Slight Heart blood deficiency
Whitish, moist coating	Normal

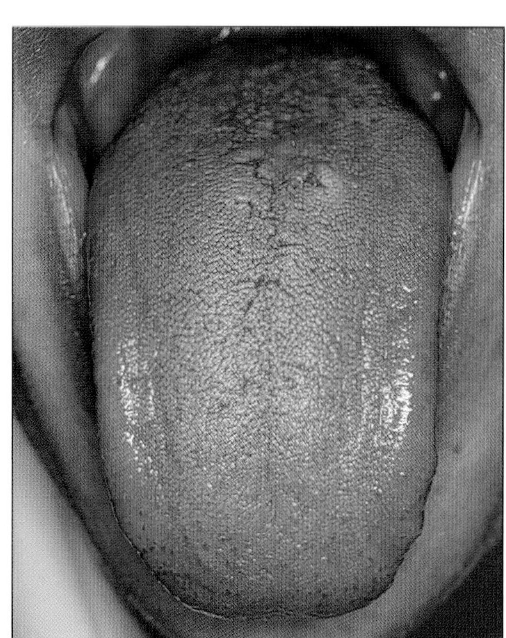

Fig. 7.1.1.2
Female
32 years old

Symptoms

Sighing, tightness of the chest
Depressive moods
Tiredness
Lack of appetite

Western diagnosis

None

Background to disease

Feelings of guilt

Tongue description	Chinese diagnosis
Red	Heat in the blood
Curled-up, red edges	Liver qi constraint with Liver heat
White, moist coating	Normal

Fig. 7.1.1.3
Male
42 years old

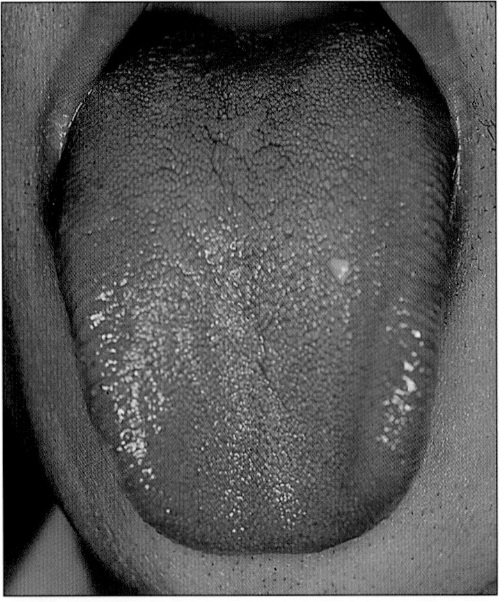

Symptoms

Restlessness
Irritability
Sleeping problems
Bloated abdomen
Feeling of pressure under the ribs
Fatigue

Western diagnosis

Hepatitis C

Background to disease

Unknown

Tongue description	Chinese diagnosis
Reddish	Developing heat
Reddish, slightly swollen edges	Heat in the Liver
Indented edges	Liver qi stagnation
Reddish center with thinning coating	Heat in the Stomach with the onset of Stomach yin deficiency
Swollen center	Retention of phlegm in the Stomach
White, greasy coating	Accumulation of dampness

Fig. 7.1.1.4
Female
63 years old

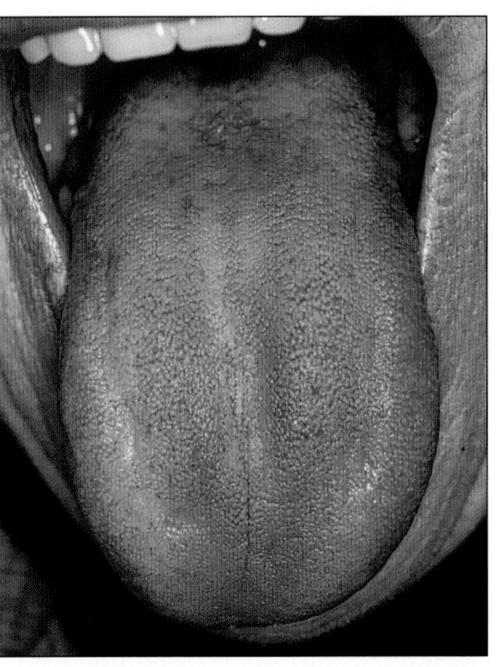

Symptoms

Pain of the entire body
Pain and sensitivity with pressure in the limbs
Stomach pains
Epigastric fullness
Long-lasting headaches
Irritability

Western diagnosis

Fibromyalgia, fibroadenomas in the breast, migraines

Background to disease

Abuse of painkillers and laxatives, dissatisfaction with personal relationships

(Patient died three years later of carcinoma of the liver)

Tongue description	**Chinese diagnosis**
Reddish	Normal
Long	Constitutional heat in the Heart
Red, curled-up edges and yellow, greasy, thick coating on the posterior third	Liver qi constraint with Liver heat, retention of damp-heat in the Liver and Gallbladder
Curled-down tip	Heat from deficiency in the Heart

Symptoms

Hoarseness
Feeling of a lump in the throat
Cough with thick phlegm
Inner tension, nervousness

Western diagnosis

Polyps on vocal cords

Background to disease

Existential angst
Severe demands at work
Irregular eating habits

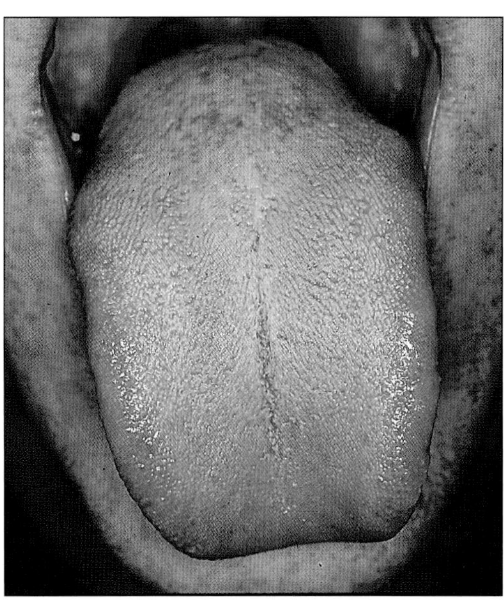

Fig. 7.1.1.5
Male
42 years old

Tongue description	**Chinese diagnosis**
Pale red	Normal
Curled-up edges	Liver qi stagnation
Deep central crack with whitish yellow coating	Retention of phlegm in the Stomach
Reddish tip	Heat in the Heart
Whitish yellow, slippery coating, slightly thicker on the left side	Retention of damp-heat in Liver and Gallbladder

Symptoms

Difficulty falling asleep and sleeping through the night
Irritability and feelings of anger
Restlessness
Nausea, lack of appetite
Tiredness

Western diagnosis

Insomnia

Background to disease

Emotional problems resulting from separation, alcohol abuse, and a hectic lifestyle

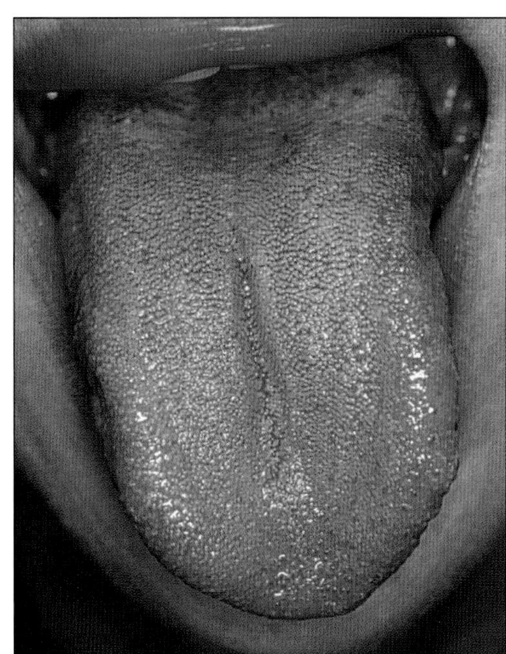

Fig. 7.1.1.6
Female
30 years old

About this case history

This case is a good example of how quarrels and disappointment can exacerbate Liver qi constraint and thereby engender heat and fire, which in turn agitates the spirit.

CASE HISTORY Prior to her first treatment the patient had not slept for three nights. She had no appetite and had not eaten for three days. She was irritable because her girlfriend had left her. Although tired, she was unable to fall asleep. She reported that although she drank a lot of alcohol to "knock herself out," it didn't work. Even before the separation, her sleep had been poor. In times of emotional tension she suffered from difficulty in falling asleep as well as sleeping through the night. She grew bored easily and therefore loved changes in all areas of her life; this developed into a hectic lifestyle. She constantly changed girlfriends, and her relationships were always short-lived. She partied a great deal, which meant that she drank a large amount of alcohol. Her pulse was fast and wiry.

Analysis. The curled-up tongue edges signal long-standing stagnation of Liver qi. Anger and fits of rage, triggered by the departure of her girlfriend, led to an implosion of the already constrained qi, and engendered Liver fire. This diagnosis is confirmed by the fast and wiry pulse. Since the emotional crisis of the patient is of recent origin, the edges of the tongue do not yet show a red discoloration.

The intensity of heat in the Liver[1] is exacerbated by the regular use of alcohol and has resulted in irritability and restlessness. In this case, the upward-rising Liver heat has agitated the spirit to such an extent that the patient has developed a severe sleeping problem. The ensuing heat in the Heart is reflected in the reddish tip of the tongue.

Alcohol not only heats the Liver but also causes an accumulation of damp-heat in the Liver and Gallbladder. The whitish yellow coating, slightly thicker on the left side of the tongue, hints at this disease pattern. This condition of excess in the Liver and Gallbladder impairs the normal activity of the Stomach and Spleen, which manifests in nausea and a lack of appetite.

An additional tongue sign—the deep crack in the center of the tongue that is covered by a whitish yellow, greasy coating—suggests a constitutional tendency toward developing phlegm-heat in the Stomach and Heart. When fire and phlegm obstruct the Heart and Stomach, the texture of the coating covering a midline crack will become yellow and dry or greasy. This tongue sign is frequently seen in cases of serious mental problems. In this case, the coating is neither yellow nor extremely greasy. Yet this sign is still noteworthy because it suggests that the patient may be in an early stage of phlegm-fire, which can lead to harassment of the spirit. Repeated cycles of insomnia may be considered as the first sign of this process.

Pathomechanism

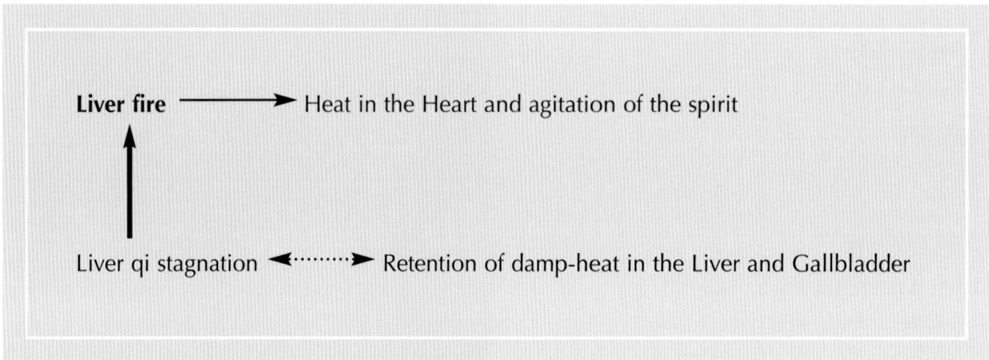

Treatment strategy. Clear the Liver fire, regulate the Liver qi, and calm the spirit.

The patient was treated with acupuncture. In the first treatment, a draining technique was used at HT-7 *(shén mén)* to calm the spirit, and at LR-2 *(xíng jiān)* and LR-3 *(tài chōng)* to clear the Liver fire and regulate the Liver qi. Following the treatment, the patient slept well for three nights. This treatment was repeated, and she slept well for a week. She grew much calmer and was no longer angry.

7.1.2 Liver Fire and Ascending Liver Yang and Associated Tongue Signs

Discriminating between Liver fire and ascending Liver yang on the basis of the tongue signs alone will not be entirely accurate; tongue diagnosis should only be formulated in conjunction with the other signs and symptoms and an educated guess as to its etiology. Both disease patterns are characterized by a strong ascending movement of heat and yang to the head. Both patterns manifest with similar symptoms: headache, dizziness, tinnitus, and irritability. Liver fire is a pattern of excess marked by the development of intense heat with such symptoms as a strong, bitter taste in the mouth, red face and eyes, and a propensity to outbursts of anger. These symptoms are more pronounced in cases of Liver fire than in cases of ascending Liver yang. Additionally, Liver fire injures and dries the body fluids, resulting, for example, in dry stools and thirst (Fig. 7.1.2.4).

By contrast, ascending Liver yang is characterized by a root of deficiency but a manifestation of excess. Like Liver fire, cases of ascending Liver yang also display symptoms such as temporal headache, dizziness, or tinnitus. However, there are differences between the two patterns. First, the symptoms are much more pronounced in cases of Liver fire. Second, with ascending Liver yang, the history would also include symptoms of deficiency such as night sweats (Fig. 7.1.2.5), which are indicative of Kidney yin or blood deficiency. Thus, disease patterns leading to ascending Liver yang can be distinguished from those responsible for Liver fire in that the former are rooted in deficiency such as Kidney yin or blood deficiency, chronic illness, excessive sexual activity, or overtaxation of the patient's physical and/or emotional resources; the symptoms should reflect this mixed pattern. By contrast, Liver fire will present with a pattern of excess, such as rage, suppressed anger, or the overconsumption of fatty foods and alcoholic beverages, as part of the etiology (Figs. 7.1.2.4).

These differences are also manifested by the tongue signs.

Tongue signs

- red edges of the tongue body with a yellow and greasy tongue coating: Liver fire (Fig. 7.1.2.4)

  Liver fire also injures the fluids, and thus the tongue coating is often dry. The yellow color and the thickness of the coating denote a pattern of excess. The coating will often cover the entire tongue body. Fig. 7.1.2.4 is a good illustration. The patient in that case had been an alcoholic for years, and also had unsatisfactory personal relationships that were partly responsible for his emotional problems. The thick, yellow coating and the red tongue body reflect the presence of the interior heat and damp-heat that contributed to his mental illness. It is important to emphasize that in cases of Liver fire, the presence of a yellow tongue coating is of more importance to the diagnosis than curled-up, red edges on the tongue, which may or may not be present.

- red or reddish edges of the tongue with noticeable red spots along their entire length are indicative of the presence of heat or fire in the Liver.[2]

As previously noted, the pattern of ascending Liver yang stems from deficiency, such as Kidney yin or blood deficiency.

- red tongue body with no coating, coating without a root or peeled appearance: Kidney yin deficiency with ascending Liver yang (Fig. 7.1.2.5). Here the edges of the tongue are not curled-up. Instead they are swollen, which is another sign denoting a pattern of excess of the Liver.

When doing tongue diagnosis it is important to pay attention to signs of excess and deficiency, especially in relation to the tongue coating. In Fig. 7.1.2.5 the peeled coating, together with all the other symptoms, reflects the weakening of the Kidney yin. By contrast, the thick, yellow (non-peeled) coating in Fig. 7.1.2.4. signifies a condition of excess, confirming the diagnosis of Liver fire.

Tongue description	**Chinese diagnosis**
Pale red	Slight blood deficiency
Swelling at the sides with red points	Ascending Liver yang
Slight notch at the tip with red points	Heart blood deficiency with heat in the Heart

Fig. 7.1.2.1
Female
44 years old

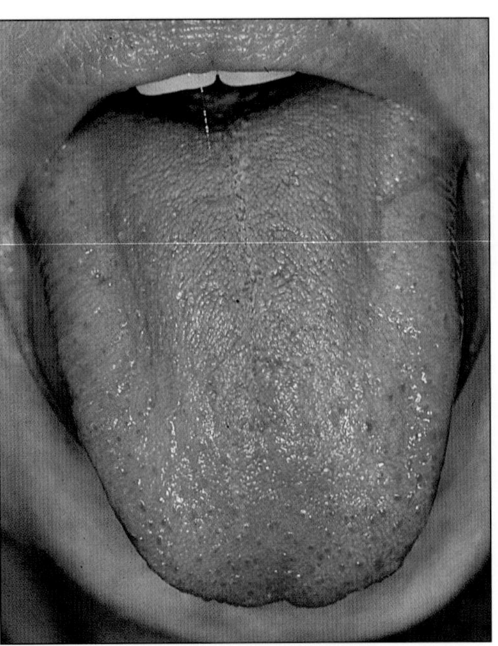

Symptoms

Panic attacks
Waking at night with palpitations and sweating, nightmares
Trembling of the head with rest
Shortened menstrual cycle with emotional stress
Exhaustion

Western diagnosis

None

Background to disease

Long-standing emotional problems

Tongue description	**Chinese diagnosis**
Pale red, wide, thin, dry tongue body	Injury to fluids from heat
Curled-up edges, very red edges in the anterior third, red points at the side	Liver qi constraint and heat in the Liver transforming into Liver fire
Slightly yellow, old, greasy coating	Long-standing damp-heat in the Liver and Gallbladder
Rootless coating at the root	Onset of Kidney yin deficiency

Symptoms

Hot feet
Tremors
Tension and restlessness that rise from the bottom of the patient to the top
Palpitations
Nausea
Diarrhea
Headaches at the forehead and temples

Western diagnosis

Heroin withdrawal

Background to disease

Heroin addiction

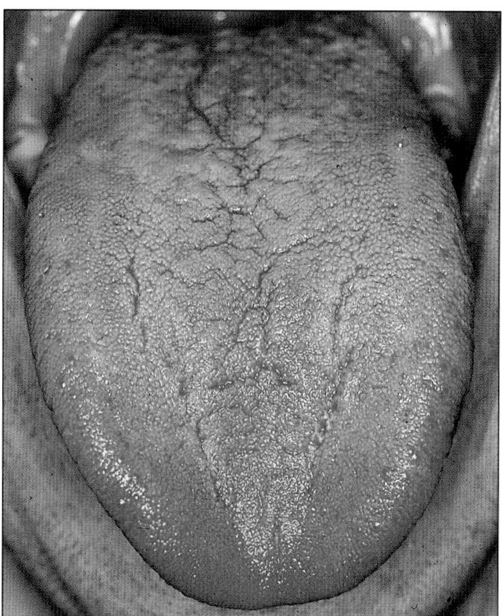

Fig. 7.1.2.2
Male
28 years old

Tongue description	**Chinese diagnosis**
Red, swollen tongue body	Damp-heat in the Liver and Gallbladder
Red sides with red points	Liver fire
Midline crack over the entire tongue body	Constitutional heat in the Heart
Yellow, thick, dry coating	Accumulation of phlegm-heat in the Stomach

Symptoms

Sudden, one-sided, right facial pain
Purulent secretion from the right eye
Conjunctival redness
Facial redness
Nausea
Bitter taste in the mouth
Restlessness
Insomnia

Western diagnosis

Heroin addiction
Fibroadenoma in the right breast
Trigeminal neuralgia

Background to disease

Heroin and alcohol addiction
Lack of sleep

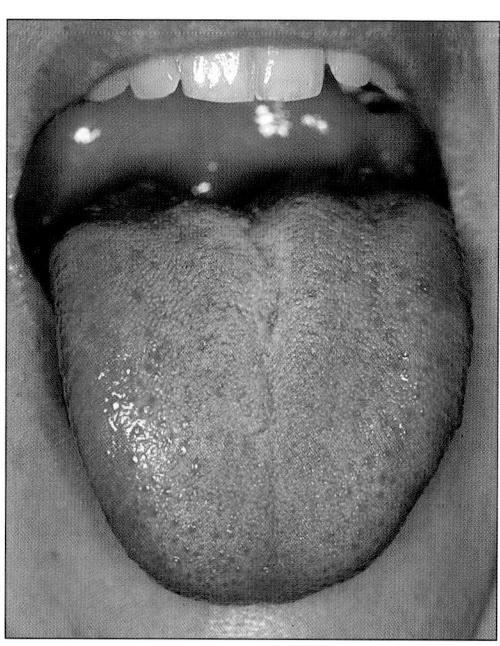

Fig. 7.1.2.3
Female
36 years old

Tongue description	Chinese diagnosis
Red with yellow, thick, greasy coating	Liver fire
Deep red, slightly bluish edges	Heat in the Liver with stasis of blood
Thin, vertical crack in the center covered with a yellow, greasy coating	Phlegm-fire in the stomach

Fig. 7.1.2.4
Male
45 years old

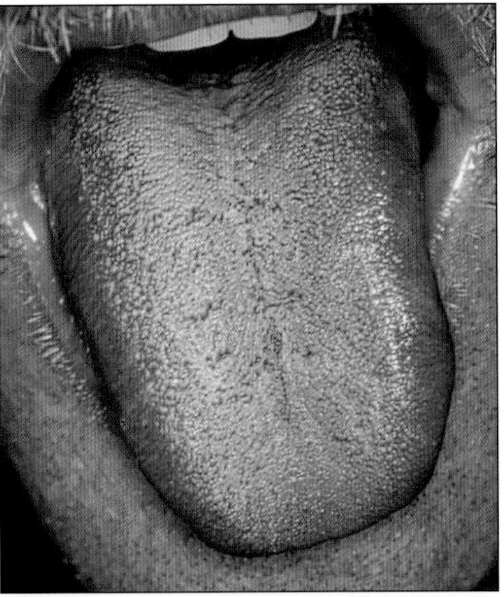

Symptoms

Restlessness
Inner agitation
Impotence
Strong thirst
Dryness of mouth
Insomnia

Western diagnosis

Bipolar disorder

Background to disease

Excessive consumption of alcohol for 16 years, smoking for 20 years, long-standing emotional problems

Tongue description	Chinese diagnosis
Red	Kidney yin deficiency
Slightly swollen edges	Ascending Liver yang
Indentation of the tip	Heart blood and yin deficiency
Rootless coating	Kidney yin deficiency

Fig. 7.1.2.5
Female
49 years old

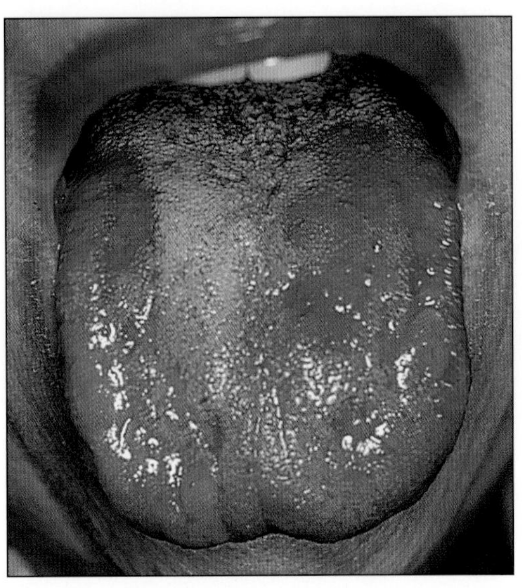

Symptoms

Loud, high-pitched tone in both ears
Diminished acuity of hearing
Irritability
Night sweats
Difficulty sleeping through the night
Nightmares

Western diagnosis

Acute loss of hearing

Background to disease

Excessive demands at work

About this case history

The tongue depicted in Fig. 7.1.2.5 highlights the difference between a pattern of Liver fire and ascending Liver yang. The coating has no root and thus suggests a pattern of deficiency.

CASE HISTORY The patient experienced three episodes of sudden hearing loss over an 18-month period. Four days prior to coming to the clinic, she woke up with diminished hearing. Her doctor gave her infusions, which did not help. Instead, it left her with a loud whistling tone in both ears, which made her extremely irritable. Two days prior to the acute onset of her symptoms she had a serious argument with some of her students, which left her troubled. She had worked for 20 years at a school for psychologically disturbed children but was beginning to lose her enthusiasm for her profession and felt constantly overtaxed.

During the previous six months she had been waking at around 3 A.M. and had difficulty falling back to sleep. When she did sleep through the night, she would have terrible nightmares that were accompanied by strong night sweats. She was always tired and stressed as a result of the lack of sleep. She noticed that the children irritated her more and more. She felt unhappy as she could not see a way out of her situation. Her menstruation, appetite, thirst, and digestion were normal. Her pulse was wiry and rapid.

Pathomechanism

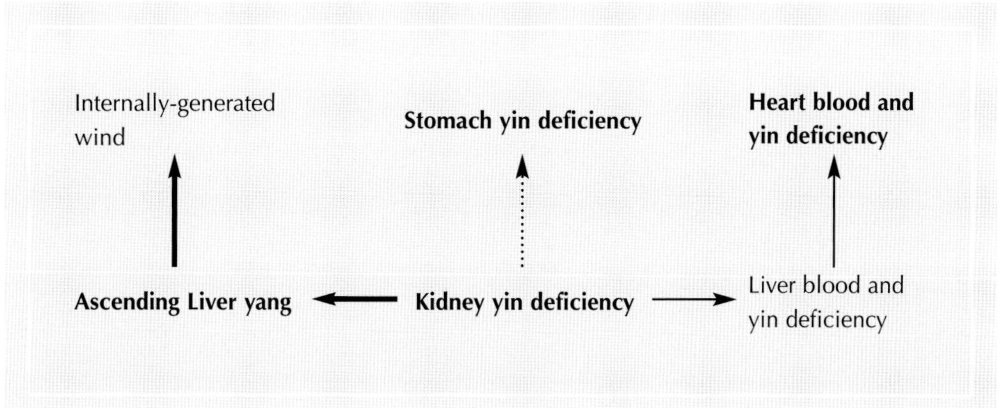

Analysis. The excessive demands of work, as well as emotional demands, have diminished the strength of the patient's Kidney yin. The severity and chronic nature of the patient's weakened constitution are reflected in the color of the tongue body and the nature of the coating, especially since a deviation from the normal pale red tongue body color develops, as a rule, over the space of many years (with the exception of those illnesses caused by pathogenic heat).

The tongue body of this patient shows different shades of red. The red in the center of the tongue is more intense than the color on the anterior third. The edges of the tongue are distinguished by an orange-red shade. This suggests a slow development of Kidney yin deficiency, and may reflect incipient deficiency of the Stomach, Heart, and Liver yin. The different shades of red suggest that the deficiency occurred at different times. Parts of the tongue body appear to be smooth like a mirror, indicating partial atrophy of the papillae as a result of Stomach yin deficiency. The combination of the Stomach yin and Kidney yin deficiency is responsible for the insufficient tongue coating and the extensive peeled area.

In this case, the yin deficiency has led to insufficient nourishment of Heart yin, which has become too weak to keep the yang inside and to anchor the spirit at night. The occasional night sweats are characteristic of Kidney yin deficiency, which is unable to draw the protective qi inside at night. Long-term Kidney deficiency can weaken the Kidney essence, which, in turn, aggravates the deficiency of blood. The indentation at the tip of the tongue reflects Heart blood as well as Heart yin deficiency. The tongue body lacks sufficient substance to maintain its normal shape. The Heart blood has probably also been weakened by the constant worrying and excessive demands of work.

A pattern of Kidney yin deficiency implies deficiency of Liver yin. This pattern is responsible for the failure of the ethereal soul to be properly housed by the Liver yin, causing nightmares. These violent dreams can also be the first sign of excessive yang.

When yin loses control over yang, it may induce the Liver yang to ascend. Here, this movement was so intense—reflected in the wiry and rapid pulse[3]—that it generated the internal movement of wind. This accounts for the sudden, acute, and partial loss of hearing. Internal wind and ascending Liver yang impair the provision of nourishing blood, yin, and essence to the ears, resulting in the loss of hearing. The inner stress caused by the patient's arguments with her students is responsible for her renewed loss of hearing. It is possible that the anger and quarrelling instigated the movement of what was already unstable yang. The swollen tongue edges reflect a long-standing disturbance of the Liver. This sign, together with the red, peeled tongue body and the other symptoms, indicates a pattern of ascending Liver yang.

In this case, the tongue diagnosis is helpful in establishing a differential diagnosis. In clinical practice, the sudden loss of hearing is often attributed to Liver fire or damp-heat in the Liver and Gallbladder. These patterns are accompanied by a yellow, greasy tongue coating, which is not found here. However, if ascending Liver yang is the result of Kidney yin deficiency, the tongue will reflect both the pattern of deficiency—the peeled coating—as well as the pattern of excess—the red, swollen tongue edges.

Treatment strategy. Extinguish the inner wind, anchor the yang, calm the spirit, and nourish the Kidneys and Liver.

For seven days the patient took a modified form of Gastrodia and Uncaria Decoction *(tiān má gōu téng yǐn)* with the addition of Magnetitum *(cí shí)*. She was simultaneously treated with acupuncture at the following points: GV-24 *(shén tíng)* to calm the spirit and extinguish inner wind from the head, GB-13 *(běn shén)* to calm the spirit and eliminate inner wind, GB-2 *(tīng huì)* to open the ears and eliminate inner wind, LR-2 *(xíng jiān)* (draining method) to subdue Liver yang, LR-3 *(tài chōng)* (neutral method) to strengthen the Liver yin and eliminate wind, and KI-3 *(tài xī)* to strengthen the Kidney yin. This treatment reduced the ringing in her ears by 80 percent, and after 10 days she was fine. Further treatment to strengthen her constitution was then undertaken.

7.1.3 Tongue Signs Associated with Internally-Generated Wind

Symptoms that occur suddenly and are characterized by trembling and tremors, spasms, vertigo, muscle tics, sudden numbness, or convulsions reflect the internal movement of wind. An illness caused by internally-generated wind can leave serious damage in its wake. However, there are a few warning signs that signal its approach, one of which being a constantly moving tongue: when extended, it moves from one side to the other. Alternatively, the patient will be unable to extend the tongue fully, and will retract it, only to extend it again.

A noticeably stiff tongue body that is very red or is covered with a thick, greasy coating also reflects the formation of internally-generated wind (Fig. 7.1.3.5). This is an important tongue sign, especially in conjunction with other appropriate symptoms.

Clinically, internally-generated wind frequently occurs in those with long-term deficiency of Kidney yin, which can lead to the ascending of Liver yang. Sudden loss of consciousness, spasms, or the sudden deviation of an eye and mouth are characteristic signs. As a rule, the tongue body is red and dry because of the underlying deficiency of Kidney yin.

Internal wind can also arise from externally-contracted heat from excess. This will cause illnesses that are characterized by high fever. The heat penetrates into the blood level and causes skin rashes, like the petechia that appears during the course of meningitis. The internally-generated wind is responsible for convulsions or rigidity of the neck. The tongue is also deviated and frequently presents with red, raised points that denote heat in the blood and the presence of toxic heat (Fig. 9.1.6).

Tongue signs

- deviated tongue body: internally-generated wind (Fig. 7.1.3.1)
- deviated, red, dry tongue body: internally-generated wind with underlying Kidney yin deficiency (Fig. 7.1.3.5)
- deviated, pale tongue body: internally-generated wind with underlying Liver blood deficiency (Fig. 7.1.3.2)

  The symptoms are less severe in deficient-type internally-generated wind than in the excess type and include numbness of the extremities, tics, and slight tremor of the head and hands.
- a pale, deviated tongue can also occur in the case of externally-contracted wind-cold that blocks the channels in the face, possibly causing facial paralysis. When wind-phlegm causes dizziness, numbness, headaches, or even wind-stroke, the tongue may deviate and be covered with a thick, greasy coating.

Tongue description	**Chinese diagnosis**
Reddish, slightly blue, *stiff* tongue body	Kidney yin deficiency and blood stagnation obstructing the channels
Deviated with yellow, greasy coating	Wind-phlegm blocking the channels
Notch at the tip	Heart blood deficiency

Symptoms

Extreme stiffness and pain of both elbows and the right knee
Fatigue
Depressive moods

Western diagnosis

Degenerative joint disease with involvement of multiple joints
Early stage in atrophy of various muscle groups

Background to disease

Physical overexertion at work
Repressed emotions

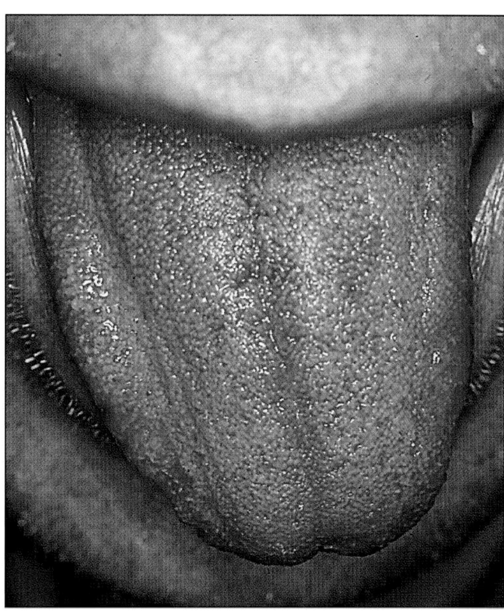

Fig. 7.1.3.1
Male
35 years old

Tongue description	**Chinese diagnosis**
Pale, swollen, teeth marks	Spleen qi deficiency (accumulation of dampness)
Pale edges	Liver blood deficiency
Deviated	Internally-generated wind
Thin, greasy, yellowish coating	Accumulation of damp-heat in the middle burner

Fig. 7.1.3.2
Female
35 years old

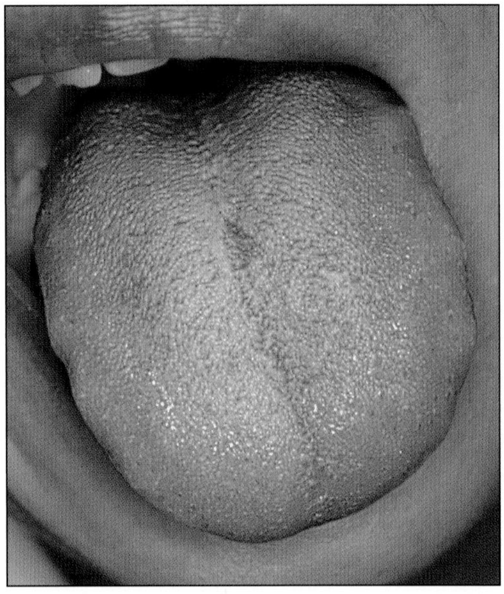

Symptoms

Inability to move right arm and leg
Numb feeling
Mental confusion
Epigastric fullness
Nausea
Lack of appetite

Western diagnosis

Cerebral apoplexy
Hemiplegia

Background to disease

Occurred after severe fall on the head
Extreme physical and mental demands of looking after her mentally and physically handicapped child

Tongue description	**Chinese diagnosis**
Pale, deviated	Blood deficiency with internally-generated wind
Yellow, greasy coating in the center of the tongue	Heat in the yang brightness *(yáng míng)* channel

Fig. 7.1.3.3
Male
59 years old

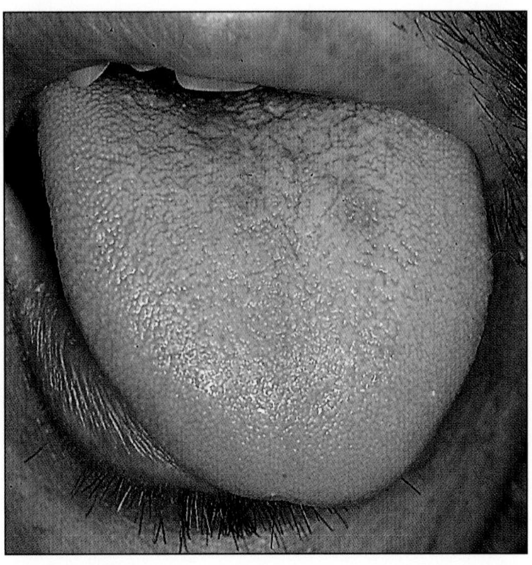

Symptoms

Right-sided hemiplegia
Loss of memory
Constipation
Epigastric fullness

Western diagnosis

Stroke

Background to disease

High blood pressure for 15 years
Physically overworked

Tongue description	**Chinese diagnosis**
Red, swollen with *dark yellow coating at the sides of the tongue*	Retention of damp-heat in the Liver and Gallbladder
Rootless coating at the center of the tongue	Stomach yin deficiency
Deviated	Internally-generated Liver wind

Symptoms

Slight left-sided facial paralysis
Paralysis of the left arm
Irritability
Restlessness
Urgent urination, burning sensation with urination

Western diagnosis

Stroke
Prostatitis

Background to disease

High blood pressure for 15 years

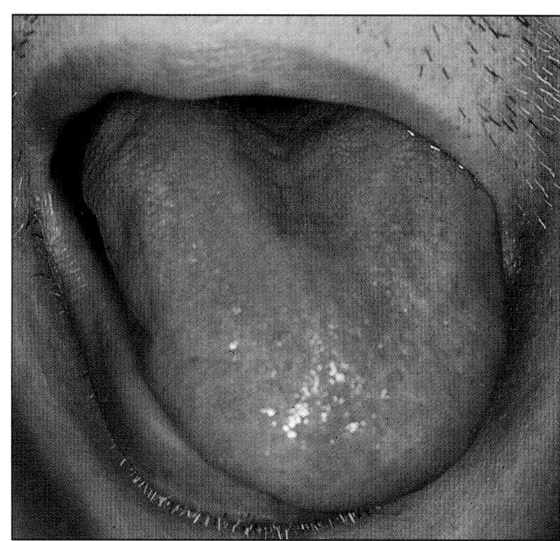

Fig. 7.1.3.4
Male
69 years old

Tongue description	**Chinese diagnosis**
Red, deviated	Kidney yin deficiency with ascending Liver yang and internally-generated Liver wind
Red in the anterior third	Heat in the upper burner
Yellow, rootless, greasy coating	Onset of injury to the fluids
Right-sided, dirty yellow, thick, greasy coating	Long-standing retention of damp-heat in the Gallbladder

Symptoms

Dizziness
Slight hemiplegia
Constipation
Restlessness

Western diagnosis

Stroke

Background to disease

High blood pressure for many years

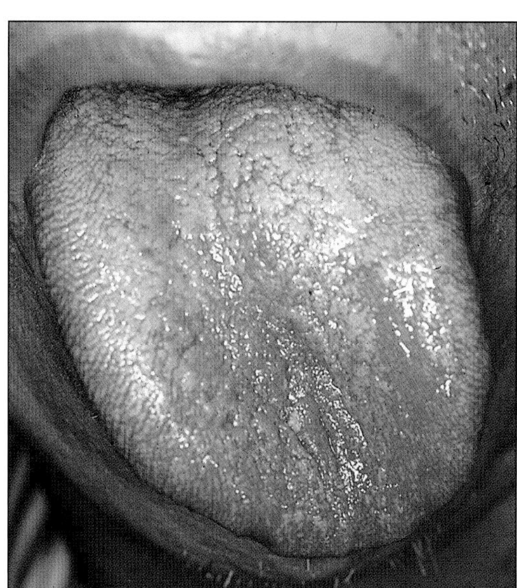

Fig. 7.1.3.5
Male
66 years old

7.2 Tongue Signs Associated with Deficiency

7.2.1 Tongue Signs Associated with Liver Blood Deficiency

From the perspective of Chinese medicine, the term 'blood deficiency' does not refer to the quantity of blood or the number of blood corpuscles. Rather, the term implies that blood cannot perform certain functions, such as nourishing the Heart or housing the spirit. A diagnosis of blood deficiency is therefore not to be equated or associated with anemia. Having said this, blood deficiency may be so deep that, on a material level, iron deficiency may occur. However, a diagnosis of blood deficiency can be made even in the absence of a shortage of blood or one of its physical components. It may exist simply as a secondary pattern resulting from Spleen qi deficiency or a weakness of Kidney essence. Therefore, treatment strategies that are merely concerned with nourishing the blood will only provide short-term relief of the symptoms.

As the term is used in Chinese medicine, blood is a form of qi. Blood is denser and more sluggish than qi. Blood nourishes the qi while qi moves the blood. Thus blood is reliant on qi for its dynamic flow. Blood is also closely connected with Kidney essence, which, via the bone marrow, participates in the production of blood. From this relationship, blood derives its 'material' character, which manifests, for example, in its ability to moisten the skin and nourish the hair. As a further example of its material nature, in cases of blood deficiency, the stools become dry and difficult to pass.

With the exception of serious blood loss, for example, during surgery or severe, long-lasting menstrual bleeding, blood deficiency is usually secondary to other disease patterns. Patterns of blood deficiency are, as a rule, secondary manifestations of a disease process and therefore do not appear by themselves. Rather, they appear in conjunction with patterns of qi, yin, or Kidney essence deficiency, or even blood stasis.

Tongue signs

The edges of the tongue reflect the quality of Liver energies.

- pale edges of the tongue body: Liver blood deficiency (Fig. 7.2.1.1)

  In cases of Liver blood deficiency, this area of the tongue is not sufficiently supplied with blood, and the degree of its paleness will reflect the depth of the pattern. However, this tongue sign will tell you nothing about the origin of the Liver blood deficiency. With respect to tongue diagnosis, this information can only be obtained from an analysis of the form, color, and texture of the tongue body.

  Blood is stored in the Liver. Lying down to rest enables the blood to return to the Liver.[4] The Liver is responsible for the circulation of blood in relation to the individual's level of physical activity. In addition, the Liver blood nourishes and moistens the muscles, sinews, and tendons. In clinical practice, this mechanism can be observed during or after an acupuncture treatment. After resting for 30 minutes, the paleness of the tongue edges will be reduced because resting has allowed the blood to return to the Liver where it is stored.

The presence of pale edges is an important sign. In addition to physical complaints, Liver blood deficiency can also lead to emotional problems since it is the function of the Liver blood to nourish and anchor the ethereal soul. Undernourishment of the ethereal soul may impair the patient's feeling of well-being and cause a 'deficiency' in the patient's visions, ideas, and plans for self-fulfillment.

If Liver blood deficiency leads, for example, to Heart blood deficiency, then sleeping problems may emerge and the intensity of mental symptoms may grow stronger. In this case, there will be additional tongue signs, such as an abnormal shape to the tip of the tongue (see Ch. 6).

The development of heat from deficiency may be exacerbated by a pattern of Liver blood deficiency that has injured the yin. This combination frequently leads to heat from deficiency in the Heart, which manifests in emotional problems and disturbed sleep. This pathomechanism would result in a tongue with a reddish tip and pale edges.

Tongue description	**Chinese diagnosis**
Pale and wide	Spleen qi deficiency
Thin	Blood deficiency
Pale edges	Liver blood deficiency
Curled-up edges	Liver qi stagnation
Small cracks in the anterior third and center	Injury to the Lung and Stomach yin

Symptoms

Constant headache, occasional migraine
Tightness of the neck and shoulder muscles
Bitter taste in the mouth
Feeling of pressure under the ribs
Irritability
Dry cough
Exhaustion

Western diagnosis

Migraine

Background to disease

Four pregnancies in the space of seven years, overworked, lack of sleep
Long-standing emotional problems, *excessive smoking*

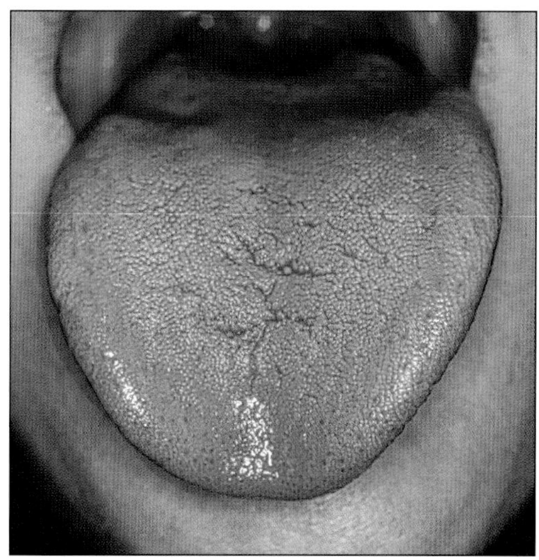

Fig. 7.2.1.1
Female
38 years old

Tongue description	Chinese diagnosis
Pale and wide	Spleen qi deficiency → slight accumulation of dampness
Pale edges	Liver blood deficiency
Thin vertical and horizontal cracks on the anterior and middle third	Stomach qi and yin deficiency
Curled-under tip	Heart blood deficiency
White, wet coating	Accumulation of fluids in the Stomach
Yellow, thin coating at the root	Slight accumulation of heat in the Large Intestine

Fig. 7.2.1.2
Female
19 years old

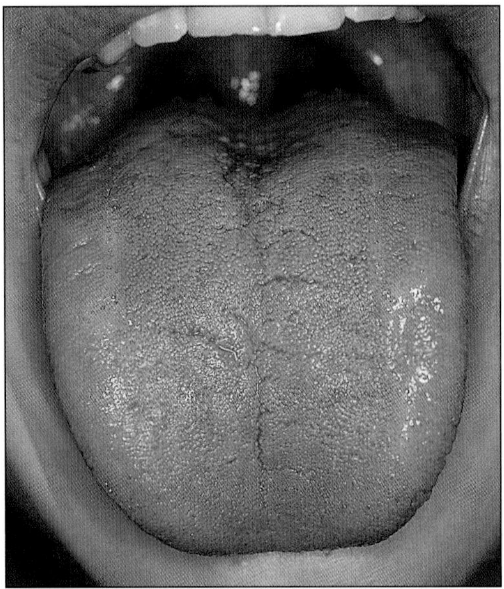

Symptoms

Constipation
Headaches
Strong thirst
Discontentment
Mood swings

Western diagnosis

Constipation

Background to disease

Anorexia nervosa between the ages of 11 and 15

Tongue description	Chinese diagnosis
Pale, especially in the anterior third	Heart blood deficiency
Pale, dry edges	Extreme exhaustion of the blood, especially Liver blood; lack of fluids
Deep red in the middle and posterior thirds of the tongue	Kidney yin deficiency with Kidney fire

Fig. 7.2.1.3
Female
38 years old

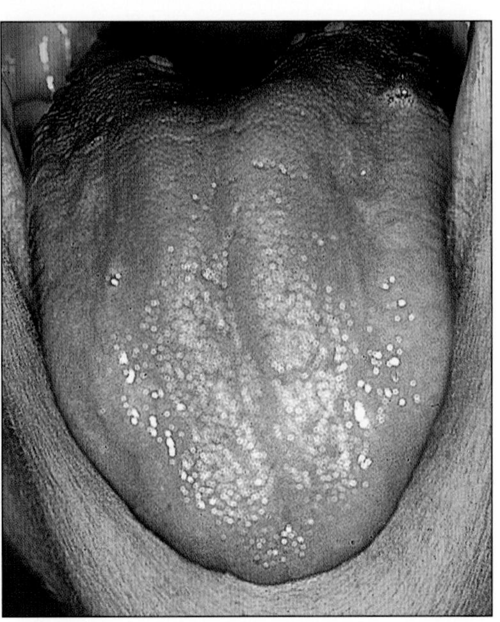

Symptoms

Fatigue
Shortness of breath
Low-grade fever
Night sweats
Severe pain in the right hypochondrium and lower abdomen
Brown urine
Weight loss to the point of emaciation

Western diagnosis

Colon cancer with metastases to the liver
Ascites

Background to disease

Condition followed chemotherapy

Tongue description	**Chinese diagnosis**
Reddish, dry, slightly thin	Stomach and Kidney yin deficiency
Pale edges	Liver blood deficiency
Long, vertical midline crack	Constitutional disharmony of the Heart
Reddish tip	Heat from deficiency of the Heart

Symptoms

Protracted, severe menstrual bleeding
Occasional night sweats
Restlessness
Depressive moods
Lack of appetite
Dryness of the mouth

Western diagnosis

Menorrhagia, menopause

Background to disease

Mental overtaxation

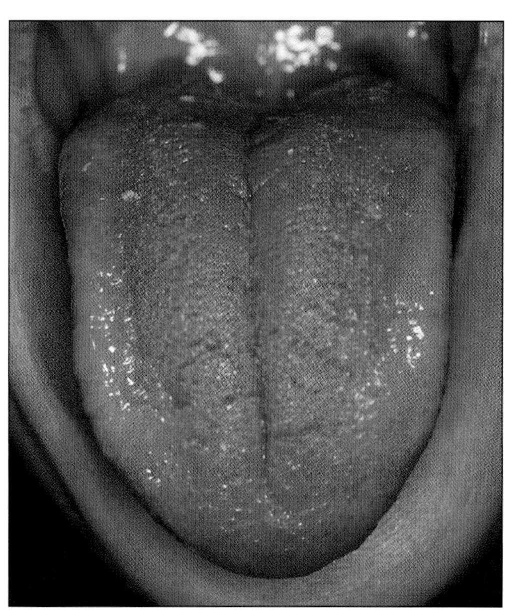

Fig. 7.2.1.4
Female
51 years old

About this case history

The results of blood loss, depriving the Liver of blood, are illustrated in the following case. The pale edges of the tongue in relation to the reddish tongue body are quite visible.

CASE HISTORY When the patient talked about her symptoms, she cried. She felt weak, exhausted, and unable to continue her work as a teacher. Her oldest son had left home, and she could not accept this change in her life. Protracted menstrual bleeding, plus her angst, led to severe exhaustion. At the time of her first treatment, she had been bleeding continuously for three weeks. The amount of blood lost was quite variable. Sometimes there was only spotting, but at other times she lost copious amounts. Medical examination revealed nothing, and her gynecologist suggested curettage. Other related symptoms were occasional night sweats and mood swings.

The patient had no appetite and therefore lost weight. When she came for treatment, she looked thin and emaciated. She was not thirsty, but at night she drank a large amount to ease her dry mouth. She felt mentally unstable. She could not imagine how to change her life. She cried a great deal and felt vulnerable. Her pulse was deficient, floating, rapid, and frail.

Analysis. The pale tongue edges, indicative of Liver blood deficiency, stand out because of the redness of the tongue body. In contrast to the preceding case histories, the blood deficiency here is not a result of Spleen qi deficiency. Rather, it is caused by protracted menstrual bleeding and an underlying weakness of the Kidney essence. If Spleen qi deficiency were involved, the entire tongue body would be pale, rather than just the edges.

The weak constitution of the patient is reflected in the red and dry tongue body. Not only is the tongue body dry, it also has no coating, an important item that suggests a deficiency of fluids and of Stomach and Kidney yin. If the texture of the entire tongue body appears dry with superficial, irregular cracks, in contrast to a smooth-looking tongue body, which is often present where there is Spleen qi deficiency with accumulation of dampness, it is caused by a

Pathomechanism

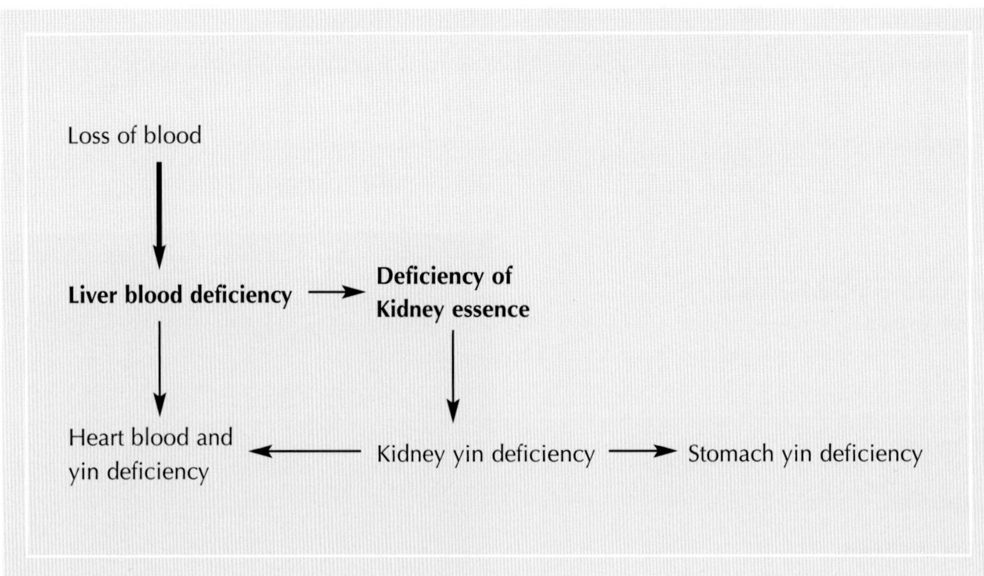

lack of fluids and /or Kidney yin deficiency. The severity of the deficiency can be determined by the redness of the tongue body.

As discussed in Ch. 6, the long, thin, vertical crack that runs along the midline of the entire length of the tongue is indicative of a constitutional disharmony of the Heart. Those with this tongue sign tend to exhibit increased emotional instability under emotional duress. The tongue body is slightly thin, which is often a sign of either blood deficiency (pale tongue body) or yin deficiency (red tongue body).

This patient had been healthy until the onset of menopause. The first symptoms set in at the age of 51. Often such symptoms are a sign of declining Kidney essence, which may give rise to deficiency of Kidney yin and/or Kidney yang. Tongue diagnosis is a useful tool when formulating a differential diagnosis in relation to climacteric symptoms, especially because it is around this time that symptoms of these deficiency patterns may occur.

A red, dry tongue is symptomatic of Kidney yin deficiency. It is this pattern that is responsible here for the protracted bleeding characterized by flooding and spotting. Kidney yin deficiency allows heat from deficiency to develop, which warms the blood. Heat in the blood interferes with the Liver's function of storing the blood. The Penetrating and Conception vessels become unstable, which is aggravated by the deficiency of Kidney yin and Kidney essence. As a result of their instability, these vessels lose their ability to restrain the flow of blood. The uncontrollable loss of blood results. The floating and rapid pulse denotes the development of heat, and the frailness of the pulse suggests an impairment of the Kidney energies.

Mental overtaxation at work, plus the 'loss' of her son, has agitated her mind, which manifests here as restlessness. The long, vertical midline crack, together with the red tip of the tongue, is an expression of heat in the Heart. Because the Heart is joined to the uterus by way of the Girdle vessel, heat in the Heart contributes to uterine bleeding. Emotional demands, which the patient feels are intolerable, intensify the heat and result in an uncontrolled and strong flow of menstrual blood.

Mental instability and mood swings are aggravated by the Liver blood deficiency, as evidenced in the pale tongue edges, because the ethereal soul is not properly anchored. Liver blood deficiency is important in the etiology of this patient's mental symptoms. If the ethereal soul and the spirit are sufficiently nourished and anchored by the blood, they will regulate and maintain an emotional balance. In this case, however, the lack of Liver blood has resulted in emotional imbalance. Another function of Liver blood is to root the Liver qi so that it can flow freely and allow an individual to react appropriately to life's changes. Although the patient wishes for changes in her life, such as terminating her professional career, she is unable to see her own needs as a positive thing. Quite the contrary, they contribute to a feeling of aimlessness and an inability to 'see' the future. Finally, the restlessness of the patient is aggravated by the deficiency of Heart blood and yin. In this case, the Liver blood and Kidney yin are not adequately supplying the Heart with blood. This destabilizes the spirit, especially in someone with a constitutional weakness.

To summarize, the Liver blood deficiency has resulted in:

- insufficient nourishment and anchoring of the ethereal soul, which manifests in the inability to find emotional balance, to have vision, and to make plans
- insufficient rooting of the Liver qi, leading to an incapacity to cope with change
- malnourishment of Heart blood, leading to depressive moods
- insufficient nourishment of the Kidney essence and the Penetrating vessel, leading to uncontrollable menstrual bleeding.

The underlying Kidney yin deficiency is responsible for her night sweats. This pattern leads to a general lack of fluids in the body, which has weakened the Stomach yin. The deficiency of yin and fluids has given rise to a dry mouth, a feeling of thirst at night, and a dry tongue body. Since heat has not yet developed in the Stomach, the patient is neither hungry nor thirsty throughout the day. The lack of nutrition, as well as the decrease in yin, has led to emaciation, resulting in further weight loss and a haggard appearance.

Treatment strategy. Clear the heat in the blood, stop the bleeding, nourish the Liver blood, enrich the Kidney yin, strengthen the Stomach yin, and consolidate the Kidney essence.

The patient was treated regularly with acupuncture. The points included ST-30 *(qì chōng)*, PC-6 *(nèi guān)*, LR-1 *(dà dūn)*, LR-8 *(qū quán)*, SP-1 *(yǐn bái)*, KI-5 *(shuǐ quán)*, and KI-8 *(jiāo xìn)*. ST-30 was used to open the Penetrating vessel, induce a feeling of well-being, and increase the appetite. KI-5 and KI-8 were used mainly because they are cleft points of the Kidney channel and Yin Linking vessel, respectively. Cleft points located on yin channels have a special effect on disorders of the blood.[5] KI-5 especially regulates the circulation of qi and blood in the Penetrating and Conception vessels. I frequently use this point to stop uterine bleeding. In addition, KI-8 clears heat and stops bleeding. The bleeding stopped after several treatments.

Follow-up: Two years later the patient developed a recalcitrant type of urticaria and dry eczema on the legs.

Endnotes

1 Chace C. *A Qin Bo Wei Anthology*. Brookline, MA: Paradigm Publications, 1997: 31. Qin Bo Wei differentiated between Liver heat and Liver fire based on their intensity and stability. Liver fire is very intense and moves strongly. By contrast, Liver heat is less intense and more stable, and is characterized by irritability and restlessness. This feeling of vexation is localized in the Heart region.

2 Ibid., 16

3 Ibid., 30.

4 Anonymous. *Su wen* [Basic Questions], edited by He W-B et al. Beijing: China Medicine Science and Technology Press, 1996: 10:61.

5 Deadman P, Al-Kafaji M, and Baker K. *A Manual of Acupuncture*. London: Chinese Medicine Publications, 1998: 345, 349.

CHAPTER 8

Tongue Signs Associated with Blood Stasis

8.1 Blue or Bluish Tongue Bodies

Blood stasis is often responsible for conditions involving pain. When the movement of blood becomes impaired or sluggish, the individual will experience a fixed, localized, sharp pain that often worsens at night or with rest. But it is important to note that blood stasis can also develop unnoticed by a person, as it happens in the formation of internal knots and lumps.[1]

The following pathomechanisms may impair and block the flow of blood, resulting in patterns of blood stagnation and/or blood stasis:[2]

- Fractures, injuries, and surgery can create an environment that leads to a pattern of blood stagnation and/or blood stasis. Injury-induced blood stasis occurs quickly but also usually disappears rather quickly. A sprained ankle that swells and then shows a bluish discoloration is a good example of acute blood stasis in the surrounding tissues. If the injury is treated inappropriately, blood stasis in the channels may develop, causing pain and stiffness. As a rule this type of blood stasis does not manifest as change of the tongue color.
- Penetration of externally-contracted cold slows the circulation of blood (Fig. 8.1.1). As a result, the flow of qi and blood in the joints becomes blocked, leading to severe joint pain and stiffness. Internal cold, arising from a deficiency of Kidney yang, may also cause blood stasis, resulting, for example, in painful menstruation or the formation of ovarian cysts.
- Patterns of heat can also contribute to the development of blood stasis. Fluids that are responsible for thinning the blood are readily injured by pathogenic heat. The blood thickens, flows sluggishly, and eventually congeals, resulting in blood stasis.

- Emotional problems, especially suppressed anger, can lead to the constraint of Liver qi. An important function of the Liver is to promote the smooth flow of qi, which is essential for transporting an adequate supply of blood throughout the body. Blood stasis can therefore develop in cases of long-standing Liver qi stagnation (Fig. 8.1.4).
- Chronic illness usually weakens the qi, blood, yin, and yang. A pattern of blood stasis may arise as a result of these deficiencies (Figs. 8.1.3). Often Heart qi and yang deficiency form the basis for a pattern of Heart blood stasis.

Despite the different causes that lead to blood stasis, in the case of the tongue it produces the same color: a bluish tinge, or blue spots or areas.

The color of the tongue body can, as a rule, accurately reflect any impairment in the movement of blood. The nature of the color is indicative of the flow of energy throughout the body. If the qi is weak, insufficient blood will be transported to the tongue, resulting in a pale tongue body. When the yang of the body is excessive and moves blood too vigorously to the head and tongue, a red tongue body may ensue. In the case of blood stasis, the movement of blood will be seriously impaired and the tongue will take on a characteristic blue tinge. This occasionally may also be seen on the lips and fingernails.

The basic color of the tongue body provides information about the cause or origin of the blood stasis. The overall color and shape of the tongue body, and the nature of the tongue coating, must also be taken into account.

Tongue signs

- pale and bluish tongue body with white, thick coating: external or internal cold leading to blood stasis (Fig. 8.1.1)
- pale and bluish tongue: qi or blood deficiency (Fig. 8.1.3)
- pale, bluish, swollen tongue body: inner cold resulting from underlying Kidney yang deficiency leading to blood stasis (Fig. 8.1.2)
- pale red and bluish tongue body with curled-up or red edges: underlying Liver qi stagnation responsible for blood stasis (Fig. 8.1.4)
- reddish-bluish tongue body with a peeled coating or no coating: Kidney yin deficiency contributing to blood stasis

Tongue description	**Chinese diagnosis**
Pale bluish	Kidney yang deficiency → blood stagnation
Slightly swollen	Accumulation of dampness
Slight indentation of the tip	Heart blood deficiency
White, greasy coating, thicker in the center	Spleen yang deficiency with retention of damp-cold[3]

Symptoms

Severe backache, stiffness of the spine, limitation of movement
Feeling of coldness in the lumbar region
Weak knees
Physical exhaustion
Lack of appetite

Western diagnosis

Deteriorated intervertebral disc

Background to disease

Hard physical work over many years, accident while skiing five years ago

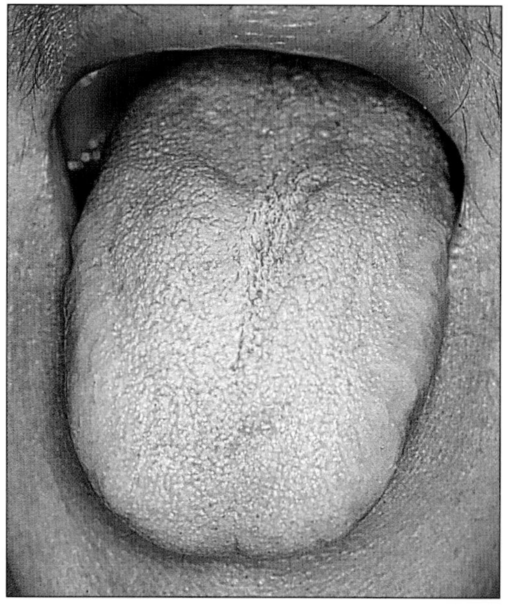

Fig. 8.1.1
Female
59 years old

Tongue description	**Chinese diagnosis**
Pale blue, swollen	Heart yang deficiency with accumulation of damp-phlegm
Intense blue discoloration in the anterior third	Heart blood stasis
Slightly deviated	Internally-generated wind
White, greasy coating	Accumulation of cold-dampness
Very distended, dark blue sublingual veins	Blood stasis in the upper burner

Symptoms

Paralysis of the left arm
Slurred speech
Racing of the heart
Exhaustion

Western diagnosis

Stroke
Hypertension
Kidney stones

Background to disease

Chronic hypertension

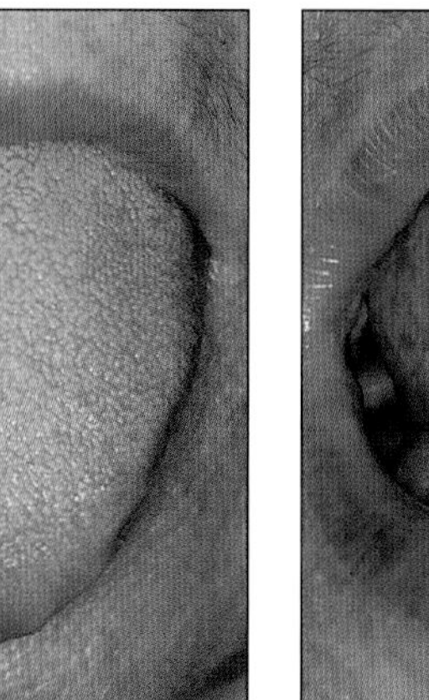

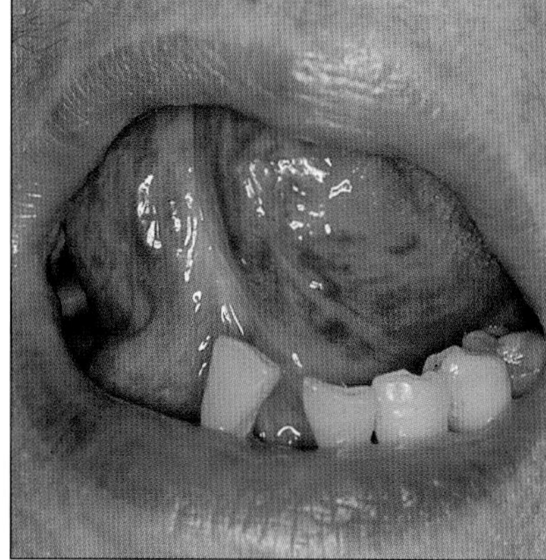

Fig. 8.1.2
Male
75 years old

Tongue description	Chinese diagnosis
Pale blue, swollen	Spleen qi deficiency with accumulation of dampness, blood deficiency and stasis
Dark blue areas	Severe Liver blood stasis

Fig. 8.1.3
Male
50 years old

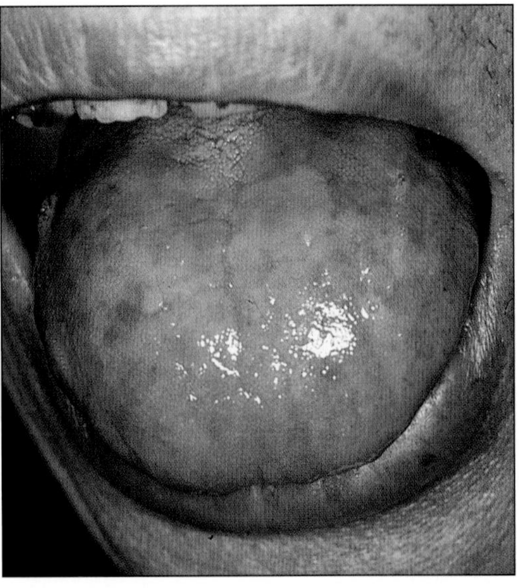

Symptoms

Caput medusae (dilated cutaneous veins around the umbilicus)
Severe weight loss
Weakness
No appetite
Edema of the lower legs

Western diagnosis

Cirrhosis of the liver

Background to disease

Unknown

Tongue description	Chinese diagnosis
Bluish red	Kidney yin deficiency with Liver blood stasis
Red sides	Liver qi constraint with heat in the Liver
Red, slightly curled-up tip	Heat in the Heart
White, slightly greasy coating	Accumulation of dampness

Fig. 8.1.4
Female
54 years old

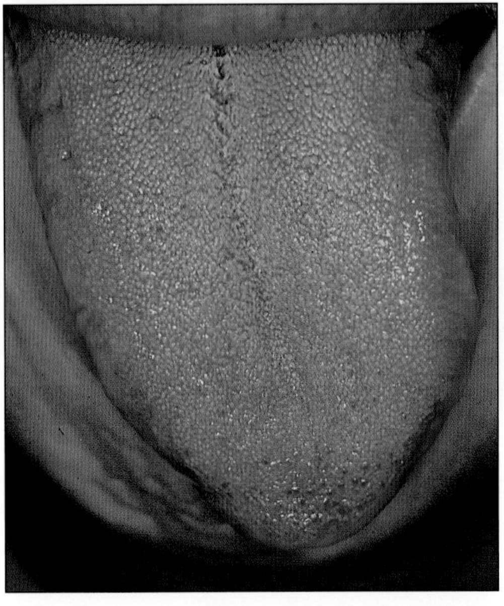

Symptoms

Edema of the left arm
Night sweats
Restlessness
Severe attacks of fear and irritability

Western diagnosis

Breast cancer

Background to disease

Condition followed radiation therapy and mastectomy
Repressed emotions

8.2 Partial Bluish Discoloration of the Tongue

Blood collects in every tissue and organ. Insufficient movement of qi through the organs, especially the Heart, Liver, Stomach, and Womb, contributes to the development of blood stasis. Occasionally, isolated bluish spots or points are visible on the tongue surface. They are a sure sign of blood stasis (Figs. 8.2.1 and 8.2.2). In this context, it is important to note that the location of the bluish spots on the tongue does not necessarily correspond to the area of blood stasis in the body.

Tongue signs

- red-blue tip of the tongue or bluish or dark red spots: long-standing heat contributes to blood stasis in the Heart
- pale bluish tongue or bluish or dark blackish spots: Heart yang deficiency leading to Heart blood stasis
- bluish discoloration on the sides of the tongue with a pale or pale red tongue body: long-standing Liver qi constraint leads to Liver blood stasis

Thus, Liver blood stasis can, on the one hand, cause sudden nosebleeds, and on the other hand, a delayed menstrual cycle. The Liver has a close relationship to the Conception and Penetrating vessels. Liver blood stasis may thus affect the functioning of these vessels, which will manifest as intense pain before and during menstrual bleeding. The same mechanism can be found in the formation of uterine fibroids, as these benign tumors correspond in Chinese medicine to congealed and stagnant blood. Distended sublingual veins and a dent at the tip of the tongue (see Section 6.1.2.) are, in my opinion, frequently seen tongue signs in women who suffer from this pathology. Interestingly enough, bluish discoloration of the sides of the tongue appears very seldom in these cases, even though this area does reflect Liver function, and the formation of uterine fibroids is strongly connected to Liver blood stasis and stagnation in the Penetrating vessel.

- red tongue body with bluish sides: heat in the Liver causing Liver blood stasis. In this case, heat thickens and clumps the blood. In patients with chronic hepatitis B or C, the sides of the tongue are frequently red and curled up because of the heat in the Liver. If the sides should take on a dark red or bluish color, the pattern of Liver blood stasis has developed in these patients. One study found that this often coincides with the beginning of cirrhotic changes in the liver cells.[4]

  Another investigation showed that blue areas on the side of the tongue point to liver pathology, but it is not possible to deduce from the appearance of blue spots that malignant tumors are present.[5] Nevertheless, one should note the intensity of the color of the blue spots as well as other signs to garner an indication of the severity of the illness.

- bluish center of the tongue: blood stasis in the Stomach

Tongue description	Chinese diagnosis
Pale and short	Spleen qi deficiency
Bluish tongue body	Blood stasis
Bluish area at one edge	Blood stasis
Slightly reddish tip	Heat from deficiency of the Heart
Light yellow, dry coating	Retention of damp-heat in the middle burner

Symptoms

Ulcer in the palate
Bluish discoloration of the nose and chin
Yellow-brownish scales inside the auricle with itchiness
Retrosternal pain on exertion
Exhaustion
Insomnia
Lack of appetite
Soft, smelly stools

Western diagnosis

Systemic lupus erythematosus

Background to disease

Abuse of caffeine, nicotine, and marijuana
Irregular lifestyle
Long-standing emotional problems
Overworked

Fig. 8.2.1
Female
33 years old

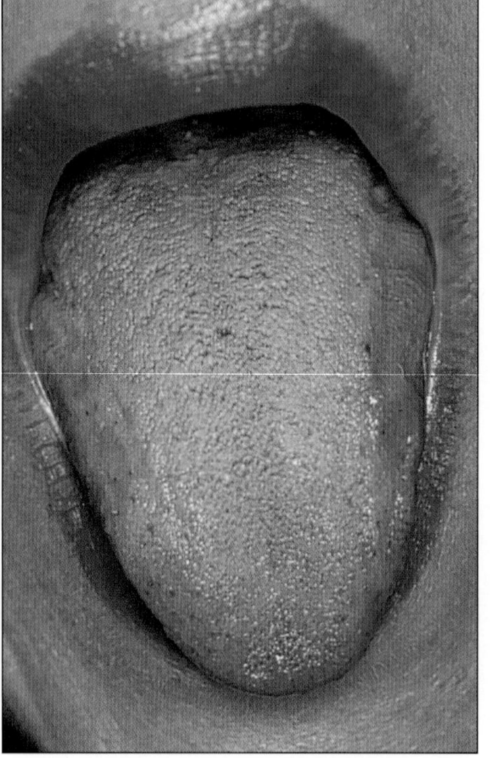

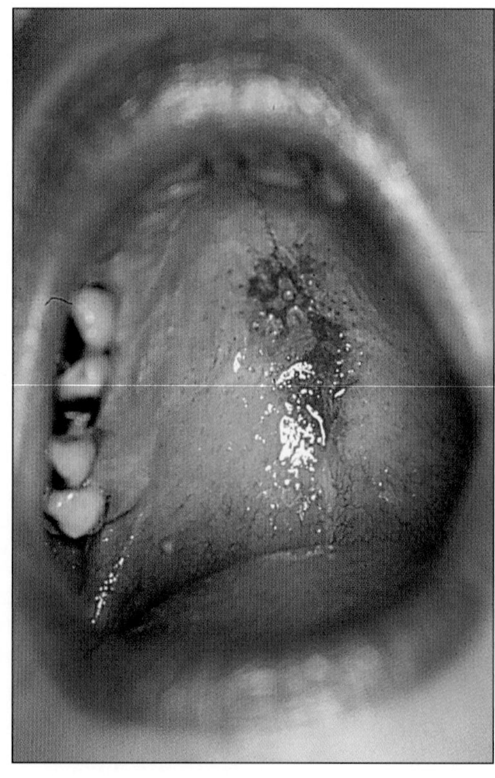

Tongue description	**Chinese diagnosis**
Pale red, bluish, slight teeth marks	Heart qi deficiency and blood stasis
Reddish blue sides on the posterior third	Heat in the Liver with blood stasis
Raised, dark red spot	Liver blood stasis

Symptoms

Constricted feeling in the chest
Shortness of breath with labored breathing and sweating, aggravated by stress and anger
Palpitations
Occasional stomach pains with epigastric fullness

Western diagnosis

Stenosis of the coronaries
Irregular cardiac rhythm

Background to disease

Excessive consumption of fatty foods
Repressed emotions

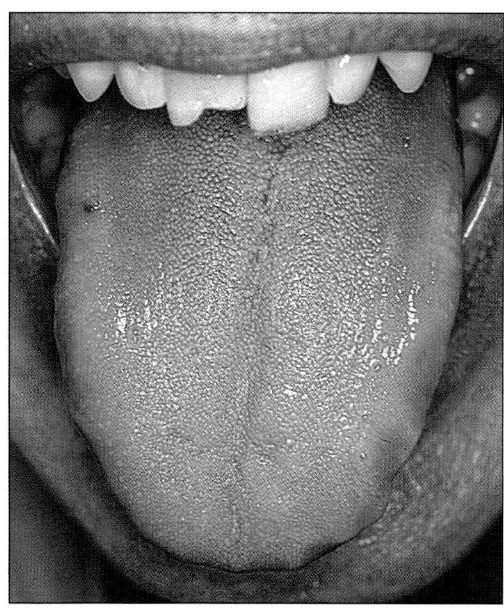

Fig. 8.2.2
Male
58 years old

Tongue description	**Chinese diagnosis**
Reddish, swollen	Retention of damp-heat in the middle and lower burners
Reddish-blue center of the tongue	Blood stasis in the Stomach
Thin vertical crack with small horizontal cracks	Slight Stomach yin deficiency
Left half of tongue swollen	Stagnation of qi, blood, and dampness in the channels

Symptoms

Heartburn
Stomach pains
Constipation or dry stools
Painful legs
Sleeping problems

Western diagnosis

Hiatus hernia
Chronic gastritis
Arterial obstruction of both lower legs

Background to disease

Excessive worry for many years
Excessive consumption of sweet and fatty foods

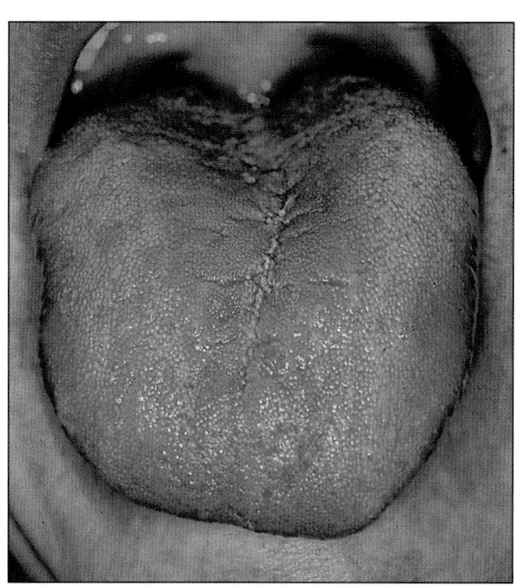

Fig. 8.2.3
Female
61 years old

Tongue description	Chinese diagnosis
Slightly pale	Spleen qi deficiency
Bluish tongue body	Blood stasis
Bluish spots on one edge	Blood stasis
Curled-up edges	Liver qi stagnation
Whitish, light yellow, greasy coating	Retention of phlegm

Symptoms

Stabbing pains in the chest
Cough with expectoration of thick, whitish phlegm
Sensation of heaviness of the body
Exhaustion
Lack of appetite
Hot lower legs and feet

Western diagnosis

None

Background to disease

Long-standing overwork
Improper Chinese herbal treatment

Fig. 8.2.4 Male 51 years old

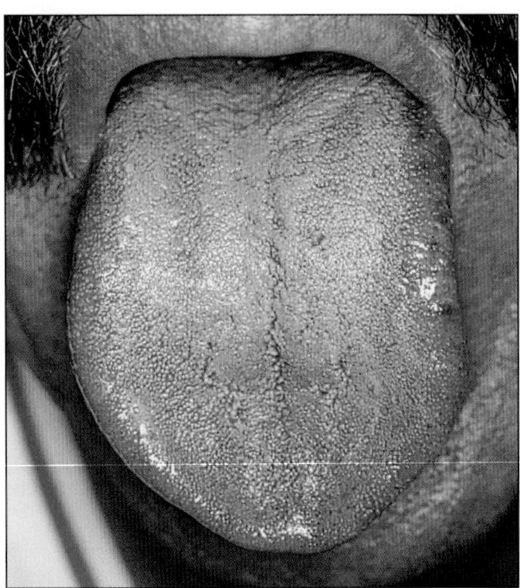

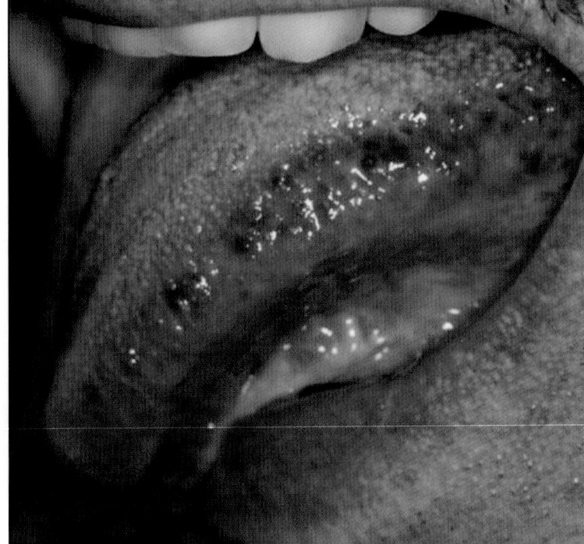

About this case history

This case was chosen not only to illustrate the outcome of improper treatment with Chinese herbs, but for the prominent markings (petechiae) at the edges of the tongue.

CASE HISTORY The patient, a massage therapist, had a strong build but was overweight. He had been taking Chinese herbs for a year to alleviate the sensation of heat in his lower legs and feet. A colleague had prescribed Six-Ingredient Pill with Rehmannia *(liù wèi dì huáng wán)*,[6] a prescription to enrich the Kidney yin. He took high doses in tablet form for about six months. During this time he felt worse. He developed a loud cough and expectorated profuse amounts of whitish, thick phlegm. He grew more and more tired, his body started to feel heavy, and his appetite declined. At the same time, he began to suffer from stabbing retrosternal pains at fairly regular intervals. There were no discernible factors that triggered the onset of this pain.

The patient's digestion was normal, although he indicated that he ate erratically and that he preferred creamy foods. He worked 14-hour days but loved his job. He would not rest and disliked holidays. He had a relaxed manner, but at the same time, there was an underlying tension. His pulse was slippery and strong.

Analysis. Hot lower legs and feet may develop from underlying Kidney yin deficiency. However, only when other signs and symptoms confirm this pattern of deficiency should Six-Ingredient

Pill with Rehmannia *(liù wèi dì huáng wán)* be prescribed. It contains rich, cloying ingredients to nourish the Kidney yin. If it is improperly prescribed, it may engender the development of phlegm, or aggravate existing phlegm, if taken for a long period of time. The misdiagnosis and subsequent treatment could have been avoided if the patient's tongue and pulse had been properly scrutinized. The tongue shows none of the characteristic signs of Kidney yin deficiency.

The curled-up edges denote constraint of Liver qi. The tongue body color is bluish and signals a sluggish movement of blood. The importance of the tongue color is underlined by numerous purple spots located on the edges, which reflect stasis of blood. It is important to note that although these spots appear at the edges, they do not automatically indicate a pattern of Liver blood stasis.

The episodic, sharp, stabbing pains behind the sternum are an indication of Heart blood stasis. Liver qi stagnation is often responsible for the development of blood stasis. How much the constraint of Liver qi is affecting the patient's attitude toward life, or vice versa, cannot be clearly determined. His work ethic does not allow him to truly relax, and this attitude constrains the free flow of qi.

Eventually the constraint of Liver qi will injure the Spleen, affecting the Spleen's transportive and transformative functions. As a result, phlegm will form, and this process is strengthened by the excessive consumption of phlegm-producing foods. In addition, taking rich Chinese herbs, in heavy doses, for a long period of time further aggravated this pathology. Phlegm impairs the circulation of yang qi, making it unable to expand. Phlegm collects in the interior and engenders heat; the patient's hot lower legs and feet are linked to this pathomechanism, not to that of Kidney yin deficiency. The sensation of heaviness in the body also originates from the accumulation of phlegm, which impairs the circulation of nutritive and protective qi through the muscles and body.

The tongue coating is whitish and greasy, reflecting the presence of phlegm. This finding is supported by the slippery pulse. There is an adage: "The Spleen produces phlegm; the Lungs store phlegm." Phlegm follows the qi and blocks the downward-directing action of the Lungs, resulting in a cough with thick phlegm. The accumulation of phlegm in the upper burner impairs the circulation of Heart yang, and subsequently of Heart blood. Together with the underlying Liver qi stagnation, this is responsible for the Heart blood stasis and resulting retrosternal pain.

The patient's exhaustion stems from chronic overwork and this contributes to the Spleen qi deficiency, which is responsible for his occasional loss of appetite. The Spleen qi deficiency,

Pathomechanism

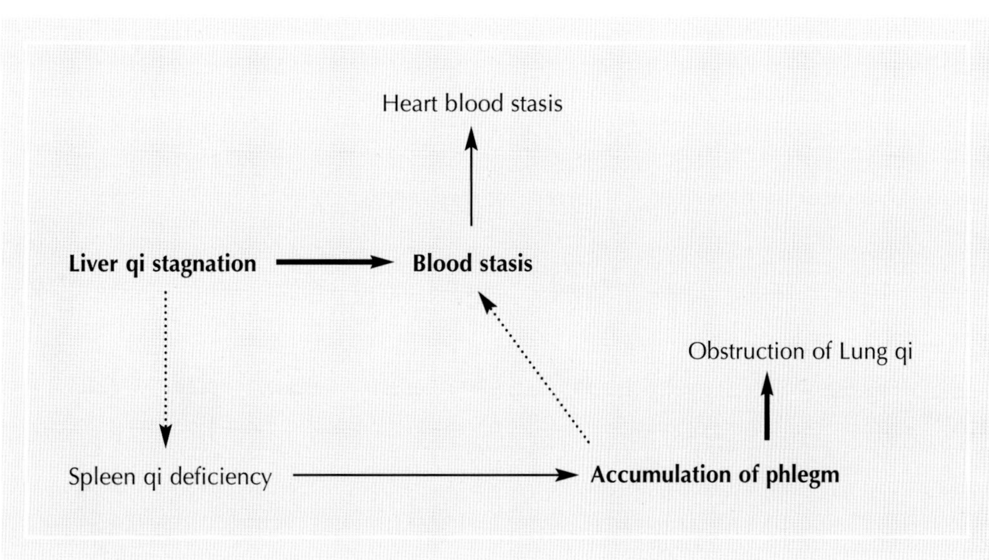

however, is not serious, which is reflected in the patient's ability to work 14 hours a day. In addition, his tongue does not have any signs that would indicate this pattern.

All the tongue signs primarily reflect a condition of excess. The spots at the edges, as well as the bluish discoloration, denote blood stasis; the curled-up edges indicate Liver qi stagnation; and the greasy coating signals an accumulation of phlegm. The only symptom associated with Heart blood stasis is the retrosternal pain. The regular occurrence of this pain underlines the necessity to consider all the aspects contributing to the development of blood stasis. The findings from the tongue are extremely important and must be taken into account when formulating a treatment strategy. Tonification is not the issue here; rather, the central concern is the transformation and elimination of phlegm and the regulation of qi and blood.

Treatment strategy. Transform the phlegm, regulate the Liver qi, invigorate the blood, and stop the coughing.

For two weeks the patient was prescribed Two-Cured Decoction *(èr chén tāng)* with the addition of Trichosanthis Fructus *(guā lóu)*, Inulae Flos *(xuán fù huā)*, Platycodi Radix *(jié gěng)*, Salviae miltiorrhizae Radix *(dān shēn)*, and Curcumae Radix *(yù jīn)*. He then felt better. The coughing and production of phlegm had decreased significantly. There was no retrosternal pain, he felt his energy returning, and his feet were less hot. The tongue body lost its bluish discoloration, but the bluish spots did not change. After three months of treatment with Chinese herbs and acupuncture, the patient felt very good. His feet were no longer hot, his appetite had normalized, he lost eight pounds, and his cough and chest pains had disappeared. However, the bluish spots on the tongue were still visible.

Three years later he returned for treatment, but burning feet were no longer a problem. He was very depressed and unhappy with his relationship. The petechiae on the tongue had almost disappeared.

8.3 Sublingual Veins

Examination of the sublingual veins is not mentioned in the classical literature. Evaluation of their significance in diagnosis is based on research that has occurred in China over the last thirty years. Clinical observation has shown that changes in the appearance of sublingual veins correlate to certain medically-defined illnesses, including coronary heart disease, cor pulmonale, high blood pressure, hepatitis, and cancer.[7]

With many patients, even if they suffer from severe organic illness, the surface of the tongue may be completely normal, which implies that the tongue body does not always reflect the severity of an illness. Even when the tongue does not show any significant pathological change, a pattern of blood stasis is often reflected by pathological deviations in the sublingual veins, especially when blood stasis plays a major role in the illness (Figs. 8.2.1 and 8.2.2). Examination of the sublingual veins is therefore essential in order to determine a pattern of blood stasis.

As previously noted, the tongue surface can be divided into three zones. Deviations in any of these zones may indicate disharmonies in a particular organ. It is tempting to do the same for the sublingual veins. However, the research does not provide any solid correlation between specific zones on the sublingual veins and particular organs. Nevertheless, in a lecture some years ago, Prof. Zhang Bo Li stated that "If the sublingual veins reach the tip of the tongue, it is often indicative of heart disease."[8] Distended sublingual veins appearing during the course of heart disease are frequently mentioned in contemporary literature. This corresponds to the findings of Western medicine where distended sublingual veins are explained as the result of a reduced backflow of venous blood during, for example, right-heart insufficiency.[9]

When examining the nature of the distended sublingual veins, assumptions concerning the localization of the blood stasis in the body should only be made after many years of clinical experience. In the interest of the patient, the practitioner should be very cautious. At this point, I want to emphasize that the mere existence of distended sublingual veins is *not* an automatic indication of severe organic disease.

Normal sublingual veins, which are situated lateral to the frenulum under the tongue, have a light blue color. They are thin, and their lengths should not measure more than three-fifths of the entire length of the underside of the tongue.[10]

In order to examine the sublingual veins, the patient should be asked to curl the tip of the tongue lightly upward, and, without great exertion, gently touch the palate. The length, form, color, and degree of distention of the veins should be noted. The appearance of small venules as well as red capillaries that may cover the underside of the tongue should also be noted. Some pathological manifestations of distended sublingual veins include:

- very long and blue (Figs. 8.3.1)
- light blue, thick, and soft (Fig. 8.3.5)
- dark blue, thick, and strongly filled (Fig. 8.3.2)
- winding, uneven, and filled with varicose-like veins (Fig. 8.3.3)

Different grades of severity can be used when evaluating the nature of the distention and length of the sublingual veins:[11]

- only slightly filled and slightly blue
- only filled in the proximal part
- filled over the entire length of the underside of tongue
- extremely filled and dark blue

The presence of pathologically-changed sublingual veins in general reflects a pattern of blood stasis. Sublingual veins that are darker and thicker are of greater consequence. There is general agreement that distended sublingual veins in the elderly are less significant than in the young.

When blood stasis and phlegm unite, the veins often look soft and thick; occasionally, they will have a shiny appearance (Fig. 8.3.5). If the blood stasis has developed as a result of heat in the body there will be dark blue, distended veins or red capillaries at the edges of the underside of the tongue. Red capillaries, especially when they appear to be slightly raised, denote pathological heat in the interior of the body.

The presence of a dark petechia—a nonraised purplish-red spot lateral to the sublingual veins—is an indication of active heart disease or of masses. Occasionally, small, distended venules that branch off from the sublingual veins are seen. They can indicate a profound pattern of blood stasis (Fig. 8.3.1).

To summarize, the shape, length, color, and degree of distention of the sublingual veins, as well as the age of the patient, must be considered when interpreting the extent of a possible pathology that includes blood stasis. The sublingual veins do not necessarily reflect an active or even serious disease process (see Fig. 8.3.2) and should always be viewed in the context of the other signs and symptoms.[12] From the perspective of Chinese medicine, it must be emphasized that any statement about the formation of lumps, or even cancer, cannot be made on the basis of tongue diagnosis alone.

Tongue description	Chinese diagnosis
Pale red	Normal
Slight teeth marks	Accumulation of dampness
Red points at the tip	Invasion of heat[13]
Light yellow, greasy, thick coating	Retention of phlegm with transformation of phlegm-heat in the Stomach
Dark blue, thin, distended sublingual veins with singular stasis spots	Blood stasis

Symptoms

Pain in the thoracic and lumbar spine
Exhaustion
Weight gain
Feeling of fullness in the abdomen
Depressive moods
Lymphatic edema of the left arm

Western diagnosis

Breast cancer with bone metastases

Background to disease

Long-standing repressed emotions
Excessive consumption of fatty foods

Fig. 8.3.1
Female
52 years old

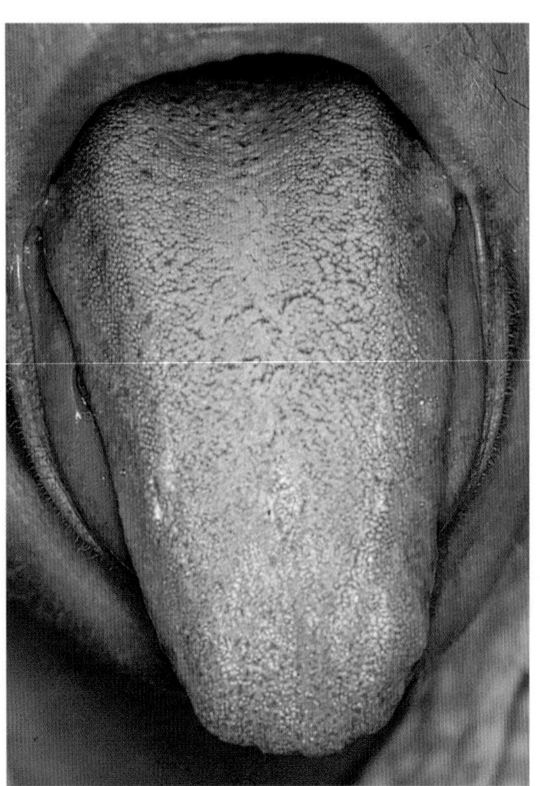

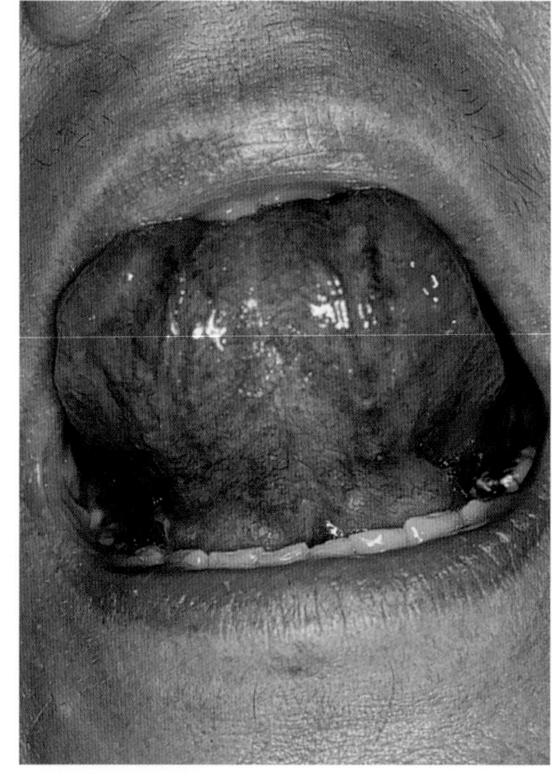

Tongue description	**Chinese diagnosis**
Pale	Spleen qi deficiency
Slightly pale edges	Liver blood deficiency
Deep depression at the root	Deficiency of Kidney essence
Blue, distended sublingual veins	Blood stasis

Symptoms

Sweating during the day and night
Hot flushes
Sleeping problems
Strong thirst
Weight gain

Background to disease

Hysterectomy to remove uterine fibroids
Taking of estrogen between the ages of 45 and 52
Condition after chemotherapy and radiation
Side effects of antiestrogens
Overwork

Western diagnosis

Breast cancer, hypercholesterolemia, hyperlipidemia

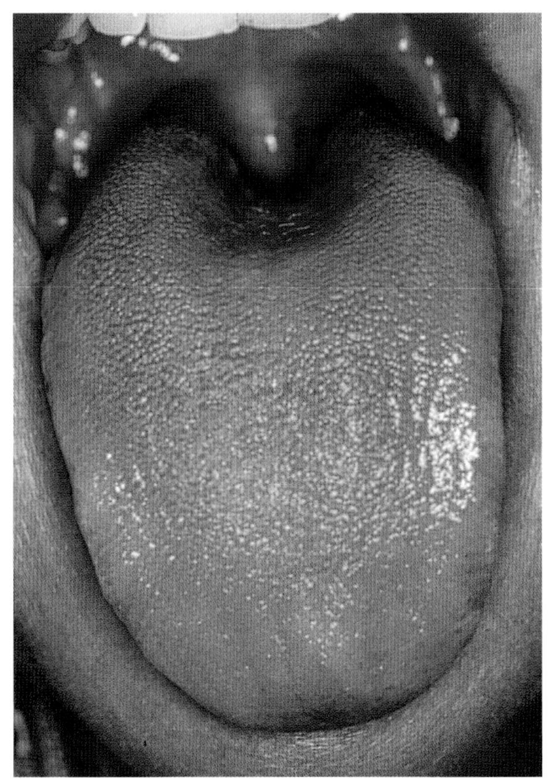

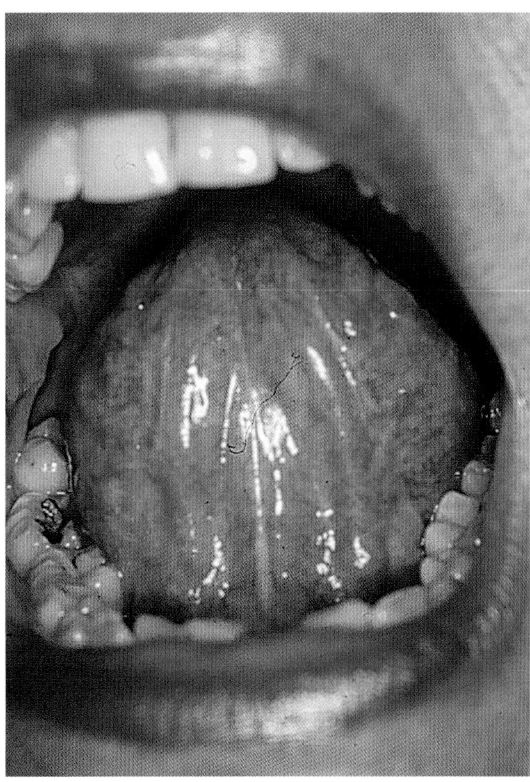

Fig. 8.3.2
Female
53 years old

Tongue description	Chinese diagnosis
Pale	Spleen qi deficiency
Slightly reddish tip	Heat in the Heart
Slight indentation of the tip	Heart blood deficiency
White, greasy coating	Accumulation of phlegm
Blue, distended, varicose sublingual veins	Blood stasis

Symptoms

Strong pains in the chest
Feeling of tightness in the chest
Difficulty breathing and shortness of breath
Exhaustion
Difficulty falling asleep

Western diagnosis

Angina pectoris

Background to disease

Sixty years of hard physical labor

Fig. 8.3.3
Female
80 years old

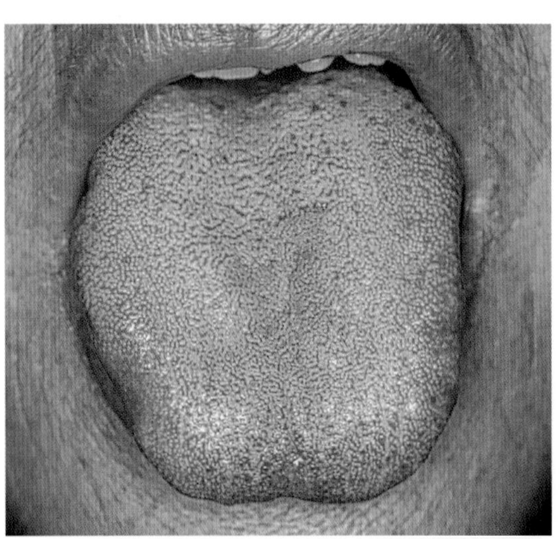

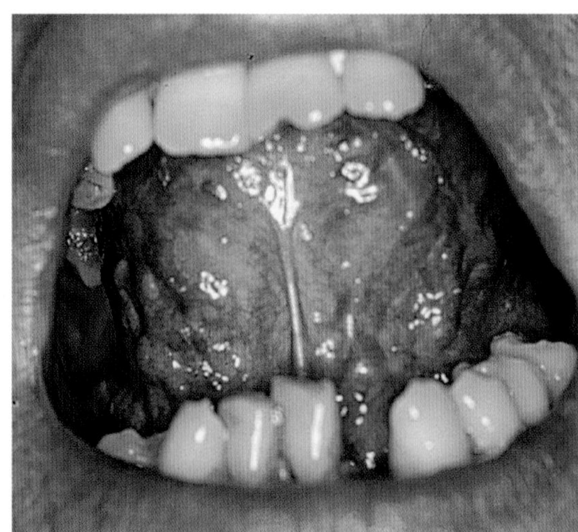

Tongue description	Chinese diagnosis
Dark red, small, *shiny*	Lung, Stomach, and Kidney yin deficiency
Dark purple sublingual veins with dark spots	Severe blood stasis in the upper burner

Symptoms

Dry cough
Night sweats
Low-grade fever, intense feeling of heat in the body
Labored breathing and shortness of breath
Exhaustion

Western diagnosis

Chronic bronchitis
Emphysema

Background to disease

Heavy smoking for 60 years

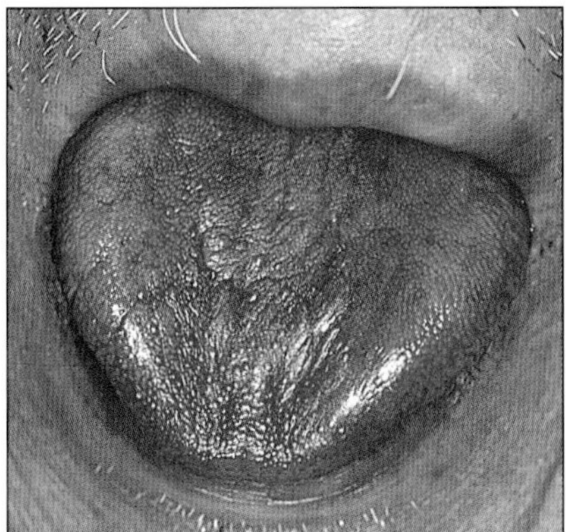

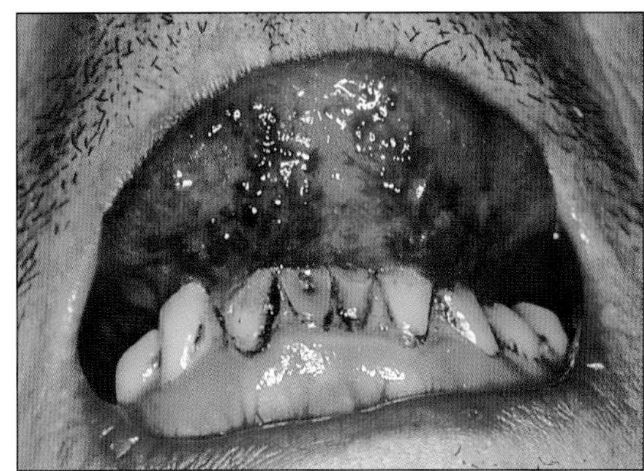

Fig. 8.3.4
Male
83 years old

Tongue description

Red tongue body

Red edges

Whitish coating in the center and yellow, thick, and greasy coating toward the root

Well-defined peeled areas in the coating

Blue, distended, shiny sublingual veins

Chinese diagnosis

Developing heat

Liver fire

Retention of damp-heat in the Liver and Gallbladder

Heat in the Stomach, Heart fire[14]

Blood stasis with retention of damp-heat

Symptoms

Pain and pressure under the right rib
Yellow discoloration of the sclera
Smelly diarrhea
Restlessness
Fits of anger

Western diagnosis

Gilbert's disease[15]

Background to disease

Family history of Gilbert's disease, abuse of alcohol

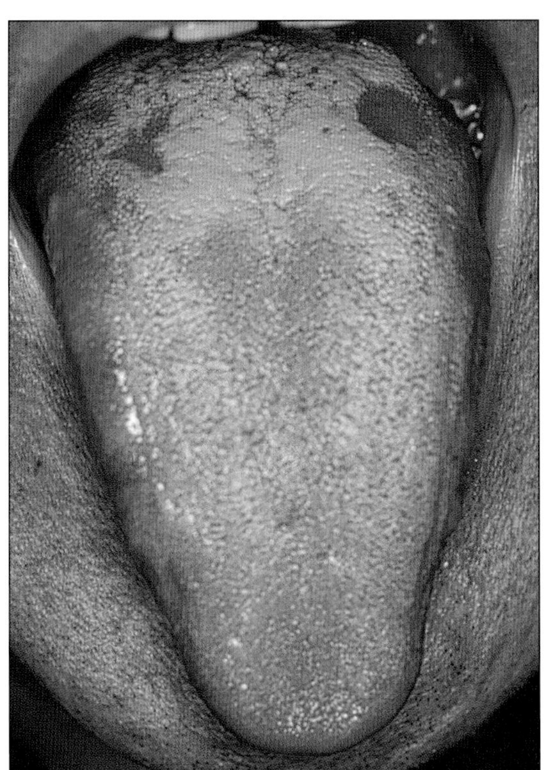

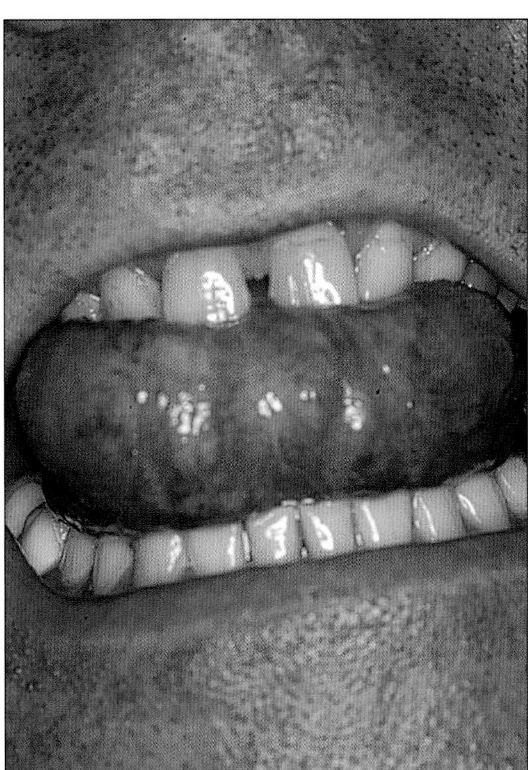

Fig. 8.3.5
Male
52 years old

About this case history

Liver fire is, in this patient (Fig. 8.3.5), responsible for the development of damp-heat as well as for Liver blood stasis. Here the distended sublingual veins have a very distinct shiny appearance, which very often is a telltale sign for hyperlipidemia.

CASE HISTORY The patient was diagnosed with Gilbert's disease. He complained of daily pains and a feeling of pressure in the right hypochondriac region. His liver enzyme levels were not elevated, but his bilirubin was raised. This manifested in a yellow discoloration of the sclera. The patient felt quite sick because of the feeling of pressure in the epigastric region. He also had daily diarrhea, which was very smelly.

The patient was dissatisfied with his personal and professional life. He occasionally experienced fits of anger and rage, and was always irritable. He calmed himself with alcohol. His appetite, thirst, and sleep were normal. His pulse was full and floating.

Analysis. Two cases of Gilbert's disease had occurred in the patient's family. Its symptoms are essentially diffuse epigastric pain, yellow discoloration of the sclera, and occasional lethargy. In Chinese medicine the yellow discoloration of the sclera is attributable to the accumulation of damp-heat in the Liver and Gallbladder. Because of this family history, it is possible that the patient has a constitutional disposition to damp-heat. The yellow, thick coating, which mainly covers the posterior third of the tongue, reflects an accumulation of damp-heat.

According to the classic tome on eye diseases,[16] yellow discoloration of the sclera may be caused by the following mechanism: "This is [caused by] the poison of wine. Wine can stimulate yang [qi]. If one drinks without moderation, the spleen conduit will receive dampness and this will harm both the liver and the gallbladder. This [in turn] incites the fire, and the fire harms the lung conduit. The white part of the eye is associated with the lung. This way an excess of wine causes the white part of the eyes to become yellow or red. [Too much] wine induces the blood to harm the liver. The liver receives the heat of the blood which rises from [there] upward toward the eyes. The eyes receive the heat-poison of the wine … and become yellow or red."

While this passage refers to the effects of overindulgence in alcohol, in this case the genetic predisposition of the patient makes it worse. Accumulation of damp-heat in the Liver and Gallbladder obstructs the flow of qi and blood in their corresponding channels, causing the localized pain and feeling of pressure under the right rib. This pattern is strengthened by the patient's alcohol abuse. Damp-heat and alcohol engender Liver fire, which in turn furthers the development of Liver blood stasis. Since the Liver fire injures the body fluids, the blood is not sufficiently thinned and becomes more viscous, which impairs its movement.

Pathomechanism

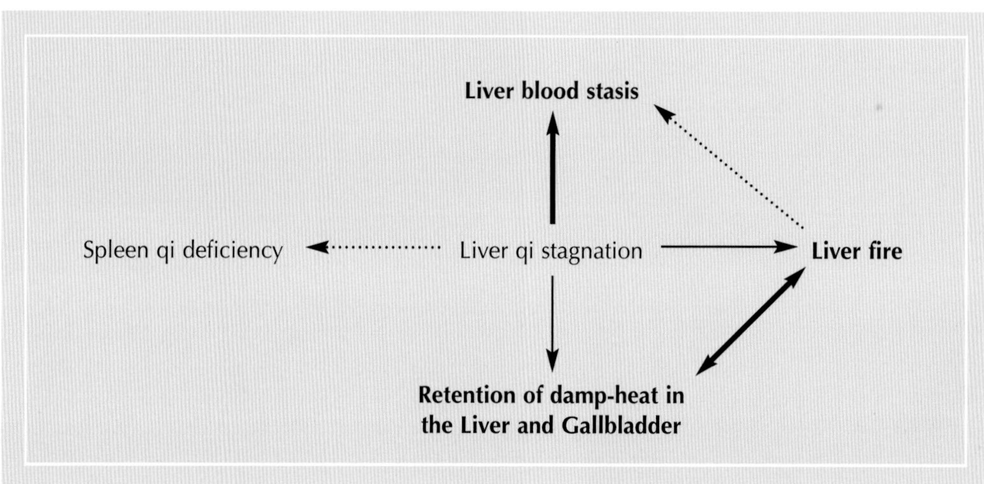

The sublingual veins are distended only at the proximal end of the underside of the tongue. In this case, they are strongly filled and shiny, signaling the presence of damp-heat. The combination of the localized, constant pain and the sublingual veins probably denotes an early stage in the development of blood stasis. This tongue sign is noteworthy since it underlines the need to invigorate the blood during treatment. In addition, the underside of the tongue is very red, which reflects the intense internal heat.

The well-defined peeled areas in the coating at the root of the tongue signal the presence of intense internal heat. This may also be interpreted as a sign of Heart fire. Pathogenic heat is also reflected in the red edges of the tongue, characteristic of Liver fire. The restlessness of the patient is due to Liver fire attacking the Heart.

The patient's discontent and irritability suggest stagnation of Liver qi, which is another causative factor here in the development of Liver fire. In this case, the patient's irritability leads to fits of anger and rage. This behavior occurs frequently when constrained Liver qi evolves into Liver fire. The full and floating qualities of the pulse reflect the excessive nature of the condition. The constraint of Liver qi and the accumulation of damp-heat impair the digestive functions of the Spleen and Stomach qi, which results in the feeling of pressure in the epigastric region. In addition, the damp-heat sinks into the lower burner where it is responsible for the soft, smelly stools.

Treatment strategy. Drain the fire from the Liver, drain the damp-heat from the Liver, Gallbladder, and lower burner, and regulate and invigorate the Liver qi and blood.

A modified version of Coptis Decoction to Resolve Toxicity *(huáng lián jiě dú tāng)* was prescribed with the addition of high doses of Curcumae Radix *(yù jīn)*. The patient took the decoction for three weeks and felt much calmer. His diarrhea, however, had improved only slightly. He is continuing with the treatment.

Endnotes

1 See Li N-M. *Zhong guo she zhen da quan.* Beijing: Xueyuan Publishing Company, 1994:1190. The appearance of a blue tongue is found in the following illnesses: colon cancer, liver cancer, stomach cancer, cirrhosis of the liver with ascites, and malignant tumors in the peritoneum.

2 "When the movement of blood in the channels and collaterals is merely impaired or sluggish, but not yet at a standstill, the condition may be termed blood stagnation (*xuè zhì*). However, if for various etiological reasons the flow of blood becomes more completely blocked or static, the condition is termed blood stasis (*xuè yū*)." Bensky D and Barolet R. *Chinese Herbal Medicine: Formulas & Strategies.* Seattle: Eastland Press, 1990: 311.

3 An alternative interpretation of this coating is obstruction of the channels and collaterals by externally-contracted damp-cold.

4 See Chen Z, Chen M-F. *The Essence and Scientific Background of Tongue Diagnosis.* Long Beach, CA: Oriental Healing Arts Institute, 1989:38. An investigation was described wherein 76 patients with primary liver cell carcinoma were examined. The orthodox medical findings were compared with TCM diagnosis. From a Chinese medical point of view, the cause of disease was diagnosed as mainly Liver blood stasis. In 59 of these patients (77%), the tongue showed the so-called 'Liver cancer line,' a bluish or crimson line located at the sides of the tongue, or bluish patches on the tongue.

5 Li, 1202. An investigation was described whereby patients were included in a study if they had bluish spots or patches at the sides of their tongues, suffered from an organic liver illness, or were ill from a malignant disease. Subjects included those with acute and

chronic hepatitis, cirrhosis of the liver, liver cell carcinoma, or metastases of the liver. In all cases of acute hepatitis, no bluish discoloration was found. Ten percent of patients with chronic hepatitis had them. However, 40% of the patients with liver cell carcinoma and 100% (three patients) of the patients with metastases of the liver had bluish areas. Those who suffered from malignant diseases other than in the liver did not have the blue discoloration, and only 0.9% of those with non-malignant diseases showed the discoloration.

6 *Chinese Herbal Medicine: Formulas & Strategies*, 263.

7 Li N-M. *Zhong guo she zhen da quan* [Compendium of Chinese Tongue Diagnosis]. Beijing: Xueyuan Press (1994): 1370. Chen Z and Chen M-F. *The Essence and Scientific Background of Tongue Diagnosis*. Long Beach, CA: Oriental Healing Arts Institute, 1989: 96-97.

8 Prof. Zhong Bo Li, "Diagnosis of Sublingual Veins in Chinese Medicine." Lecture presented at the 31st Congress for TCM in Rothenburg, Germany, 2001.

9 Beaven DE and Brooks SE. *Color Atlas of the Tongue in Clinical Diagnosis*. London: Wolfe Medical Publications, 1988.

10 Prof. Zhong Bo Li, ibid.

11 Ibid.

12 This volume presents pictures and case histories where patterns of blood stasis play a role in the development of cancerous illness (Figs. 4.1.2.9, 8.3.1, 8.3.2). The tongue bodies of these patients do not show blue spots or areas. One may therefore conclude that disease processes are not necessarily reflected on the tongue body. In some, a pattern of blood stasis is signaled by distended sublingual veins.

Knots and lumps are always a manifestation of the gathering or accumulation of 'material.' Blood stasis, and the accumulation of phlegm, are important factors in their formation. The tongue body often indicates which of the two is more important in the disease process, or it may point to the root of the disease. Blood stasis, and the accumulation of fluids or phlegm, are manifestations of a disease, while the root is either stagnation of qi and yang deficiency, Kidney yin deficiency, or pathogenic heat.

The third factor involved in the formation of malignant lumps is the presence of heat toxin. It penetrates to the deepest layers, including the internal organs of the body. Viral infections can contribute to the development of heat toxin, for example, the hepatitis C virus can cause liver cell carcinoma, HIV can lead to Kaposi sarcoma, and HPV can cause carcinoma of the cervix.

13 The patient had just finished a course of radiation therapy directed toward the left breast. Occasionally, radiation therapy results in heat signs in the anterior third of the tongue body.

14 Chen M-L et al. *Gu jin tu shu ji cheng, yi bu quan lu* [Collection of Writings Past and Present: Complete Medical Section], vol. 5. Beijing: Peoples Medical Publishing House, 1995: 84.

15 Also called Gilbert's syndrome. It is an inborn error of bilirubin metabolism with apparently no liver damage or hematologic abnormalities.

16 Anonymous. *Essential Subtleties on the Silver Sea, Yin hai jing wei*, translated by Kovacs J and Unschuld P. Berkeley: University of California Press, 1998: 305.

CHAPTER 9

Tongue Signs Associated with Heat Disorders

Externally-contracted wind-heat enters the body through the nose and mouth. The symptoms include fever, sore throat, headaches, and thirst. Often acute, externally-contracted wind-heat penetrates directly into the Lungs where it impairs the Lung qi, which manifests in a cough. At the onset of such an illness, the tongue has a thin white or yellow coating. A floating, rapid pulse is another sign of wind-heat attacking the outer protective layer of the body. Tongue diagnosis is extremely helpful in acute disorders that result from wind-heat or epidemic heat. As a rule, pathogenic heat, especially when it penetrates to the inside, manifests as a yellow discoloration of the tongue coating and/or as red points on the tongue body. The location and degree of redness of the red points and papillae are noteworthy. In this context, the anterior third of the tongue body reflects the condition of the upper burner, the middle third reflects the condition of the middle burner, and the posterior third reflects the condition of the lower burner.

9.1 Red Points at the Tip of the Tongue

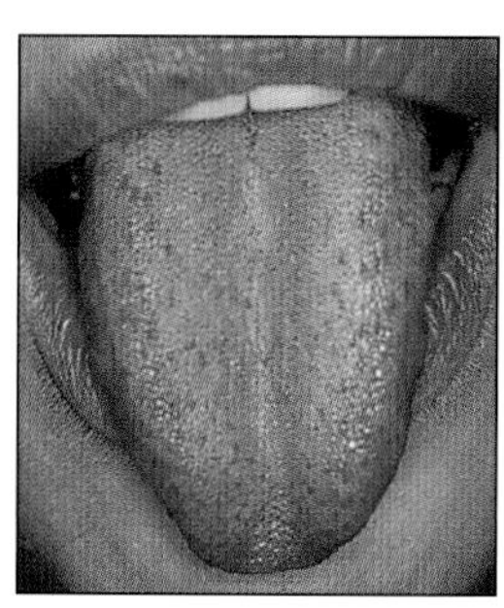

Fig. 6.1.4.6

Red points at the tip of the tongue can be a sign of externally-contracted wind-heat or toxic heat. These red, 'rough-grained' points often herald the beginning of a cold, and are occasionally visible one or two days before the onset of the illness. They should not be confused with points that reflect heat in the Heart. In the latter case, the points tend to be positioned very closely to each other, rather like fine-grained sand, are less raised, and are of a light red color; they can, however, evolve to a deep red color (Fig. 6.1.4.6). By contrast, the red points associated with external wind-heat or toxic heat tend to be bigger, more raised, and of a darker red color. And because they are positioned wider apart from each other, the points have a rough-grained look. While the points indicating heat in the Heart are only visible at the tip of the tongue, those indicative of externally-contracted wind-heat extend over the entire anterior third of the tongue. And if heat toxin is present, they may extend even further, occasionally covering the entire tongue body.

Tongue signs

- reddening of anterior third of the tongue or red points: strong wind-heat pathogen (Fig. 9.1.6)

  Bright red points in this area indicate the rapid development of a severe sore throat and an infection of the upper respiratory tract (Fig. 9.1.1). In this example, the red points remain only in the anterior third and do not expand toward the middle portion of the tongue; their distribution, as well as the fresh red discoloration, denotes an acute disorder that has not yet penetrated deeply.
- red points spreading to the middle portion of the tongue body (Fig. 9.1.3) or over the entire tongue body (Fig. 9.1.5): intense external heat with transformation into heat toxin

  Bright red points on the anterior third of the tongue are frequently found in people suffering from allergic rhinitis and/or allergic asthma (Fig. 9.1.8). Often, these red points emerge weeks before an actual acute spell. Occasionally they remain for months without acute symptoms being present. Here, the tongue sign indicates a remnant of heat that can be triggered when pathogenic factors invade the body.
- very red, big, and raised or thorn-like points: accumulation of heat toxin (Fig. 9.1.6)

  Since this type of heat is considerably stronger and often more aggressive than externally-contracted wind-heat, the tongue signs are accordingly more pronounced.
- red points distributed over the entire tongue body: accumulation of heat toxin (Fig. 9.1.5)
- red points with a yellow, greasy tongue coating: damp-heat or phlegm-heat contribute to the development of heat toxin (Fig. 9.1.7)

In general, red points on the tongue are important signs denoting heat in different layers of the body. Their degree of redness, size, texture, and location are important, as is the underlying color of the tongue. If red points appear on a red tongue body, as opposed to a pale tongue body, a more rapid development of heat in the deeper layers (i.e., in the organs) and subsequent injury to fluids should be expected. Red points and a yellow, thick, greasy coating point toward the development and transformation of heat into heat toxin.

In Fig. 9.1.2, the red, raised points are more significant than the slightly pale and swollen tongue body since the color and shape of the tongue body relate to the underlying constitution of the patient and not to the acute disorder. Evaluation of the constitution, however, is still important as it may determine how quickly the pathogenic factors will penetrate into the deeper levels and the extent to which they might injure the fluids.

A comparison of Figs. 9.1.1 and 9.1.5 highlights the differences that can be found in the appearance of the red points. The patient in Fig. 9.1.1 has an acute sore throat and difficulty swallowing. The disorder is not yet severe, as shown by the red points that are only located in the anteior third of the tongue, and are not raised. In Fig. 9.1.5, the red points are raised and distributed over the entire tongue body, indicating a greater intensity and deeper penetration of the pathogenic heat.

Tongue description	**Chinese diagnosis**
Pale, swollen	Spleen qi deficiency with blood deficiency and accumulation of dampness
Red points at the tip and anterior third	Acute, externally-contracted wind-heat

Symptoms

Fever
Sore throat
Severe pain upon swallowing
Cough

Western diagnosis

Acute cold

Background to disease

Lack of sleep
Overwork

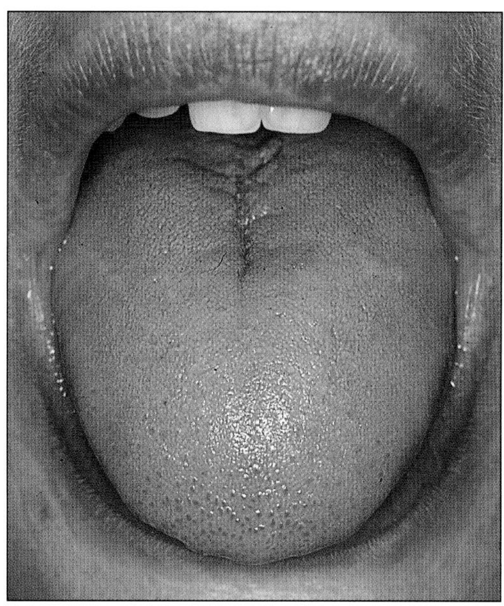

Fig. 9.1.1
Female
37 years old

Tongue description	**Chinese diagnosis**
Pale red	Normal
Thin	Slight blood deficiency
Red points on the anterior third	Acute, externally-contracted wind-heat
White, thin, and moist coating	Early, superficial stage of warm-febrile disease

Symptoms

Sore throat with difficulty swallowing
Red throat
Slight headache
Feeling of malaise
Fear of the illness

Western diagnosis

None

Background to disease

Lack of full recovery from previous infections
Inclined to overwork
Unresolved emotions regarding death of family members

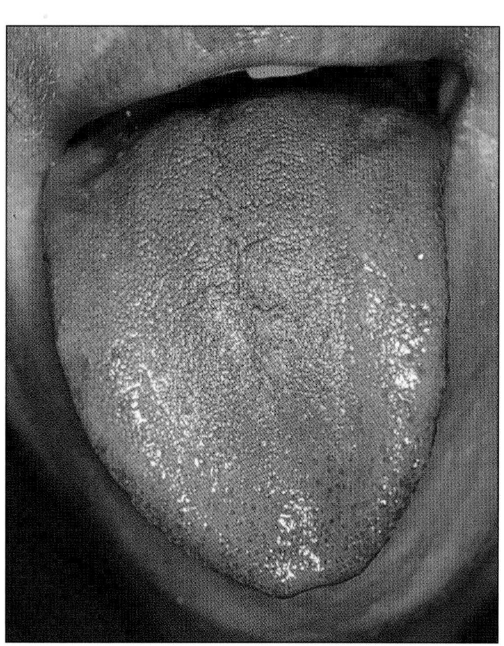

Fig. 9.1.2
Female
37 years old

Tongue description	Chinese diagnosis
Pale, swollen, teeth marks	Spleen qi deficiency (accumulation of dampness in the middle burner)
White and thick in the center with light yellow coating	Accumulation of damp-phlegm
Bright red, raised points at the tip and sides	Acute, externally-contracted wind-heat, damp-heat transforming into toxic heat

Fig. 9.1.3
Female
32 years old

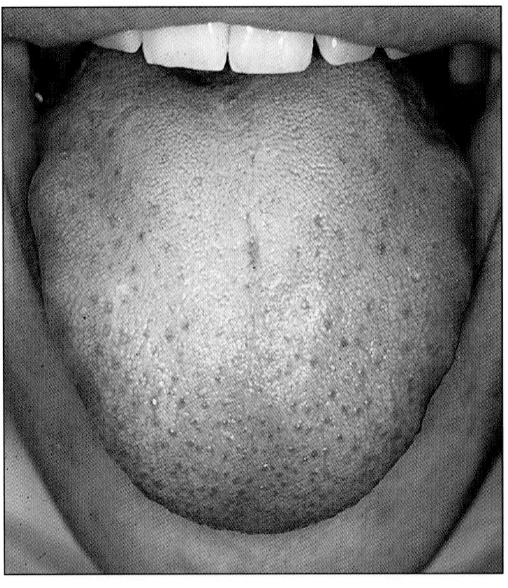

Symptoms

Severe sore throat with strong feeling of malaise
Tendency to catch colds
Cough with yellow, thick phlegm
Exhaustion

Western diagnosis

Chronic tonsillitis

Background to disease

Excessive physical training as a dancer
Dancing in cold working conditions while sweating
Irregular eating habits
Excessive consumption of raw foods

Tongue description	Chinese diagnosis
Red, swollen	Heat in the blood and accumulation of dampness
Deep vertical crack in the center of the tongue with light yellow, dry coating	Stomach yin deficiency with heat in the Stomach
Two localized, rootless, round patches[1]	Heat in the Stomach, penetration of heat toxin into the center of the tongue
Deep red, raised points at tip and red points at the sides	Accumulation of heat toxin

Fig. 9.1.4
Female
29 years old

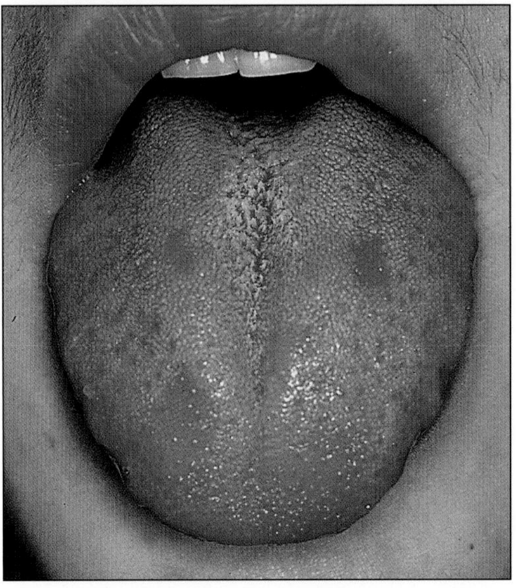

Symptoms

Frequent formation of furuncles with pus and blood
Muscle aches
Night sweats
Tiredness

Western diagnosis

Lead poisoning

Background to disease

Lead poisoning

Tongue description	Chinese diagnosis
Pale red, swollen	Slight Spleen qi deficiency (accumulation of dampness)
Light red and brownish raised points over the entire tongue body	Accumulation of heat toxin
White, thin coating at the sides, light yellow, thick coating in the center	Externally-contracted dampness penetrating to the interior
Yellow, greasy coating at the root	Retention of damp-heat in the lower burner

Symptoms

Nonspecific feeling of malaise
Burning of the tongue
Occasional feelings of internal cold
Tiredness
Inner tension

Western diagnosis

None

Background to disease

Possible food poisoning by crabmeat

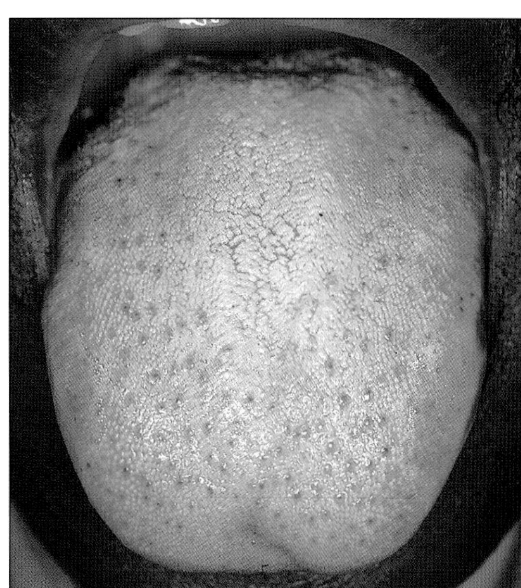

Fig. 9.1.5
Male
31 years old

Tongue description	Chinese diagnosis
Pale red	Normal
Deviated	Internally-generated wind
Pointed shape with red tip	Heat in the Heart
Red, big, raised points at the anterior third and the sides	Long-standing toxic heat lodging in the interior, possibly Liver fire
Light yellow, thick, greasy coating	Accumulation of phlegm-heat

Symptoms

Severe headaches at the vertex that worsen upon exertion
Tight neck muscles
Inner restlessness

Western diagnosis

None

Background to disease

Condition arose after contracting viral meningitis in 1968 and 1988

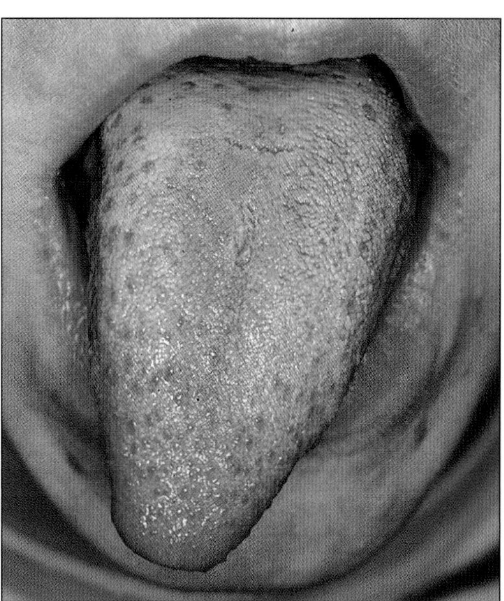

Fig. 9.1.6
Female
31 years old

Tongue description	Chinese diagnosis
Pale red, bluish	Blood stasis
Pale patches at the sides	Liver blood deficiency
Red points over entire tongue body	Long-standing heat toxin lodging in the interior
Red, big, slightly raised points on the anterior and middle thirds	Long-standing accumulation of heat toxin
Dark yellow, dry coating	Accumulation of damp-heat in the lower burner transforming into heat toxin

Fig. 9.1.7
Female
39 years old

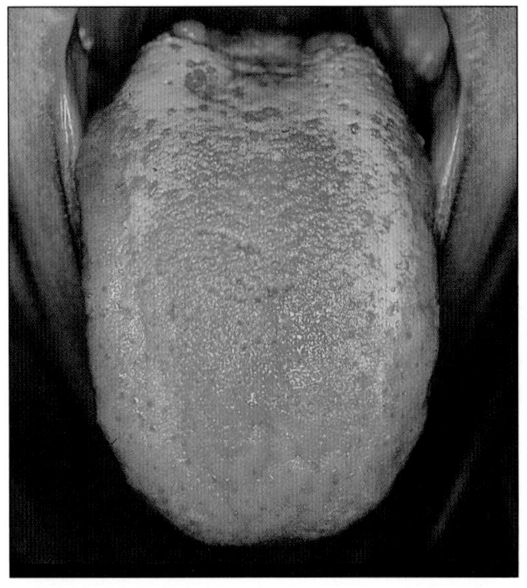

Symptoms

Explosive, foul-smelling diarrhea after eating
Nausea
Thick, yellow vaginal discharge
Extremely profuse menstrual bleeding
Short menstrual cycle

Western diagnosis

Suffered 15 years from anorexia nervosa
Underweight

Background to disease

Prolonged sexual abuse in childhood
Many operations due to injuries of the genitals
Abuse of nicotine, black tea, and chocolate

Tongue description	Chinese diagnosis
Red	Heat in the blood
Red, raised, large points in the anterior and middle third	Acute, externally-contracted wind-heat
Whitish, thin, and dry coating in the center	Onset of injury to the fluids

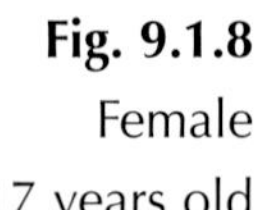

Fig. 9.1.8
Female
17 years old

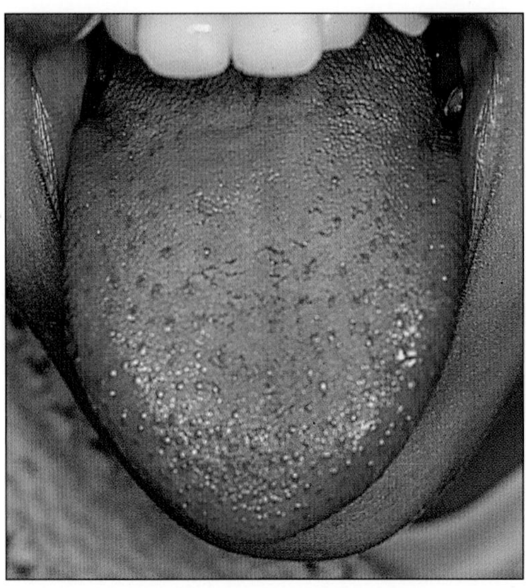

Symptoms

Difficulty breathing, tightness of the chest
Shortness of breath
Red, itchy eyes
Sneezing fits
Blocked nasal breathing

Western diagnosis

Allergic rhinitis, allergic asthma

Background to disease

Family history of allergies

CASE HISTORY Three years prior to visiting the clinic, the patient developed an allergic reaction to cats; prior to that incident, she never had such a reaction. A thorough medical work-up revealed allergies to various grasses, animal hair, and house mites. Allergic rhinitis was a common trait in her mother's family, and her condition began when her parents were divorcing, which had made her very sad. The initial symptom was sneezing that turned into a runny nose. The nasal secretion was white and slightly viscous. Slowly, the symptoms of the patient worsened. Frequently, her nose felt dry, her nasal breathing was blocked, and she developed a persistent, irritable, dry cough. She complained of tightness in the chest and difficulty breathing. Her symptoms were only relieved when she used bronchodilators. She also suffered from red, itchy eyes.

At the age of 16, a gynecologic examination revealed that she had an unusually small uterus and underdeveloped ovaries. She was given hormones that induced her first menstruation. In the main, she felt quite well. Her pulse was floating and rapid.

Analysis. This case is an example of an attack by wind-heat that impairs the Lung function of inducing the qi and fluids to descend and disperse. The raised, red points in the anterior and middle part of the tongue reflect the strength of the external wind-heat. Since the red points extend as far as the center of the tongue, they can be clearly differentiated from those that merely indicate a disturbance associated with the Heart. Acute heat is signaled by the fresh red color of the points, and its intensity is reflected in the quality of the raised papillae. The coating is whitish, thin, and dry, and covers the middle part of the tongue body. The location of the coating indicates that the heat has started to penetrate into the body, causing the fluids to dry up.[2] The dry consistency of her nasal passages confirms this finding.

External wind penetrates the nose and disturbs the function of the Lungs, which causes the sneezing fits. Red, itchy eyes result from wind-heat attacking the head. Initially, the patient's allergies and condition were characterized by a disruption of Lung qi that manifested as a white, viscous nasal secretion. As her condition worsened, the nasal passages became dry and the nasal breathing became impaired. The penetration of wind-heat, and the impairment of Lung qi, led to heat from constraint, which affected the nose. Therefore, the nose, an 'offshoot' of the Lungs, became congested.[3] Over the long term, heat in the Lungs injures the the fluids and yin. This, in combination with the blocked Lung qi, contributes to the nasal congestion.

As her condition worsened, the patient suffered from a dry, stubborn, and irritable cough. There are two possible mechanisms for the development of this cough:

1. Heat attacked the Lungs and injured the fluids, resulting in a dry cough. Because she simultaneously experienced difficulty breathing, the cough can be seen as a precursor to asthma, thus underlining the severity of the blockage of Lung qi.
2. In a healthy body, the Kidneys receive qi and fluids from the Lungs. The Kidneys then return 'steam' to moisten the Lungs. Disruption of this mechanism, whereby insufficient moisture reaches the Lungs, will lead to a dry, irritable cough. In this case, the labored breathing and tightness of the chest are caused by the blockage of qi in the chest and Lungs.

Pathomechanism

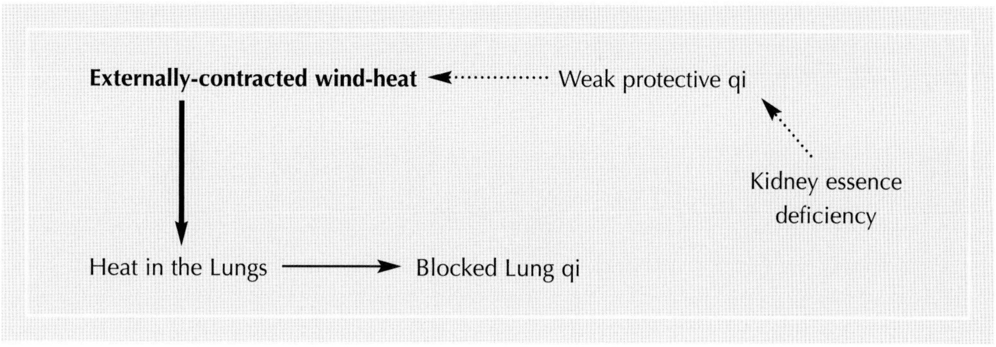

Externally-contracted wind-heat ◄······· Weak protective qi

↓ (Externally-contracted wind-heat → Heat in the Lungs)

Kidney essence deficiency ····► Weak protective qi

Heat in the Lungs ——► Blocked Lung qi

Frequently recurring attacks of externally-contracted factors eventually weaken the protective qi and destabilize the exterior. Thus, the patient grew more sensitive and reacted more quickly when exposed to grass, house mites, or animal hair.

The family disposition to allergies and the underdevelopment of the patient's reproductive organs reflect a weakness of Kidney essence. Specifically, the Kidneys nourish the uterus, which is one of the six extraordinary hollow organs that store essence.[4] Kidney essence and protective qi reach and supply different areas of the body via the extraordinary vessels, especially the Governing, Conception, and Penetrating vessels. Since the protective qi is rooted in the Kidneys, deficiency of Kidney essence can also contribute to an unstable exterior.

The onset of the allergic rhinitis is most informative. It occurred when the patient was 14 years old. Around this time the Kidney energy typically strengthens in preparation for the menarche.[5] The patient's parents separated during this time, causing her great distress. Sadness disperses qi. The allergies started when her emotional state was especially unstable. This directly affected her Lung qi, and subsequently her protective qi. This condition was then aggravated by the insufficient unfolding of Kidney essence.

Treatment strategy. Release the wind-heat, eliminate the heat from the Lungs, unblock the nose, and stabilize the exterior.

At first, a modified version of Xanthium Powder *(cāng ér zǐ sǎn)* was prescribed, with the following additions: Mori Cortex *(sāng bái pí),* Lonicerae Flos *(jīn yín huā),* Forsythiae Fructus *(lián qiào),* Peucedani Radix *(qián hú),* and Tribuli Fructus *(cì jí lí).* After three weeks, Xanthii Fructus *(cāng ěr zǐ)* was replaced by Liquidambaris Fructus *(lù lù tōng)* to open the nose, and by Lilii Bulbus *(bǎi hé)* to moisten the Lung yin. After taking the modified decoction for three months, the patient was much improved. She had only a slight allergic reaction to cats. Later on, Jade Windscreen Powder *(yù píng fēng sǎn)* was added to the prescription. During the past three years, she has rarely suffered from labored breathing, tightness of the chest, or any of her other allergy symptoms.

9.2 Damp-Heat and Associated Tongue Signs

A yellow, thick, greasy tongue coating that covers the tongue indicates the presence of damp-heat (see also Ch. 10).

The quality of the coating can be used to determine the relative strength of the dampness and heat: If the dampness predominates, the coating will be more greasy, and if the heat predominates, the coating will be more yellow and/or dry. If the coating appears to be dirty yellow in color, the damp-heat has been present for a long time in the body and is often located in the yang brightness *(yáng míng)* channels.

Externally-contracted pathogenic damp-heat can cause acute illnesses, especially in the summer and in hot, damp, tropical climates. Damp-heat can penetrate into the protective and qi levels and cause fevers that worsen in the afternoon, headaches, a feeling of heaviness in the body, and general body aches. At the onset of such a disease, the tongue coating remains white. If the pathogenic influence is strong or penetrates further into the interior, the coating will change and appear more yellow and greasy. This is especially noticeable in the center of the tongue.

Spleen qi deficiency also leads to the formation of damp-heat. The fluids accumulate and are transformed into dampness. The internally-generated dampness, in turn, obstructs the qi mechanism in the middle burner. This can impair the Stomach's function of moving the impure parts of digested foods downward. The accumulation of dampness and the stagnation of qi in the middle burner give rise to heat. This process is more likely to occur in those who favor fatty, fried, and spicy foods. The use of alcohol also contributes to this process. If the accumulation of damp-heat is due to underlying Spleen qi deficiency, the tongue body will be pale or pale red, and the yellow, greasy coating will most likely be located in the root (or the posterior third) of the tongue.

Damp-heat can collect throughout the body. Because of its heavy nature, it has a tendency to gather in the lower burner where it impairs the flow of qi. Damp-heat often affects the Intestines and Bladder. Characteristic tongue signs of this pathology are a yellow, greasy, thick coating in the posterior third that is interspersed with big red points (Fig. 9.2.4).

By itself, tongue diagnosis is not a very precise instrument for identifying the location of the damp-heat when the symptoms include recent-onset burning sensation when urinating, dark, turbid, and scanty urine, or strong-smelling, burning diarrhea. The presence of the yellow, greasy thick coating in the posterior third of the tongue only confirms the presence of damp-heat; it does not identify its location, that is, in the Bladder or Intestines. This information can only be obtained by combining tongue diagnosis with pulse diagnosis and a differentiation of the other symptoms. In the middle burner, damp-heat causes a sensation of fullness in the epigastrium and abdomen as well as abdominal distention. When it affects the Stomach and Intestines, the symptoms include foul-smelling diarrhea or constipation. Again, the tongue coating is yellow, thick, and greasy, especially in the center of the tongue, reflecting the accumulation of damp-heat in the Stomach.

When dampness is transformed into phlegm it will be stored in the Lungs. The formation of phlegm-heat in the Lungs can be attributed either to fire 'brewing' the fluids that have become stagnant owing to underlying Spleen qi deficiency, or to externally-contracted heat that has lodged in the Lungs. Phlegm and heat interfere with the downward-moving action of the Lung qi, resulting in a loud cough with copious, yellow phlegm. Here, the coating is again yellow and greasy, and occasionally the anterior third of the tongue is swollen.

The Liver and Gallbladder are especially vulnerable to accumulation of damp-heat. All the above mentioned factors as well as Liver qi constraint can lead to accumulation of damp-heat in the Liver and Gallbladder channels, or just the Gallbladder channel. The tongue coating is also yellow, thick, and greasy. An interesting variation is presented by the appearance of bilateral lines on each half of the tongue, which is indicative of damp-heat (heat dominant) in the Liver and Gallbladder (Fig. 9.2.7).

In addition, in the case of rheumatic illness painful obstruction *(bì)* disorders that are characterized by swollen and hot joints, the tongue coating is often yellow and greasy.

A swollen, red, or dark red tongue is also indicative of damp-heat, although this is less frequently seen. This type of tongue is, however, quite common in those who consume a lot of alcohol or fatty foods. The heat is responsible for the redness, and the dampness is responsible for the swollen tongue body.

Tongue description ------------------------ **Chinese diagnosis**

Tongue description	Chinese diagnosis
Red	Heat in the blood
Red points over the entire tongue body	Constrained pathogenic heat in the interior
Yellow, thick coating	Retention of damp-heat transforming into heat toxin

Fig. 9.2.1
Female
39 years old

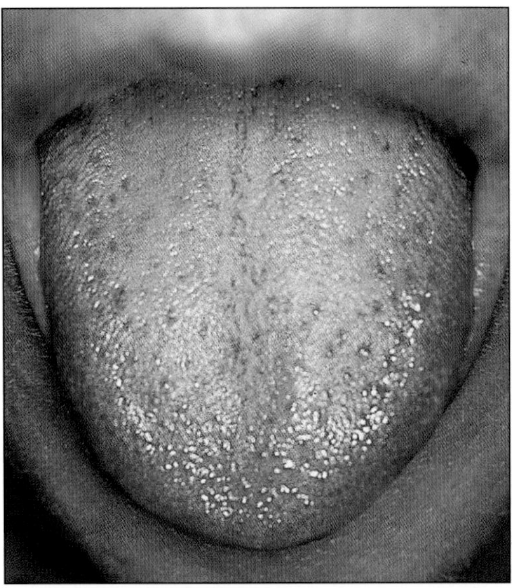

Symptoms

Swelling, redness, and deformation of the metacarpal, metacarpalphalangeal, and metatarsal joints
Wandering pain
Epigastric fullness and pain

Western diagnosis

Chronic rheumatoid arthritis
History of Chlamydia infection

Background to disease

Family history of rheumatoid arthritis
Bacterial infection
Overwork

Tongue description ------------------------ **Chinese diagnosis**

Tongue description	Chinese diagnosis
Red, slightly swollen, wet	Heat developing with accumulating dampness
Yellow, thick, greasy coating with red points at the root	Retention of damp-heat in the Bladder

Fig. 9.2.2
Female
30 years old

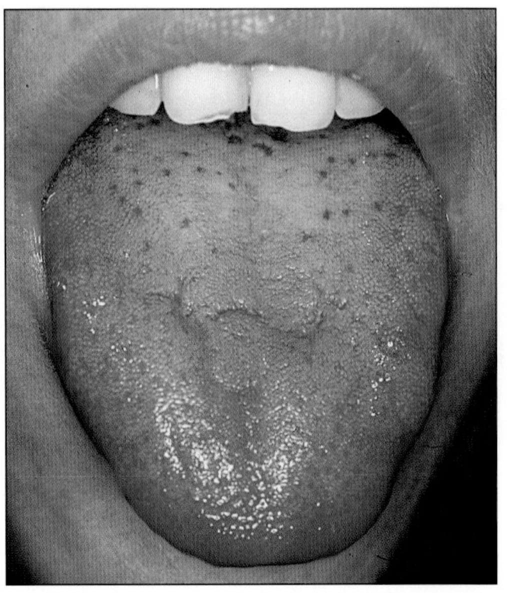

Symptoms

Frequent burning sensation with urination
Smelly urine
Sneezing fits
Itchy eyes
Mouth ulcers
Inflamed gums

Western diagnosis

Chronic urinary tract infection
Allergic rhinitis

Background to disease

Long-standing emotional problems
Excessive consumption of raw and dairy foods

Tongue description	**Chinese diagnosis**
Red, long	Constitutional heat in the Heart
Vertical crack in the center of the tongue	Stomach yin deficiency
Light yellow, thick, greasy coating over the entire tongue body	Retention of damp-heat
Light yellow, thick coating with red points on the posterior third	Retention of damp-heat in the lower burner transforming into heat toxin

Symptoms

One-sided swelling of Bartholin's gland
Pain in the genitals
Yellow vaginal discharge
Inner restlessness

Western diagnosis

Chronic Bartholinitis

Background to disease

Excessive sexual activity together with excessive use of alcohol
Emotional problems

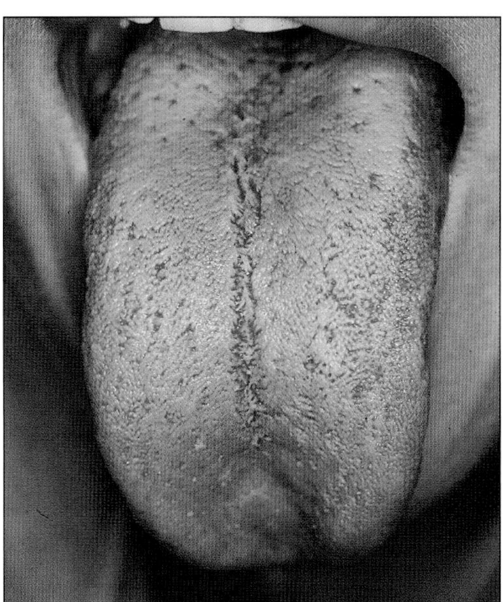

Fig. 9.2.3
Female
32 years old

Tongue description	**Chinese diagnosis**
Pale red, swollen, slightly wet, teeth marks	Spleen qi deficiency (accumulation of dampness)
Yellow, thick coating with red points at the root	Retention of damp-heat in the Large Intestine and genitals
Slight notch at the tip	Slight Heart blood deficiency

Symptoms

Itching and burning in the vagina
Swelling and redness of the labia
Smelly, soft stools
Foul-smelling flatulence
Tiredness
Strong inner tension

Western diagnosis

Acute candidiasis

Background to disease

Condition followed frequent use of antibiotics
Long-standing emotional problems

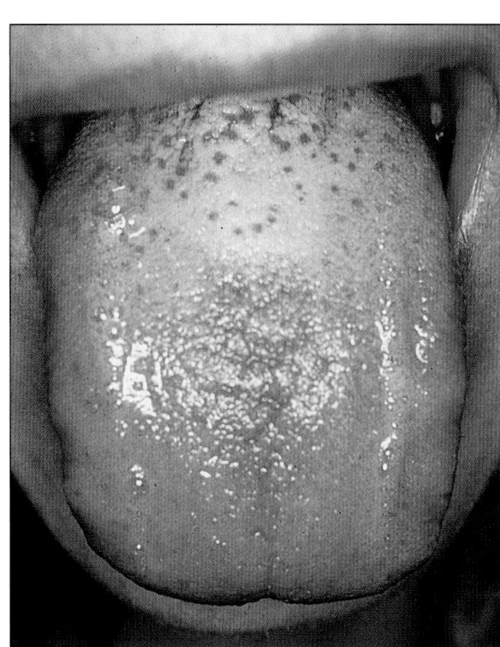

Fig. 9.2.4
Female
28 years old

Tongue description ------------------------- **Chinese diagnosis**

Pale, very swollen, teeth marks — Spleen qi deficiency (accumulation of dampness)

Thick, dry, dirty yellow coating — Accumulation of heat toxin in the three burners

Fig. 9.2.5
Female
52 years old

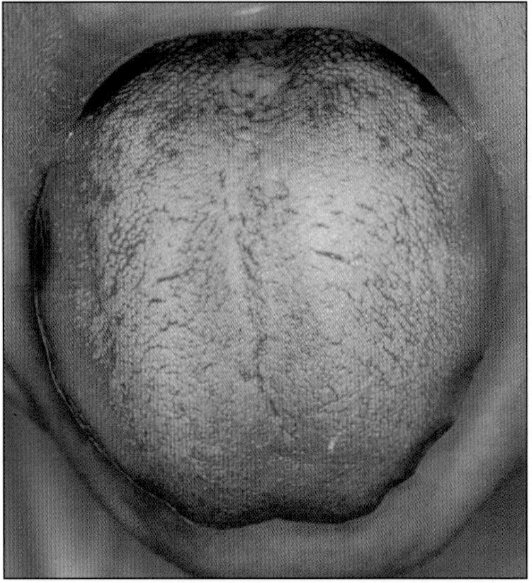

Symptoms

Red, swollen, inflamed, and bleeding gums
Purulent ulcerations
Severe facial pain
Red face
Sweating
Thirst
Feeling of malaise
Overweight

Western diagnosis

Necrotizing ulcerative gingivitis

Background to disease

Insufficient dental care and treatment
Alcohol abuse
Excessive consumption of sweet foods

Tongue description ------------------------- **Chinese diagnosis**

Pale red, wide — Accumulation of damp-heat

Brownish yellow, thick, dry coating over the entire tongue body — Retention of damp-heat and phlegm in the three burners

Fig. 9.2.6
Female
58 years old

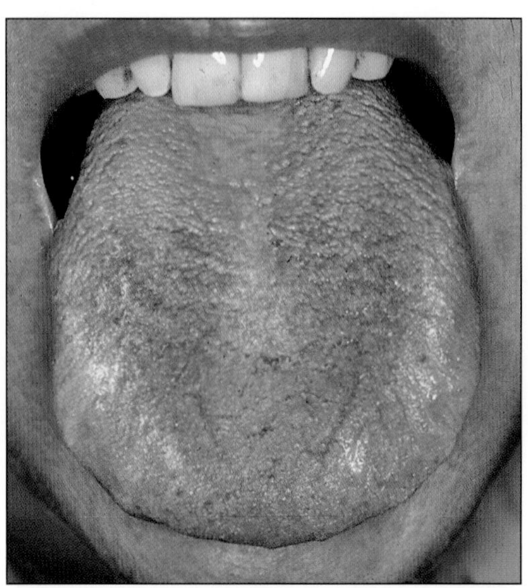

Symptoms

Diffuse, dull pain throughout the entire body
Exhaustion
Mental confusion
Soft, smelly stools
Inability to sleep through the night
Itchy skin

Western diagnosis

Chronic urticaria

Background to disease

Excessive physical and mental demands due to personal problems

Tongue description	**Chinese diagnosis**
Pale	Spleen qi deficiency
Swollen sides in the middle third, slight teeth marks	Spleen qi deficiency → accumulation of dampness
Yellow, one-sided coating	Retention of damp-heat in the Gallbladder
Thin crack in the anterior third	No associated pathology

Symptoms

Dizziness
Feeling of pressure and distention in the ears
Mucus in the throat
Flatulence and epigastric fullness
Depressive moods

Western diagnosis

None

Background to disease

Irregular eating habits
Excessive consumption of cold foods
Onset of condition followed an acute chill

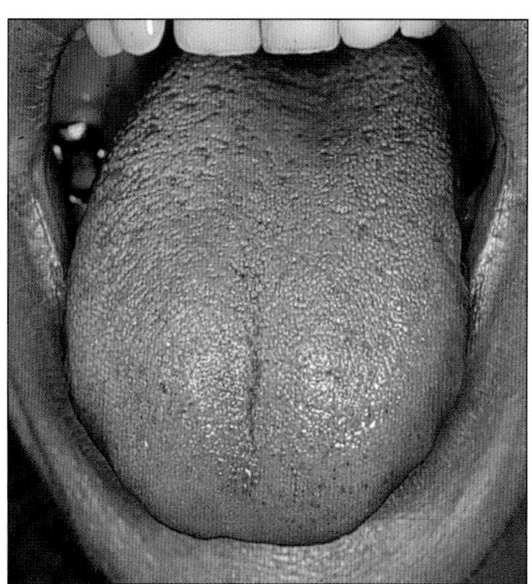

Fig. 9.2.7
Female
43 years old

CASE HISTORY The patient experienced dizziness and had a feeling of pressure and distention in both ears. She also felt that there was mucus lodged in her throat. Medical examinations did not turn up anything. She assumed that the symptoms were connected to a chill she had caught three months before; she was now sensitive to drafts.

After eating, she suffered from epigastric fullness that was relieved only by passing gas, which had become a real problem. She had little appetite and ate irregularly. Because of her digestive problems, she preferred to eat light foods such as curd and yogurt. Her pulse was wiry and sinking.

Analysis. The tongue body and coating reflect two coexisting but different pathologies. The tongue body shows the underlying constitution: Spleen qi deficiency with an accumulation of dampness. The tongue coating represents the acute disease process and provides an important sign: the yellow, right-sided coating signals the development of heat in the lesser yang channels. The symptoms began three months after she had contracted a chill. The pathogenic factor is now lodged in the half-interior, half-exterior stage, as reflected in the one-sided yellow coating. The patient's aversion to drafts may be an expression of the half-exterior aspect of this stage. However, if the lesser yang stage were still dominated by wind and cold, then the coating would be white and one-sided, not yellow and one-sided. The yellow coating reflects the development of heat in the lesser yang channels.

Heat in the Gallbladder rises, resulting in dizziness and a feeling of pressure in the ears. The Gallbladder and Triple Burner channels encircle the ear, and this accounts for their frequent involvement in acute disorders with this pattern.

Underlying Spleen qi deficiency has caused an accumulation of dampness, as reflected in the swollen sides on the middle part of the tongue. The pale tongue body and the sinking pulse also suggest this deficiency. Her digestive symptoms appear after eating. Retention of dampness in the middle burner blocks the qi mechanism, resulting in epigastric fullness and flatulence. These symptoms are exacerbated because the Gallbladder qi has attacked the Stomach, reflected in the wiry pulse, and the Spleen, resulting in a lack of appetite.

Pathomechanism

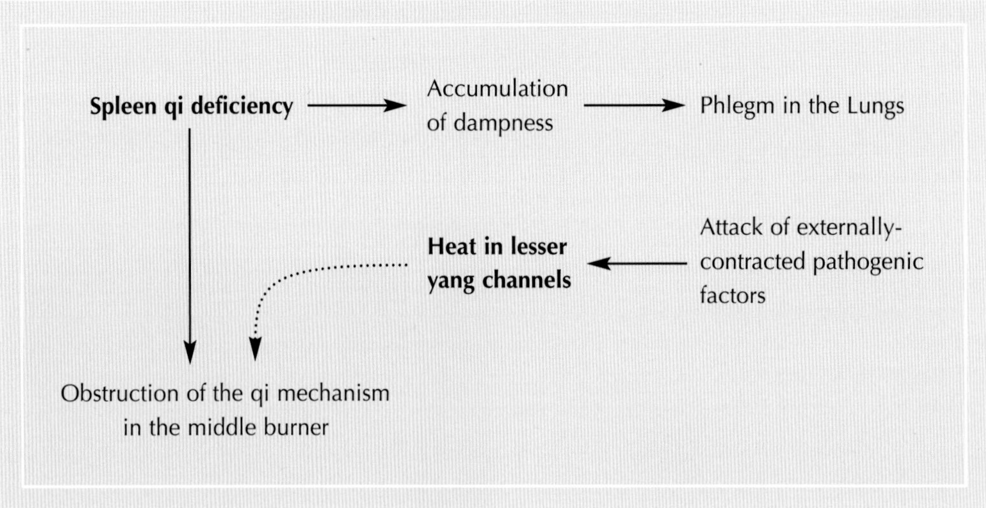

The excessive consumption of dairy and cold foods engendered dampness, which has accumulated and transformed into phlegm that is stored in the Lungs. In this case, the phlegm is lodged in the throat. The thin, vertical crack is not relevant to the diagnosis, as there are no symptoms indicative of Lung yin deficiency.

Treatment strategy. Harmonize the disorders of the lesser yang stage, strengthen the Spleen qi, drain the dampness, and transform the phlegm.

A modified version of Minor Bupleurum Decoction *(xiǎo chái hú tāng)* was prescribed, with the addition of Chrysanthemi Flos *(jú huā),* Uncariae Ramulus cum Uncis *(gōu téng),* and Acori tatarinowii Rhizoma *(shí chāng pǔ).* After taking this decoction for three weeks, the dizziness and feeling of pressure in the ears were much reduced, as were her digestive problems. The patient changed her eating habits and felt much better.

CASE HISTORY A butterfly erythema was the first sign of the illness eight years before. The onset of the systemic lupus erythematosus, as evidenced by skin lesions, was very sudden. Prior to this illness, the patient had been healthy. Cortisone tablets were prescribed, and the skin lesions subsequently cleared. There were no symptoms for a period of four years. Then, for no apparent reason, her wrist and ankle joints started to swell and were extremely warm and painful; these symptoms were reduced by taking anti-inflammatory medication. However, even with the medication, her joints still remained painful, especially when the weather became damp.

The illness appeared to be very aggressive. The patient now suffered from proteinuria and her blood creatinine level was elevated (1.6mg/dl). Her urine was yellow and turbid although the excreted volume of urine was normal. Her blood pressure was significantly raised (185/130mmHg), and was being controlled by medical treatment. Hypertrophy of the left heart had been found as well. At the onset of the illness, the patient took 7.5mg of cortisone orally each day, as well as several other anti-inflammatory drugs. Her main complaints were the joint pains, night sweats, and constant elevated temperature.

The patient felt very thirsty and hungry. Her digestion was normal. She considered her menstruation to be regular and problem-free, although the bleeding was heavy and it lasted for seven days, after which she felt exhausted for two days. Otherwise, her energy was good. Despite the severity of her illness, the patient seemed quite relaxed. Her pulse was notably slippery and rapid.

Tongue description	**Chinese diagnosis**
Scarlet red	Heat in the blood level
Swollen	Retention of phlegm
Red edges	Heat in the Liver
Slight indentation of the tip	Heart blood deficiency
Yellow, thick, old coating	Injury to the fluids by heat and accumulation of heat toxin
Peeled or reduced coating in areas	Onset of Stomach and Kidney yin deficiency

Symptoms

Hot, swollen joints
Pain with movement
Night sweats
Thirst and voracious appetite
Dry eyes
Feeling of heat in the body
Turbid urine

Western diagnosis

Systemic lupus erythematosus, hypertension

Background to disease

Unknown

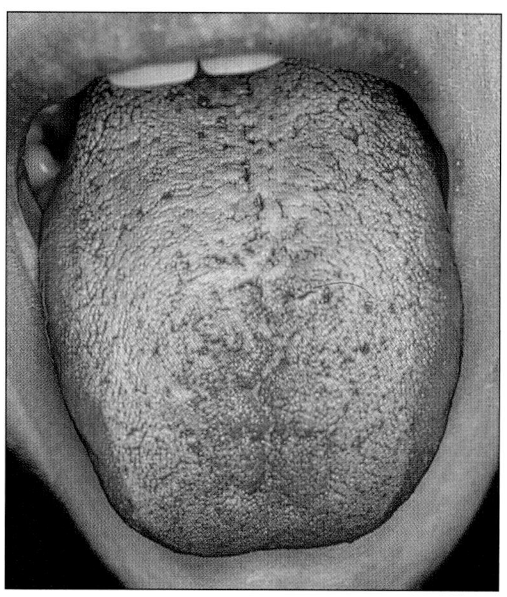

Fig. 9.2.8
Female
28 years old

Analysis. The tongue body color is scarlet red and reflects the penetration of heat to the blood level. In some circles of Chinese medicine, systemic lupus erythematosus is classified as painful obstruction syndrome. At the onset of this illness, heat penetrated to the blood level and injured the blood. In this case, the intensity of the heat and its transformation into heat toxin was reflected in the red skin lesions on the cheeks. Cortisone treatment worked quickly and eased the effects of heat in the blood. However, it did not lead to a sufficient clearing of the heat. Consequently, four years later, her kidneys, heart, and joints were affected.

The heat had been continuously suppressed, which left it simmering. In this state, it injured the fluids, blood, and yin. This process allowed heat to accumulate in the blood, channels, and collaterals. The remaining heat in the blood was responsible for the enhanced body warmth of the patient, although her skin itself was not hot to the touch. Many years ago, heat constituted the root of the illness, and the scarlet tongue body reflects this event. The ensuing deficiency of fluids and yin represented the branch of the illness. Eight years later, however, an evaluation of the root and branch of the disease mechanism must be viewed differently. Because of the chronic nature of the illness, Kidney yin deficiency is now considered the root, while damp-heat obstruction, ascending Liver yang, and the movement of internal wind are regarded as the branches or manifestations of her illness.

The dry and old tongue coating reflects the injury to the fluids by the internal heat, and the coating's yellow discoloration signals the presence of heat. The coating has disappeared entirely from the anterior third of the tongue, while on the posterior third, the coating has thinned out. The lack of coating, as well as its texture, suggest the development of Stomach yin as well as Kidney yin deficiency. Injured fluids and weakened Kidney yin are responsible for the insufficient and aged appearance of the tongue coating, as yin and fluids are necessary to sustain and form new coating. To summarize, the texture of the coating reflects the injury

Pathomechanism

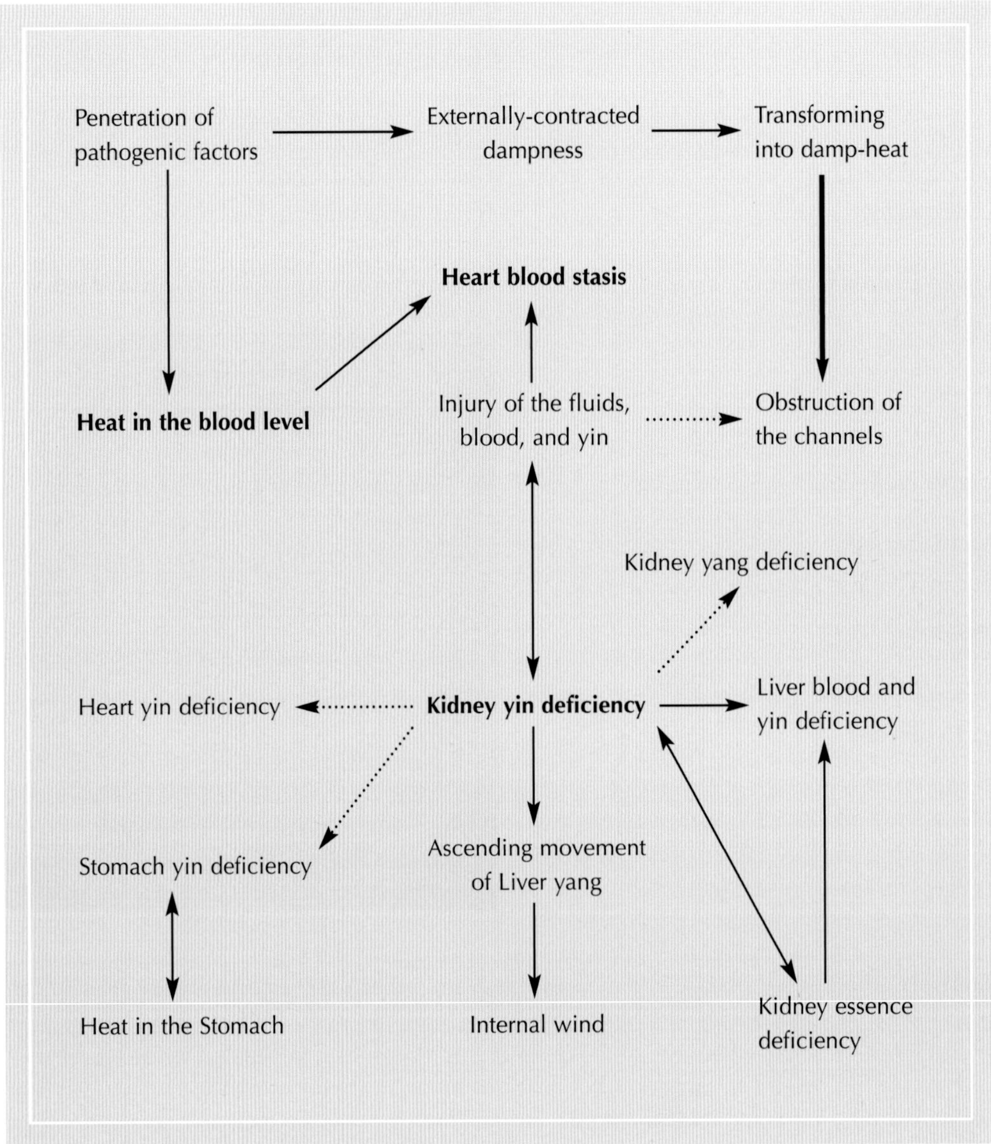

to the fluids and yin, while the scarlet red tongue body reflects the depth to which the heat has penetrated.

Heat is also responsible for the other symptoms. The patient's intense thirst and hunger mirror the development of Stomach heat and fire. Long-term use of cortisone and other anti-inflammatory drugs are believed to injure the fluids in the Stomach, which in turn engenders heat, creating a vicious circle. The hypertrophy of the left heart is possibly caused by the heat in the blood, which has scorched and congealed the blood, and led to blood stasis.[6]

Apart from her constant feeling of heat in the body, it was the night sweats and joint pains that most troubled the patient. A disharmony between water and fire is the cause of the night sweats. The weakened Kidney yin cannot control the Heart yang. The uncontrolled Heart yang is unable to store the sweat, and it leaks out. Hot, swollen joints are characteristic of damp-heat obstruction. In this case, external dampness aggravates the pain as the circulation of qi and blood in the channels, collaterals, and joints is blocked. Dampness combines with underlying heat to form damp-heat, which aggravates the obstruction of qi and blood in the channels. The warmth in the joints reflects the presence of heat, while the pain and swelling reflect the presence of dampness.

The injury to the Kidney yin has led to Liver blood and yin deficiency. Liver blood is responsible for nourishing and moistening the eyes. In this case, its deficiency has resulted in dryness of the eyes. The Kidney yin deficiency allows the Liver yang to ascend, which in turn engenders internal wind, resulting in high blood pressure. The Kidney yin deficiency also affects the Kidney essence. If both energies are exhausted, a weakness of Kidney yang will follow. As a result, the Kidneys are destabilized, preventing them from securing the essence, which is evident in the loss of protein in the urine.

The protracted menstrual bleeding is caused by heat in the blood, which impairs the Liver's function of storing blood. The blood consequently moves in an uncontrolled fashion, reflected in the heavy and protracted bleeding. Since blood is an aspect of yin, the bleeding has further weakened the Kidney yin, which accounts for the patient's exhaustion following menstruation. The monthly loss of blood, the intense sweating at night, and the loss of protein in the urine all contribute to the decline in blood, yin, and essence.

Surprisingly, the shape of the tongue body is swollen. Here this is not a sign of the accumulation of dampness due to underlying Spleen qi deficiency. Rather, it is a result of the retention of phlegm. The intense heat in the body has caused the fluids to congeal, and, eventually, the congealed fluids have been transformed into phlegm. Heat moves the phlegm, which contributes to the increased volume of the tongue. However, a pattern of phlegm is not deemed important in relation to the entire disease process. The pulse is the only other sign indicating the presence of heat and phlegm.

Treatment strategy. Nourish the Kidney yin, cool the blood, eliminate the damp-heat in the channels and joints, and remove the obstruction in the channels and joints.

A modified decoction of Anemarrhena, Phellodendron, and Rehmannia Pill *(zhī bái dì huáng wán)* was prescribed, with the addition of Sargentodoxae Caulis *(hóng téng)*, Smilacis glabrae Rhizoma *(tǔ fú líng)*, Anemarrhenae Rhizoma *(zhī mǔ)*, Lycii Cortex *(dì gǔ pí)*, and Ophiopogonis Radix *(mài mén dōng)*. Three weeks later, the patient felt better. The joint pains were much improved and she was able to lower her intake of anti-inflammatory drugs. The night sweats had improved slightly, and the level of creatinine had fallen to 0.7mg/dl. However, based on the advice she received from her medical doctors, she decided to discontinue Chinese herbal therapy. Four months later, she returned because the creatinine level was again elevated. After two more months of taking the herbal decoction, her creatinine level was again stabilized, and she again felt much better. However, once again her doctor persuaded her to discontinue taking the herbs due to their alleged toxicity.

Endnotes

1 See *Compendium of Charts and Books Past and Present: Complete Collection of the Medical Section (Gu jin tu shu ji cheng: yi bu quan lu)*. Beijing: Peoples Medical Publishing House, 1991: 5:84. Here it is noted that a tongue that looks yellow and rough and presents with a localized patch indicates heat that has penetrated deeply into the Stomach. In addition, the toxin of the pathogenic influence is located at the same depth. If Heart fire leads to inner restlessness and thirst, one should prescribe Major Order the Qi Decoction *(dà chéng qì tāng)* to guide it downward.

2 Maciocia G. *Tongue Diagnosis in Chinese Medicine*, rev. ed. Seattle: Eastland Press, 1995: 99.

3 "Lung qi has a connection to the nostrils. When the qi in the Lungs is harmonious, the nose can differentiate between fragrances and stench." Anonymous. *Huang di nei jing ling shu yi shi* [Translation and Explanation of the Yellow Emperor's Inner Classic: Divine Pivot], edited by Nanjing College of Traditional Chinese Medicine, Traditional Chinese Medicine Department. Shanghai: Shanghai Science and Technology Press, 1997: 17:158.

4 Anonymous. *Su wen* [Basic Questions], edited by He W-B et al. Beijing: China Medicine Science and Technology Press, 1996: 11:67

5 Ibid., 1:1.

6 Chen Z and Chen M-F. *The Essence and Scientific Background of Tongue Diagnosis*. Long Beach, CA: Oriental Healing Arts Institute, 1989: 30. The text describes research on patients with left heart hypertrophy that found changes in the color of the tongue in a large fraction of the people studied. As a rule, the tongue body was red, especially the tip.

CHAPTER 10

Tongue Coatings

10.1 Tongue Coatings and the Eight Principles

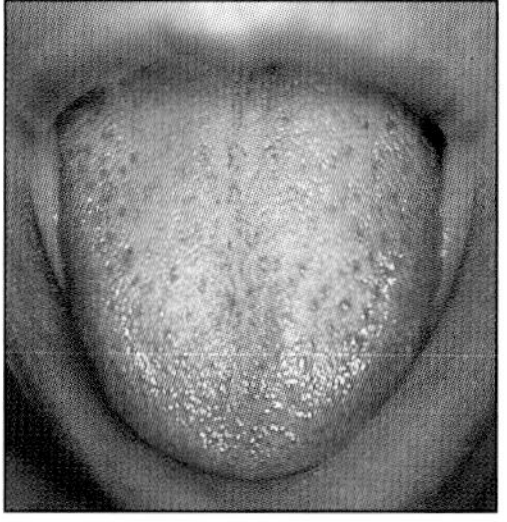

Fig. 9.2.1

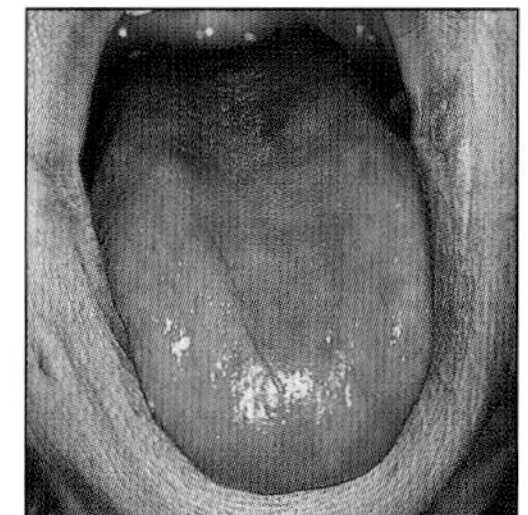

Fig. 4.1.4.3

An assessment of the coating is important in order to carry out a differential diagnosis according to the eight principles.

- Thick coating: condition of excess (Fig. 9.2.1)
- Lack of coating: condition of deficiency (Fig. 4.1.4.3)

For example, in the case of Stomach and Kidney yin deficiency, there may be an absence of a coating, often in combination with a red tongue body. By contrast, for Spleen and Kidney yang deficiency, which can lead to an accumulation of dampness, the development of this excessive disorder is manifested in a thick, white, slippery coating. The tongue body will typically be pale and swollen.

- White coating: presence of cold
- Yellow coating: presence of heat

The diagnosis of the tongue coating is of particular importance when illness is caused by externally-contracted pathogenic factors. In such cases, the coating will reflect the qualities and depth of penetration of the pathogenic factors. Thus, in the case of externally-contracted wind-cold, the coating will be white; in the case of externally-contracted wind-heat, it may be yellow.

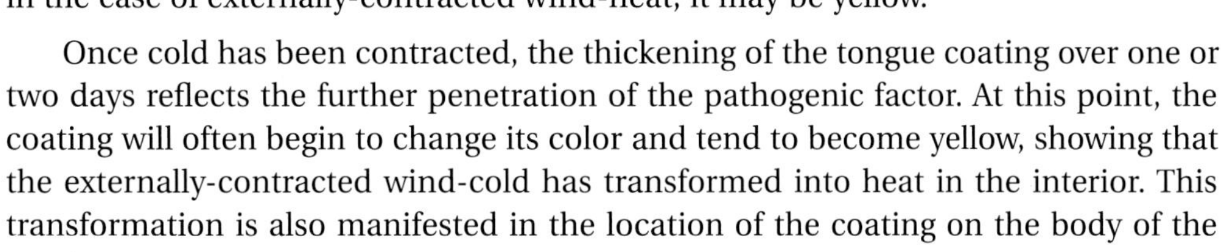

Once cold has been contracted, the thickening of the tongue coating over one or two days reflects the further penetration of the pathogenic factor. At this point, the coating will often begin to change its color and tend to become yellow, showing that the externally-contracted wind-cold has transformed into heat in the interior. This transformation is also manifested in the location of the coating on the body of the tongue:

- Tip of the tongue: reflects the exterior of the body (yang)
- Middle and posterior thirds of the tongue: reflects the interior of the body (yin)

In the case of externally-contracted wind-cold, the theory is that the coating is mainly located on the anterior third of the tongue, but in my own clinical experience, it is often not visible. It is important to realize that the coating at this stage is still quite thin. This tells us something about the location of the pathogenic factor, namely, that the illness is still in the superficial level of the body and has not yet penetrated to the interior. If this thin, white coating is also wet, it suggests that the dispersing function of Lung qi is impaired.

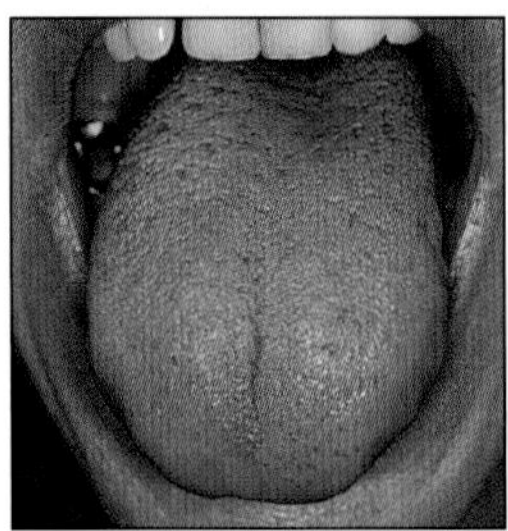

Fig. 9.2.7

If the pathogenic factor has penetrated to a deeper level, the coating will often be located in the center of the tongue. If the coating becomes yellow and dry, it suggests the formation of internal heat that is beginning to injure the fluids. Thus, the color, thickness, moisture, and location of the coating on the tongue body all provide information about a disorder caused by an externally-contracted pathogenic factor. An interesting distribution of the coating can be found in cases of acute disorders in the lesser yang (*shào yáng*) stage of the six stages of disease. A one-sided, white, slippery or wet coating on the right half of the tongue means that the pathogenic factor is half-exterior and half-interior. If this right-sided coating is dry and yellow, it represents the retention of phlegm-heat or damp-heat in the Gallbladder (Fig. 9.2.7). By contrast, a one-sided yellow coating on the left half of the tongue is indicative of heat in the Liver. Finally, yellow strips of coating on either half of the tongue signify intense damp-heat in the Liver and Gallbladder.

In general, one can say that the condition of the hollow organs (*fŭ*) is mainly reflected in the color and nature of the tongue coating.

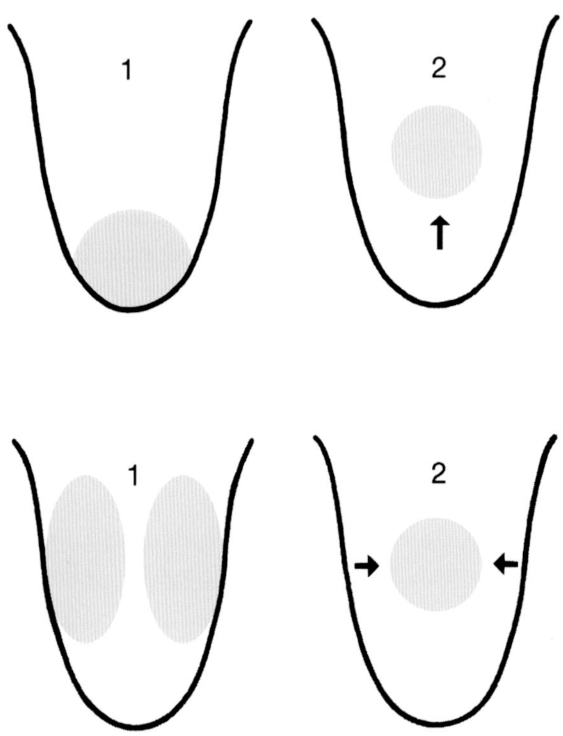

Changes to the coating due to the penetration of externally-contracted pathogenic factors. The arrow indicates the direction of the penetration from the exterior to the interior.

10.2 Different Aspects of the Tongue Coating

Excess and deficiency are reflected in the thickness of the coating. However, the coating does not identify the cause. For example, a thick coating can appear in interior as well as exterior patterns of disharmony. Among patterns caused by internal factors, dampness, phlegm, food stagnation, interior heat, and cold are most prominent. Among patterns caused by external factors, externally-contracted wind-cold, wind-heat, or summer-heat are the leading factors.

To summarize, in acute cases it is especially important to note changes in the coating. If it is thin at the onset of an illness and starts to thicken, it is always an indication of the further penetration of the pathogenic factor. If the coating becomes thinner and lighter in color, this is a clear sign that the patient is recovering. The pathogenic factor is now becoming weaker, and the protective (defensive) qi is again gaining strength.

The moisture or degree of wetness of the tongue reflects the condition of the body fluids. A normal tongue should be slightly moist, which reflects proper circulation of the fluids. A dry, wilted tongue mirrors the exhaustion of the fluids.

In this chapter we will discuss the nature of the tongue coating and its moisture. Examples of wet, slippery, greasy, rough, and dry coatings are shown in the accompanying photographs.

10.2.1 Wet and Slippery Coatings

A wet coating may indicate an accumulation of dampness caused by a deficiency of Spleen qi and yang, or of Kidney yang. Here, the tongue body is pale and swollen, and the coating is white. The wet, white, and thin coating can also indicate penetration of externally-contracted wind-cold.

If the coating appears very wet, greasy, or slightly sticky, it is described as slippery. This coating represents a further stage in the evolution of a wet coating and points to a more serious yang deficiency, especially if it is white, as this represents an accumulation of damp-cold. In this case, the tongue body color is pale. However, this type of tongue can also indicate further penetration of the pathogenic factor.

If the slippery coating appears to be of a thicker consistency and slightly greasier, it may be assumed that more dampness has accumulated. If the coating also appears to be a little sticky, the dampness is transforming into phlegm. If the coating is both yellow and slippery, the dampness is transforming into damp-heat. This type of coating is often visible where there is disharmony between the Liver and Gallbladder, or between the Spleen and Stomach.

Tongue coating

- white, moist, and thin: normal
- white, moist, and thin: externally-contracted wind-cold
- slippery: accumulation of dampness
- white and slippery: accumulation of damp-cold
- yellow and slippery: dampness transforming into damp-heat

Tongue description	**Chinese diagnosis**
Pale red, swollen	Slight Spleen qi deficiency (accumulation of dampness)
Wet, white, thin coating	Acute externally-contracted wind-cold
Thin, greasy, yellow coating in the posterior third	Retention of damp-heat in the Bladder

Fig. 10.2.1.1
Male
25 years old

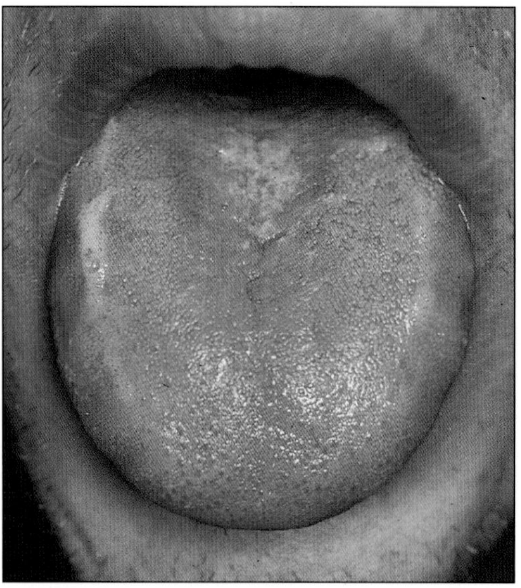

Symptoms

Generalized body aches
Headache
Heavy sensation in the body
Runny nose
Occasional burning sensation with urination

Western diagnosis

Acute cold

Background to disease

Overworked
Long-standing emotional problems

Tongue description	**Chinese diagnosis**
Pale red and swollen with wet, white, thin coating	Spleen qi deficiency (accumulation of dampness)
Depression at the root of the body	Onset of essence deficiency

Fig. 10.2.1.2
Male
33 years old

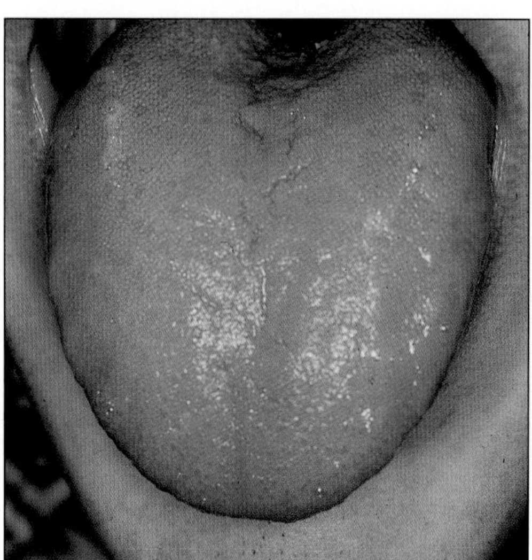

Symptoms

Tiredness
Lack of concentration
Heavy sensation in the head
Flatulence
Inner restlessness
Weakened vision

Western diagnosis

Diabetes mellitus

Background to disease

Unclear

Tongue description	**Chinese diagnosis**
Pale	Spleen and Lung qi deficiency
Swollen right half of tongue	Dampness obstructing the channels
Slippery, white, thin coating	Accumulation of damp-cold
Slight notch at the tip of the tongue	Heart qi and blood deficiency

Symptoms

Cough with white, thin mucus
Frequent urination
Lack of appetite
Dry mouth

Western diagnosis

Coronary heart disease

Background to disease

Physically overworked for many years, hard working conditions
Smoked for 40 years

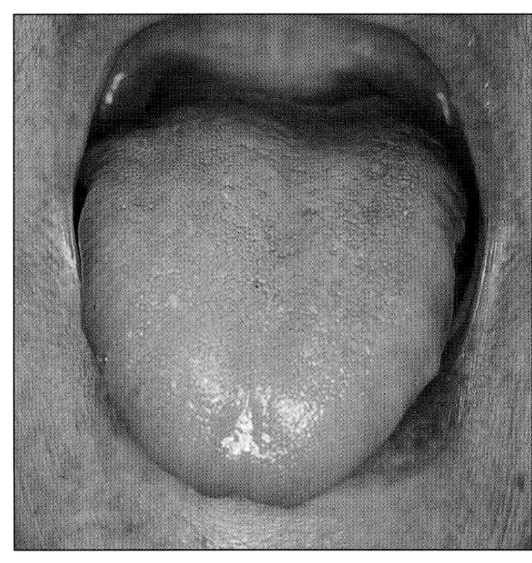

Fig. 10.2.1.3
Female
67 years old

Tongue description	**Chinese diagnosis**
Reddish, slightly contracted tongue body	Slight Kidney yin deficiency
Red points at the tip	Heat from deficiency in the Heart blood
Slippery, pale yellow coating	Acute, externally-contracted damp-heat
Yellow, thick, greasy coating in the posterior third	Onset of transformation of damp-heat into heat, and sinking of damp-heat

Symptoms

Slight fever
Acute diarrhea with foul-smelling stools
Vomiting
Stomach pains
Exhaustion

Western diagnosis

Acute summer flu

Background to disease

Inappropriate clothing
Consumption of raw foods

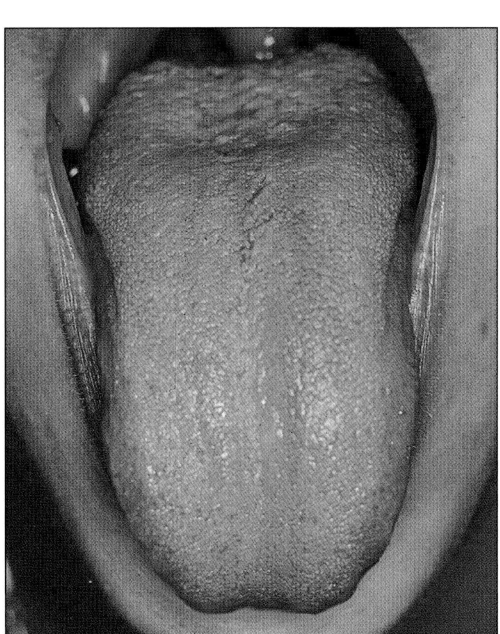

Fig. 10.2.1.4
Female
37 years old

Tongue description ------------------------- **Chinese diagnosis**

Tongue description	Chinese diagnosis
Pale red and swollen, with red sides	Retention of damp-heat in the Liver and Gallbladder
Long midline crack	Constitutional weakness of the Heart
Thick, slippery, yellow coating, especially in the center of the tongue	Retention of phlegm-heat in the Stomach, phlegm mists the Heart

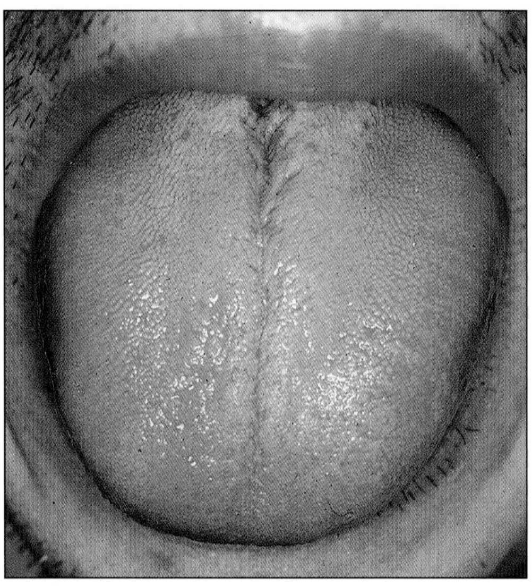

Fig. 10.2.1.5
Male
59 years old

Symptoms

Mental retardation, slow to understand
Poor hearing
Numbness of the finger tips
Smelly urine at night

Western diagnosis

Diabetes mellitus (type II)

Background to disease

Possible birth defect
Excessive consumption of sweet and fatty foods

Tongue description ------------------------- **Chinese diagnosis**

Tongue description	Chinese diagnosis
Pale red	Slight Spleen deficiency
Red points at the sides and tip of the tongue	Acute, externally-contracted wind-heat with penetration to the interior
Slippery, white, thin coating transforming into yellow coating in the center and posterior third	Externally-contracted dampness transforming into damp-heat

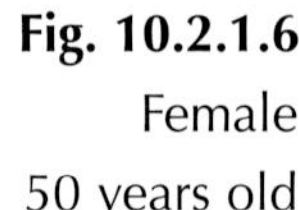

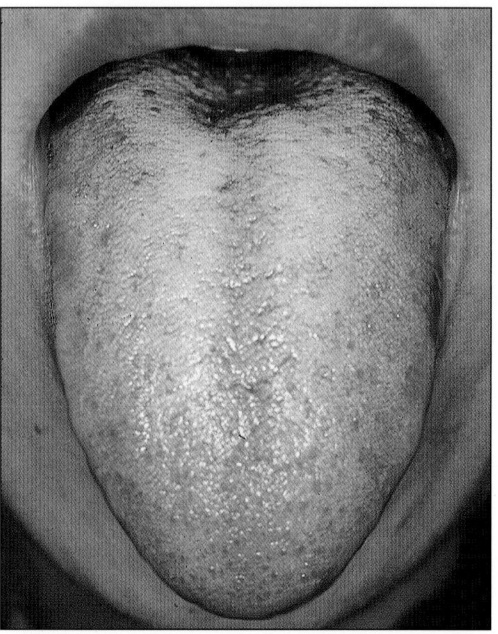

Fig. 10.2.1.6
Female
50 years old

Symptoms

Burning sensation with urination
Turbid urine
Acute episodes of diarrhea after consumption of fruit and alcohol
Runny nose
Itchy eyes
Dry cough, especially at night

Western diagnosis

Acute cystitis
Acute allergic rhinitis
Chronic sinusitis

Background to disease

Irregular eating habits

10.2.2 Greasy Tongue Coatings

As a rule, the greasy coating accompanies a yellow one. A yellow tongue coating not only reveals the penetration of an externally-contracted pathogenic factor, it also reflects internal patterns of disharmony. This type of coating is a common feature in clinical practice.

The greasy coating looks sticky and dry and is often of a thick consistency, which, in the case of an interior disease, reflects an accumulation of damp-heat or phlegm-heat given that the color of the coating is yellow. If the coating is more yellow and dry than sticky, then heat is the more dominant factor. If heat meets with an accumulation of dampness in the interior, over a period of time the heat will interact with the accumulated dampness, resulting in phlegm-heat. This process of dampness transforming into phlegm is reflected in a rough or sticky consistency to the coating. If the coating is thin and of a light yellow color, the dominant factor is accumulated dampness.

Tongue coating

- light yellow, greasy, and thick: damp-heat, dampness predominant (Fig. 10.2.2.2)
- yellow, greasy, and dry: damp-heat, heat predominant
- light yellow or slightly gray color and greasy: acute food stagnation

  In such cases, it is generally located in the center of the tongue and reflects the stagnation of qi in the middle burner. If this disharmony persists for a long time, the coating will become thicker, which is commonly associated with an aggravation of the symptoms.
- White, thick, and greasy coating: cold-dampness or cold-phlegm (Fig. 10.2.2.1)

  This type of tongue coating will be accompanied by a variety of symptoms such as a sensation of heaviness in the body, a feeling of fullness in the chest and epigastrium, or a lack of appetite.

Tongue description ---------- **Chinese diagnosis**

Reddish blue, with blue and black points — Heart blood stasis

Greasy, white, thick coating — Accumulation of cold-dampness and food stagnation

Fig. 10.2.2.1
Male
75 years old

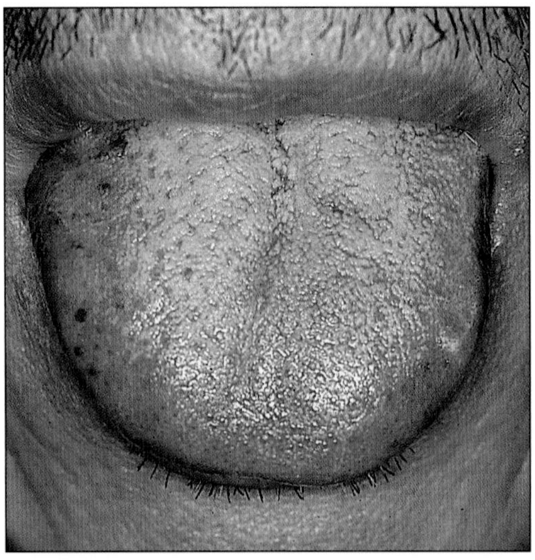

Symptoms

Feeling of fullness in chest and epigastrium
Pains in the chest
Dry cough
Palpitations
Sour taste in the mouth

Western diagnosis

Angina pectoris

Background to disease

Smoking for many years
Physically overworked

Tongue description ---------- **Chinese diagnosis**

Pale red, with red sides — Heat in the Liver

Greasy, white coating at the sides becoming yellow in the center — Accumulation of damp-heat transforming into phlegm-heat in the Stomach

Rough, dry, yellow coating in the center and posterior third — Damp-heat transforming into phlegm-heat in the Stomach

Fig. 10.2.2.2
Female
40 years old

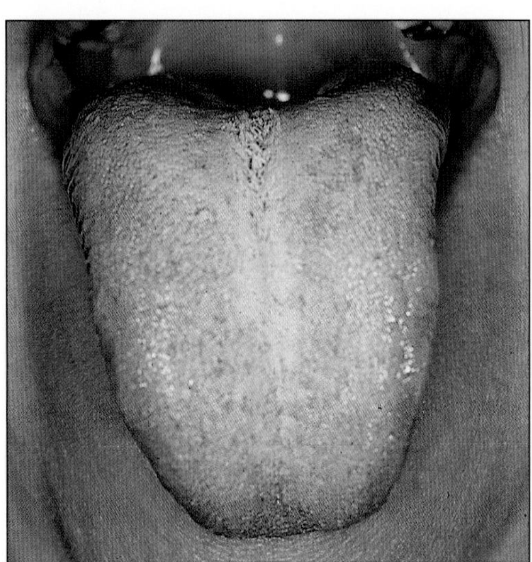

Symptoms

Constipation
Stomach pain
Feeling of fullness in the stomach
Pain under the ribs
Headache
Swollen fingers in the morning

Western diagnosis

None

Background to disease

Irregular eating habits
Frequent bouts of gastritis during puberty
Emotional problems

Tongue description	**Chinese diagnosis**
Red, slightly stiff tongue body	Developing heat with injury to the fluids
Red, slightly curled-up tip	Heat in the Heart
Whitish-yellow, greasy, thick coating in the anterior and middle thirds	Accumulation of damp-heat in the middle burner
Yellow, greasy, thick coating with thorns on the posterior third	Retention of damp-heat in the lower burner

Symptoms

Soft stools
Sensation of urgency to defecate
Occasional pellet-like stools
Smelly stools
Flatulence
Sleeping problems

Western diagnosis

None

Background to disease

Abuse of alcohol
Overconsumption of fried foods

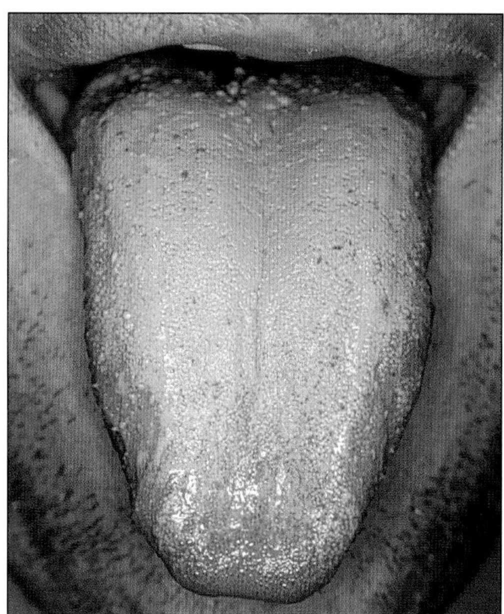

Fig. 10.2.2.3
Male
34 years old

Tongue description	**Chinese diagnosis**
Red	Heat in the blood
Indentation of edges with red points	Liver qi stagnation → Liver fire
Midline crack covered with light yellow, dry coating	Phlegm-heat in the Stomach
Red, dry center	Heat in the Stomach
Yellow coating with red points	Retention of damp-heat in the lower burner

Symptoms

Shortened menstrual cycle
Heavy menstrual bleeding
Distended and painful breasts preceding menstruation
Yellow vaginal discharge
Sneezing fits, nasal discharge
Itching palate, mucus in the throat
Restlessness

Western diagnosis

Ovarian cysts, allergic rhinitis

Background to disease

Emotional problems since puberty

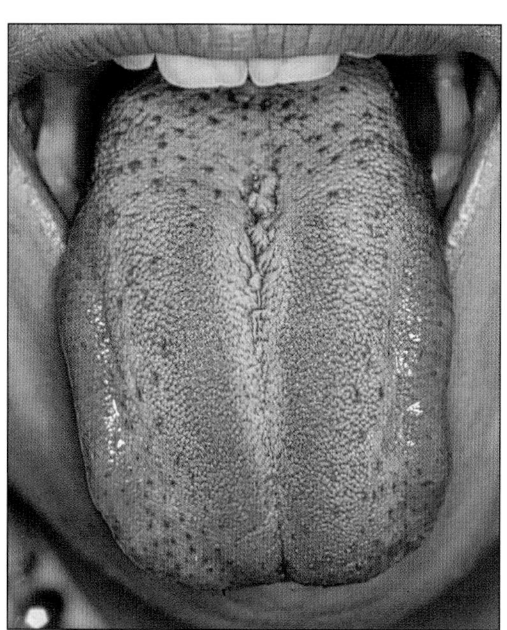

Fig. 10.2.2.4
Female
29 years old

Tongue description	Chinese diagnosis
Pale red, with curled-up edges	Liver qi constraint
Greasy, thick, yellow coating	Accumulation of damp-heat in the Liver and Gallbladder
Old, thin coating in the center of the tongue	Stomach yin and fluid deficiency

Fig. 10.2.2.5
Male
53 years old

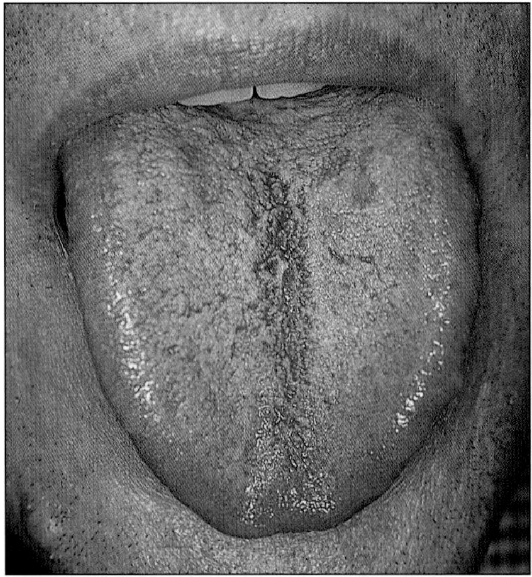

Symptoms

Severe burning pain in the left waist area and chest
Exhaustion
Lack of appetite
Severe dryness of the mouth
Rapid weight loss

Western diagnosis

AIDS
Postherpetic neuralgia

Background to disease

Viral activity
Inability to eat

10.2.3 Dry and White or Yellow Coatings

Independent of its color, a dry or rough-looking coating is always an indication of depleted body fluids. For example, a white, greasy, dry, or rough coating may suggest Spleen and Stomach qi deficiency, as well as a deficiency of fluids in the Stomach. On the one hand, owing to the weakness of Spleen and Stomach qi, there is an accumulation of dampness, giving the coating its greasy consistency. On the other hand, the deficiency of fluids in the Stomach means that the tongue is not receiving adequate moisture; the coating will therefore appear dry.[1]

If the coating is yellow and dry without being sticky or greasy, it is an indication of injury to the fluids by internal heat, which will thicken any accumulated dampness or phlegm in the interior. As a result, the coating will become rough and dry and yellow in color, all of which suggest the presence of the heat. Heat influences the movement of fluids and blood. When heat injures and dries the fluids and yin, the tongue coating will develop a dry and/or greasy texture. The presence of heat is also signaled by the yellow discoloration of the tongue coating. Both the color and texture of the coating reflect the quantity of damp-heat retained in the body, as well as its quality, that is, whether dampness or heat predominates. If the coating is more thick and moist (Fig. 10.2.1.5), dampness is predominant; if the coating is drier and more yellow (Fig. 9.3.8), heat is predominant. The distribution of the tongue coating is also important in diagnosing damp-heat. For example, damp-heat in the lower burner is reflected in a yellow, thick, and greasy coating on the posterior third of the tongue. However, the precise location of the damp-heat in the body can only be determined by observing the patient's other signs and symptoms.

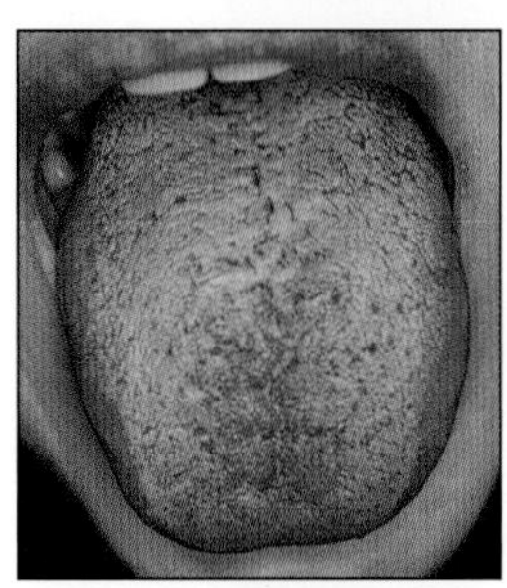

Fig. 9.3.8

Tongue description	**Chinese diagnosis**
Pale, swollen, slight teeth marks	Spleen qi deficiency (accumulation of dampness)
Dry, white coating in the anterior third and center of the tongue	Accumulation of cold-phlegm
Greasy, thick, yellow coating in the posterior third	Accumulation of damp-heat in the lower burner

Symptoms

Nausea after eating cheese
Runny or congested nose
Cough with copious amounts of mucus
Dizziness during menstruation
Backache
Frequent urination at night

Western diagnosis

Allergy to cow's milk
Allergic rhinitis

Background to disease

Excessive consumption of fruit (a minimum of 10 bananas per week)

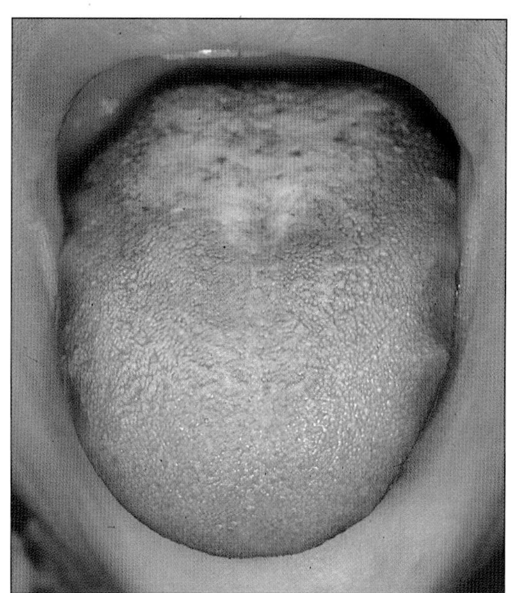

Fig. 10.2.3.1
Female
28 years old

Tongue description	**Chinese diagnosis**
Pale red	Normal
Red, raised points on the anterior third	Heat toxin in the upper burner
Dry, rough, white coating	Deficiency of fluids in the Stomach

Symptoms

Swollen cervical and inguinal lymph nodes
Stomach pains and epigastric fullness
Distended lower abdomen

Western diagnosis

Non-Hodgkin's lymphoma

Background to disease

Condition followed radiation therapy and chemotherapy

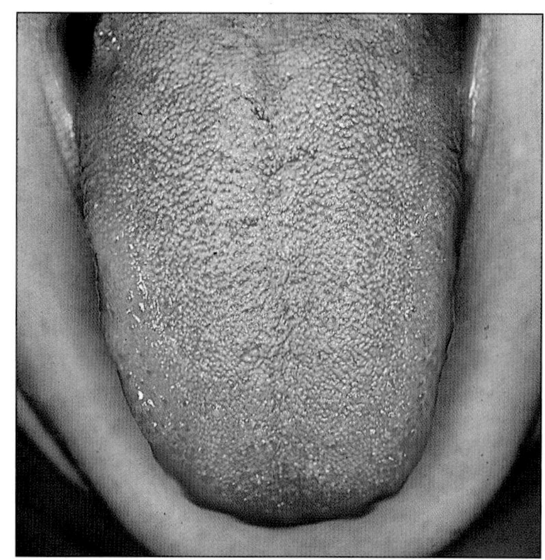

Fig. 10.2.3.2
Female
31 years old

Fig. 10.2.3.3
Female
38 years old

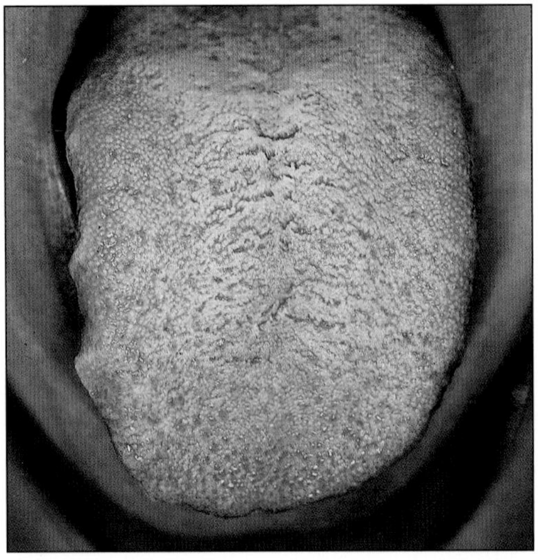

Tongue description ------------------------ **Chinese diagnosis**

Tongue description	Chinese diagnosis
Reddish, big, rough tongue body	Kidney yin deficiency with slight deficiency of fluids
Red points at the tip	Heat in the Heart
White, dry coating turning yellow toward the center of the tongue	Accumulation of phlegm, heat developing

Symptoms

Purulent stye
Red conjunctiva
Strong thirst
Constipation
Inability to sleep through the night
Inner restlessness

Western diagnosis

Chronic sinusitis
Acute conjunctivitis

Background to disease

Overworked
Lack of sleep
Long-standing emotional problems

Fig. 10.2.3.4
Female
62 years old

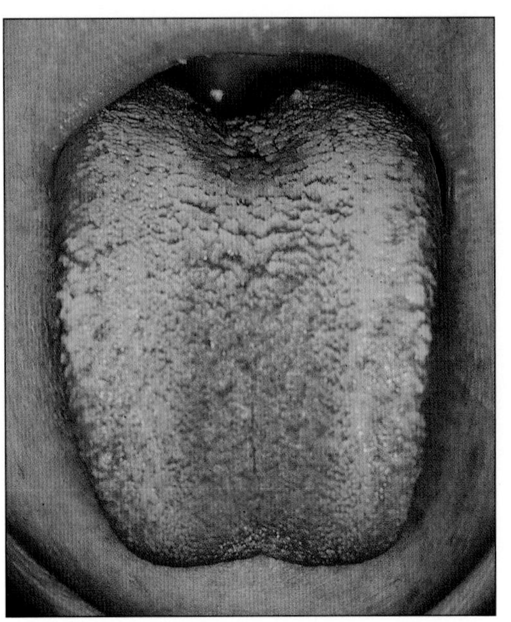

Tongue description	Chinese diagnosis
Red, dry	Kidney yin deficiency
Thick, greasy, white at the sides, *dirty yellow coating in the center of the tongue*	Accumulation of cold-dampness with blockage of qi in the middle burner, transforming to heat

Symptoms

Dizzy spells
Tingling and numbness of the arms
Pains in the shoulder and lumbar region

Western diagnosis

None

Background to disease

Excessive consumption of fatty foods
Physically overworked

Tongue description	**Chinese diagnosis**
Pale	Spleen qi deficiency
Swollen sides	Spleen qi deficiency
Red edges	Heat in the Liver
Yellow, thick, tofu-like coating	Retention of phlegm-heat

Symptoms

Bitter taste in the mouth
Insomnia
Irritability
Lack of appetite
Soft stools
Nausea

Western diagnosis

None

Background to disease

Overconsumption of fatty and spicy foods

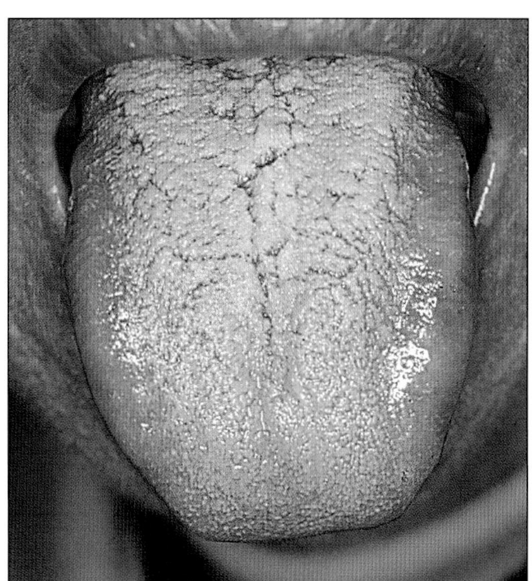

Fig. 10.2.3.5
Male
45 years old

10.2.4 Black (or Gray) Coating

A gray or black coating is often an indication of a serious illness. As a rule, it is the result of a long-standing pathology. It indicates extreme heat as well as cold patterns of disease.

If the black coating is also slippery in appearance, it reflects a deficiency of Spleen and Kidney yang with excessive internal cold. If this type of coating is only visible at the center of the tongue, while the sides show the remains of a white coating, it is indicative of Spleen yang deficiency with the accumulation of cold-dampness.

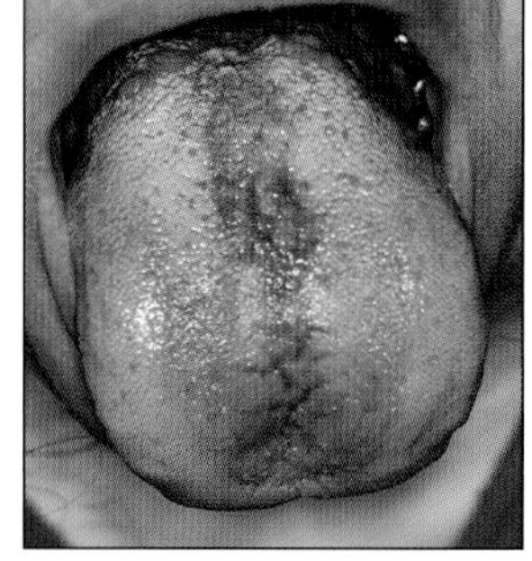

If the black coating is dry and appears cracked, it can be assumed that there is a serious development in a persisting disorder. This type of coating indicates that the yin is declining, which may lead to its separation from the yang. The patient may be in danger since the black coating reflects the development of extreme heat that can consume the body fluids. The drier and blacker the coating, the more severe the exhaustion of yin and fluids.

A yellow coating at the sides and a black, greasy coating in the center of the tongue are indicative of extreme heat in the Stomach. A persistently yellow coating reflects the long-standing retention of damp-heat. Extreme heat in the Stomach burns the fluids and causes the black, burnt-looking coating. (*See also* Ch. 11, Special Tongue Signs.)

Tongue description ------------------------- **Chinese diagnosis**

Reddish with red sides, contracted tongue body and tip — Heat in the Liver, Lungs, and Heart; injury to the yin in the upper burner

Black coating in the center and posterior third of the tongue, yellow at the sides — Long-standing heat in the yang brightness (*yáng míng*) channel with injury to the fluids

Fig. 10.2.4.1
Male
33 years old

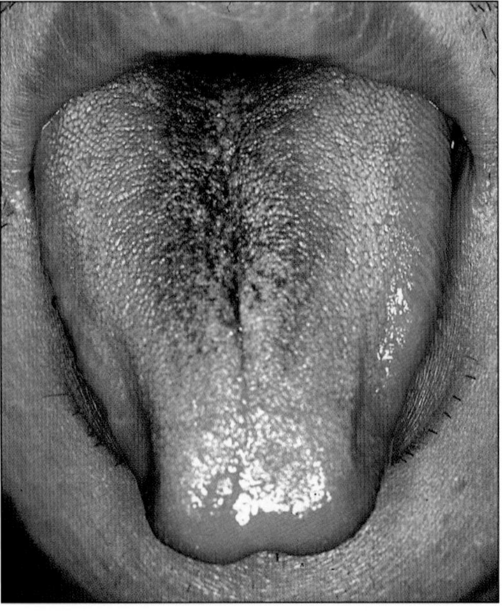

Symptoms

Pain in the throat
Dry mouth
Feeling of heat in the nose
Occasional nosebleeds
Blocked nasal passages
Headache

Western diagnosis

Carcinoma of the nasopharynx

Background to disease

Smoked for many years
Possible environmental factors (pollution)

Tongue description ------------------------- **Chinese diagnosis**

Red, swollen — Retention of phlegm-heat

Slightly pale sides — Slight Liver blood deficiency

Deviating — Movement of internally-generated wind

Black, thick, greasy coating with dirty yellow coating at the sides — Retention of phlegm-heat in yang brightness (*yáng míng*) channel

Fig. 10.2.4.2
Female
83 years old

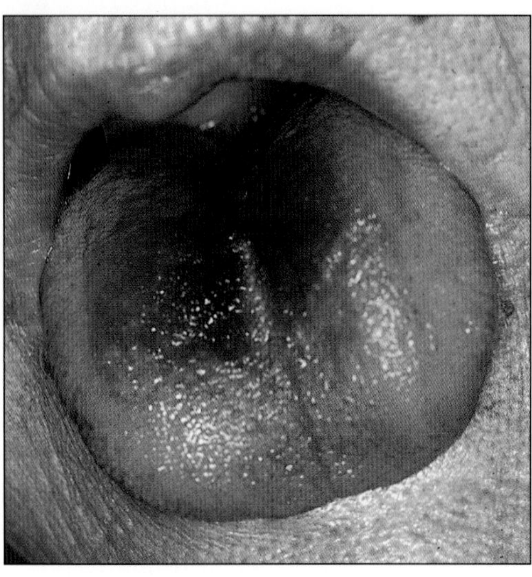

Symptoms

Slurred speech
Constipation with hard, dry stools
Loss of memory
Inability to move left arm and leg

Western diagnosis

Apoplexy with left-sided hemiplegia

Background to disease

High blood pressure for 20 years

About this case history

The following case history is a good example of a yellow, greasy coating that thickens toward the root of the tongue. This is seen quite frequently and denotes retention of damp-heat in the lower burner. In relation to the location and severity of the patient's complaints, the color and nature of the coating can contribute to an understanding of the predominance of heat or dampness, which of course will influence the composition of the herbal formula prescribed in treatment.

Tongue description	**Chinese diagnosis**
Slightly pale	Spleen qi deficiency
Slightly curled-up edges	Liver qi stagnation
Light yellow, greasy coating from the center to the root	Retention of damp-heat
Light yellow, thin coating with red points at the root	Retention of damp-heat in the Bladder

Symptoms

Burning pain before and after urination
Urinary urgency
Dark, sparse urine
Irritability
Tiredness

Western diagnosis

Acute cystitis

Background to disease

Demands of work
Excessive consumption of fruit and salads

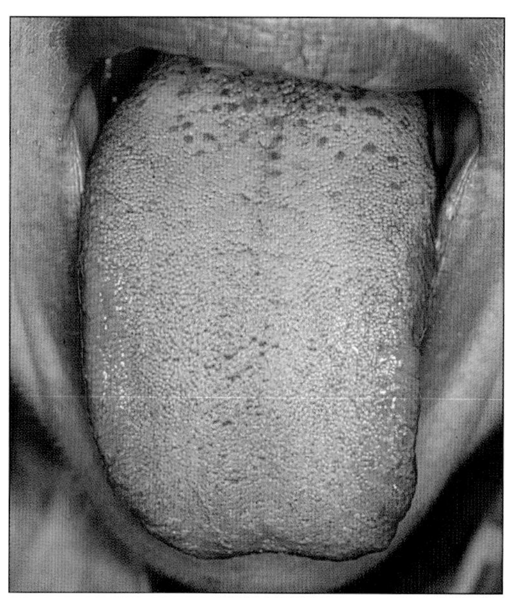

Fig. 10.2.4.3 Female 43 years old

CASE HISTORY The patient presented with acute symptoms. The evening prior to visiting the clinic she felt a drawing sensation in her bladder. She woke in the morning with strong pains and a burning sensation before and during urination. She had an urgent need to urinate, which caused pains in her lower abdomen. She passed small amounts of dark, turbid urine. She had no fever. A urine test revealed the presence of nitrates. Although she was not thirsty, she forced herself to drink a large amount of fluids. Her bowel movements were normal. This was her second bout of cystitis within three months, and she could not find a cause for this recent bout. The first infection had been successfully treated with antibiotics; it was triggered by getting cold, wet feet. In general, she felt well, although she was often tired and irritable due to her workload. Her pulse was rapid and slippery.

Analysis. This is an example of heat-induced painful urination syndrome. The acute onset, burning pain, and the urgency to urinate characterize this condition of excess in the Bladder. The degree of yellow discoloration and the greasy texture of the tongue coating implicate both dampness and heat equally in the acute bout of cystitis. The light yellow coating, by itself indicative of both dampness and heat, covers the entire tongue body. This coating has a greasy texture that reflects an accumulation of dampness, possibly caused by overconsumption of fruit and salads. The large, red papillae at the root of the tongue indicate heat in the lower burner, further implicating heat as a major factor in this case.

Pathomechanism

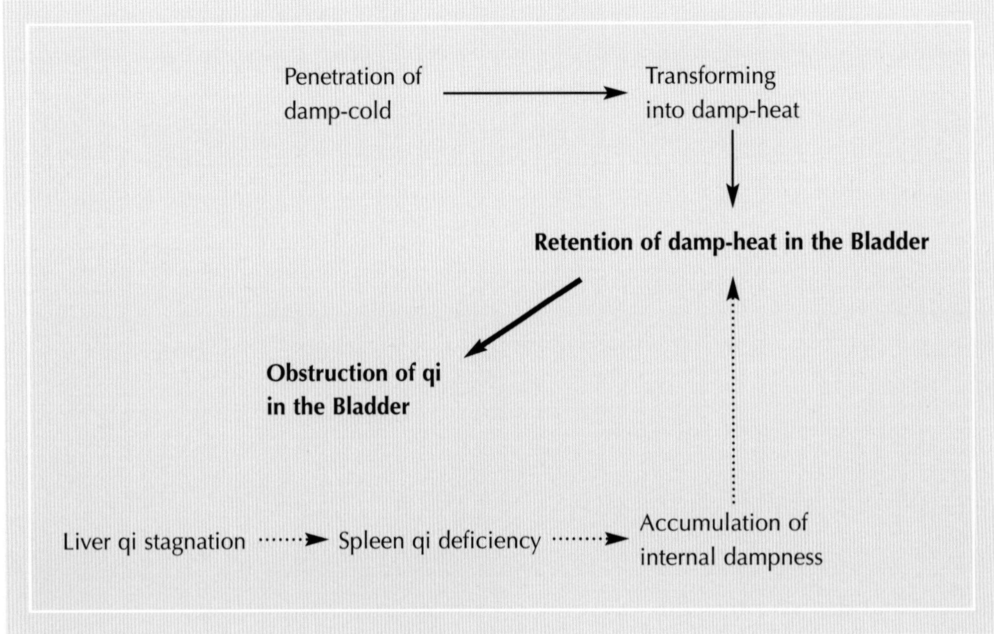

The patient complained of a drawing sensation prior to the onset of the acute infection. This reflects the effect on the movement of Bladder qi by damp-heat. The damp-heat obstructs the qi mechanism in the Bladder. The turbidity of the urine reflects the inability of the Bladder qi to transform the turbid fluids. The damp-heat in the lower burner obstructs the flow of qi, which is responsible for the pain in the lower abdomen. Heat, as reflected in the papillae and in the rapid, slippery pulse, parches the fluids, resulting in sparse and dark urine, in the sense of urgency to urinate, and in the burning sensation.

The curled-up edges of the tongue denote an underlying pattern of Liver qi stagnation. Since the patient's irritability is the only corresponding symptom, this pattern is not considered to be the cause of the acute infection, especially since the first bout of cystitis was caused by damp-cold transforming to damp-heat in the Bladder. Antibiotics, administered three months before, were effective in eliminating acute heat. However, some pathogenic factors, usually dampness and residual heat, often remain behind. In this case, it is possible that the remnants of damp-heat in the Bladder are the cause of the acute condition.

The patient's constitution is good. The tongue body does not show any significant signs apart from the curled-up edges, which indicate constraint of Liver qi. This, in combination with an inappropriate diet, may have slightly impaired the Spleen's transportive and transformative functions. Neither the tongue nor the pulse reflects Spleen qi deficiency.

Treatment strategy. Clear the heat, drain the dampness, regulate the Bladder qi, and regulate the urination.

For two days a modified version of Eight-Herb Powder for Rectification (*bā zhèng sǎn*) was prescribed. *Mù tōng* (Akebiae/Clematidis/etc. Caulis) and Dianthi Herba (*qú mài*) were removed from the formula, and Dioscoreae hypoglaucae Rhizoma (*bì xiè*) was added. For 12 hours after taking this decoction, the urge to urinate and the burning pain were reduced. However, she did have strong diarrhea. On the third day, she felt a slight drawing sensation in the bladder. A subsequent urine test was negative.

Endnote

1 Be aware that brushing one's tongue will eventually lead to a dry and rough tongue surface.

CHAPTER 11

Special Tongue Signs

This chapter will show a few extraordinary tongue signs, or those that one does not see often during one's clinical practice.

11.1 Completely Cracked Tongue

A unique type of tongue is the completely cracked tongue. Deep, wide cracks always located at the edges and sides of the tongue are a distinctive feature of this completely cracked tongue body. Despite its startling appearance, no particular disharmony or pattern of disease is associated with this type of tongue, and it often occurs in more than one family member.

Nevertheless, the cracked tongue may point to a constitutional weakness and deficiency of fluids and Kidney yin.[1]

These tongues are usually big and swollen. It is therefore important to check the tongue body color. If it is pale, it is indicative of deficiency of the blood and fluids; if it is red and completely cracked, it indicates deficiency of the yin and fluids. As a rule, this type of tongue has very little coating or no coating at all, which can be explained by the lack of fluids in general. However, it bears repeating that a person with this type of tongue does not necessarily have any serious or organic illness. From a biomedical point of view, it may point to Melkersson–Rosenthal syndrome, which is a rare neurological disorder characterized by recurring facial paralysis, swelling of the face and lips (usually the upper lip), and the development of folds and furrows in the tongue. Onset is in childhood or early adolescence. After recurring attacks (ranging from days to years in between), swelling may persist and increase, eventually becoming permanent. The cause of Melkersson–Rosenthal syndrome is unknown, but there may be a genetic predisposition. Lingua plicatae can be symptomatic of Crohn's disease or sarcoidosis.

Tongue description ---------- **Chinese diagnosis**

Pale red with cracks over the entire surface, with notches and cracks at the sides — Constitutional weakness of qi, blood, yin, and fluids

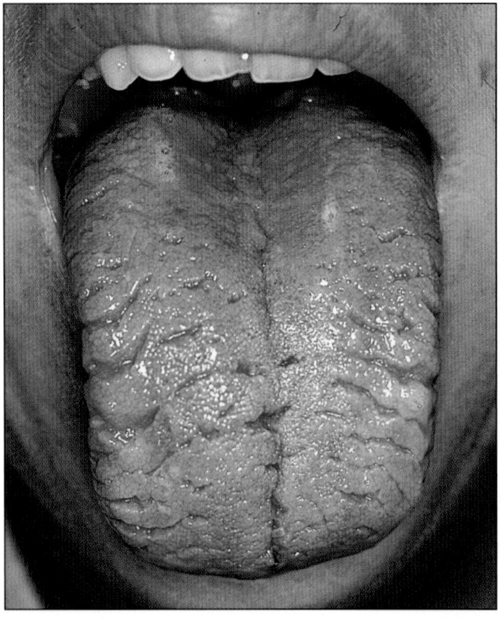

Fig. 11.1
Female
35 years old

Symptoms

Stomach pains
Heartburn
Vomiting with excitement
Feelings of fear

Western diagnosis

None

Background to disease

Overworked
Emotional problems
Constitutional weakness

Tongue description ---------- **Chinese diagnosis**

Tongue description	Chinese diagnosis
Red	Kidney yin deficiency
Reddish tip	Heat in the Heart
Deep vertical crack in the center of the tongue	Stomach yin deficiency and deficiency of fluids
Notches and cracks at the sides	Deficiency of fluids and yin
No coating	Stomach yin deficiency

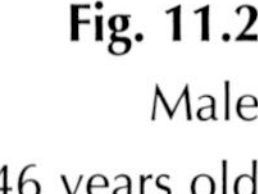

Fig. 11.2
Male
46 years old

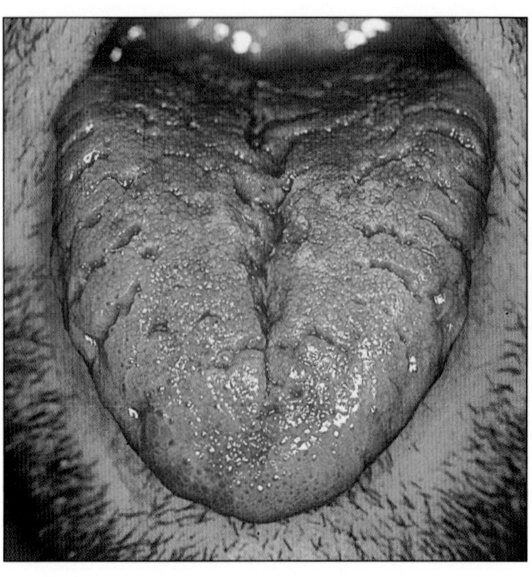

Symptoms

Impotence
Difficulty urinating, dribbling urine
Depressive moods
Irritability
Heartburn

Western diagnosis

Hypertrophy of the prostate

Background to disease

Emotional problems
Constitutional weakness

11.2 Unusual Coatings

11.2.1 Tofu-like Coating

This coating looks like tofu or soy cheese. It consists of big, rough-grained flakes that seem to lie just on the surface of the tongue. This coating can indicate extreme yang and excessive heat in the interior.

There is another interpretation of this tongue coating in the literature: "a rise of turbid substances, as in food stagnation or turbid phlegm." This means that food stagnation as well as retention of damp-heat can cause this type of coating.

Tongue description	**Chinese diagnosis**
Red, soft, slightly narrow tongue body	Kidney yin deficiency
Thick, greasy, tofu-like, pale yellow coating	Internal heat with retention of phlegm-heat

Symptoms

Cough with blood-tinged sputum
Shortness of breath
Pains in the chest
Backache
Subfebrile temperatures
No appetite

Western diagnosis

Carcinoma of the nasopharynx
Metastases to the lungs and cervical vertebrae

Background to disease

Smoked for 40 years

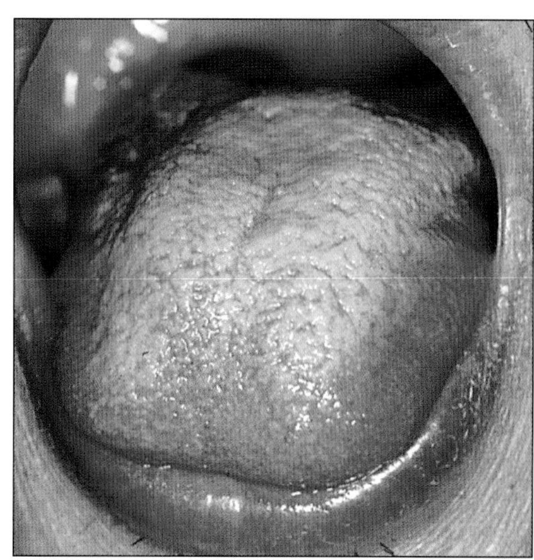

Fig. 11.2.1.1
Male
63 years old

Tongue description --- **Chinese diagnosis**

Bright red, narrow tongue body — Kidney yin deficiency with injury to the fluids

Tofu-like, pale yellow coating — Retention of damp-phlegm in the yang brightness *(yáng míng)* channel transforming into phlegm-heat, food stagnation

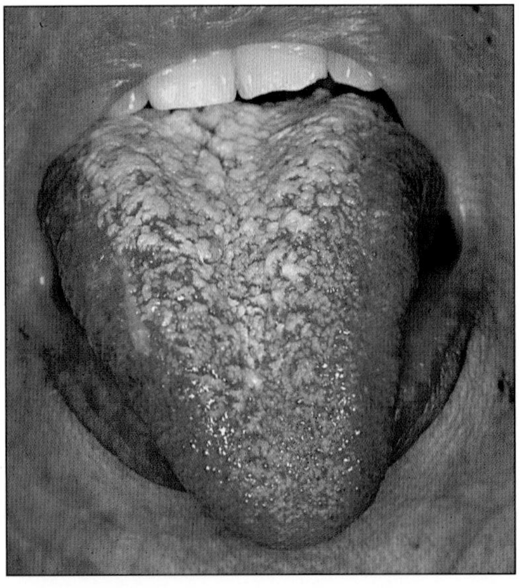

Fig. 11.2.1.2
Male
69 years old

Symptoms

Subfebrile temperatures
Pain under the right hypochondrium
Foul-smelling stools
Flatulence
Distended abdomen

Western diagnosis

Carcinoma of the large intestine, with metastases to the liver

Background to disease

Unknown

11.2.2 Black, Hairy Tongue

A black, hairy tongue in humans is a harmless condition caused by a fungus which grows on the top surface of the tongue. It is associated with the elderly, as well as with antibiotic use.[2] While black is the most common color associated with the condition, other colors are also possible. It will disappear quite quickly once the bacterial flora in the gut has been reestablished.

Tongue description --- **Chinese diagnosis**

Pale tongue body — Slight blood deficiency

Dry, yellow, patchy, black coating — Retention of damp-heat, fluids injured by antibiotics

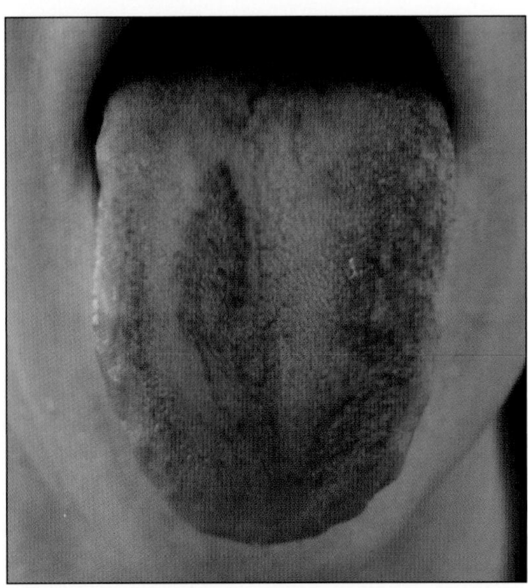

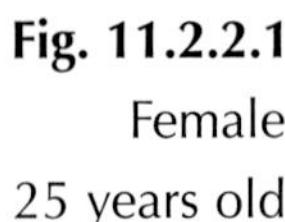

Fig. 11.2.2.1
Female
25 years old

Symptoms

Burning after urination
Urgency to urinate
Tiredness

Background to disease

Condition following acute cystitis treated with antibiotics

11.2.3 Patchy Tongue Coating

Any unusual tongue signs should be questioned. This is especially true for tongue coatings. For example, sucking a sweet or tablet can erase the coating at the center of the tongue (Fig. 11.2.3.1), falsely suggesting Stomach yin deficiency.

If patients with asthma or a serious heart condition have to use aerosols, the root of the tongue may have no fur due to the mechanical application of a spray (Fig. 11.2.3.2). In this photo, the patient suffered from angina pectoris and used aerosols frequently during the day.

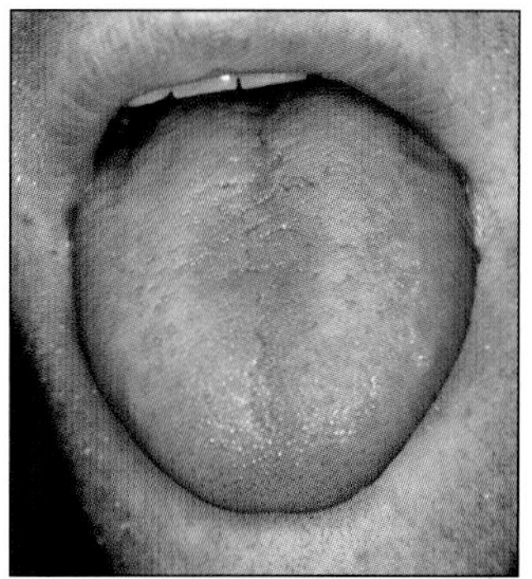

Fig. 11.2.3.1

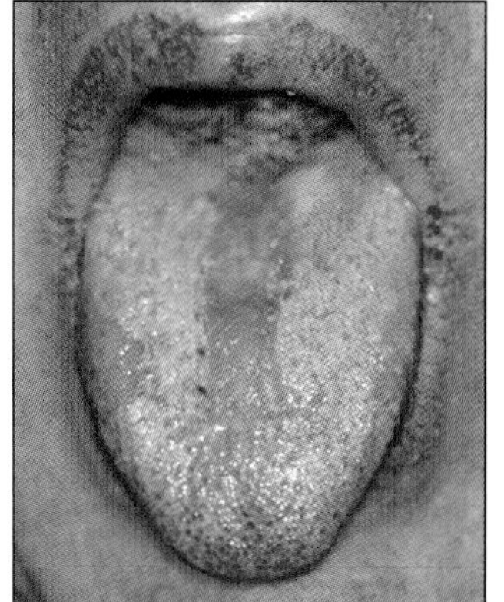

Fig. 11.2.3.2

Endnotes

1 Song T-B. *Atlas of the Tongue and Lingual Coatings in Chinese Medicine.* Beijing: Peoples Medical Publishing House and Editions Sinomedic, 1981:64.

2 Lingua villosa nigra is also reported with doxycycline use.

CHAPTER 12

Changes in the Tongue Following Treatment with Acupuncture and Herbs

The figures in this chapter illustrate changes in the color, shape, and coating of the tongue as a result of the healing process. In each case, the first photograph—designated by the letter 'a' following the figure number—shows the tongue as it appeared prior to treatment. This is followed by one or two photographs of the same tongue—designated by the letters 'b' and 'c'—subsequent to the start of treatment.

12.1 Changes in the Tongue Body Color and/or Shape

The color of the tongue body represents one of the most important aspects of tongue diagnosis. It reflects the underlying energetic condition of a person, especially the quality of their qi and blood. When both energies are strong, the tongue body has a fresh, pale red color. The condition of the yin and yang as well as the quality of blood circulation can also be determined from the color. Finally, an illness that is caused by heat or cold may also affect the color of the tongue body.

In acute illnesses, the tongue body color can change quite quickly, especially if the primary factor at the onset of the disease process is heat. High fever injures the body fluids, resulting in a sudden reddish discoloration of the tongue body. By contrast, heavy blood loss can quickly lead to a pale tongue body, denoting injury to the qi and blood. In chronic illnesses, it may take some time until the tongue body color deviates from the normal pale red. Thus, the evaluation of the tongue body color is an important tool, particularly in cases of mild or chronic illnesses, when ascertaining the underlying condition of the patient's qi, blood, yin, and yang.

In Figs. 12.1 through 12.3, the shape and/or color of the tongue body changed noticeably. In Fig. 12.1a, the tongue body was reddish when treatment began, reflecting the developing heat resulting from energetic changes that occurred during a pregnancy and that engendered such symptoms as heartburn and nausea. The treatment strategy there was to stop the development of heat by regulating the patient's energies while gently nourishing her Stomach and Kidney yin. Following treatment with Chinese herbs, the tongue body became slightly pale (Fig. 12.1b). The speed of the color change underlined the rapidity of the process by which the heat initially developed. The patient had only been pregnant for 12 weeks at the time of the first consultation.

The severe pain of the patient in Fig. 12.2 was the result of deep-seated blood stasis as reflected in the slight bluish discoloration of the tongue body in the channels and bones. The primary color of the tongue body, however, was red (Fig. 12.2a), and this sign plus the peeled tongue coating indicated a condition of Kidney yin deficiency. The initial treatment involved acupuncture to resolve the blood stasis, followed by an herbal prescription to strengthen the Kidney yin. The acupuncture relieved the pain and resulted in the disappearance of the bluish discoloration; the use of herbs resulted in a reduction in the red discoloration (Fig. 12.2b). This change in tongue color over such a short period of time is extraordinary given that the blood stasis had been present for many years. In my experience, this kind of change usually takes place after months of treatment.

The color of the tongue body should always be considered in conjunction with its shape and texture. The shape signals the presence of excess or deficiency. For example, a swollen tongue body reflects a pattern of excess the accumulation of dampness while a thin tongue body reflects a deficiency of blood or yin. The color and shape of the tongue body are needed to further discriminate between blood and yin deficiency. Generally speaking, yin deficiency will result in a tongue body that is red and thin, while a pale, thin tongue reflects a pattern of blood deficiency.

The tongue body in Fig. 12.1a is red and slightly contracted, and its texture appears to be uneven. Together, these signs suggest an injury to the body fluids by heat. Not only did the heat change the color of the tongue, it also changed its shape. At the conclusion of treatment in this case, the tongue body was still slightly swollen, while the tongue surface appeared to be more regular.

In Fig. 12.3, the main complaints consisted of irritability and a vaginal discharge. The indentations found along the edges of the entire length of the tongue body (Fig. 12.3a) were indicative of a long-standing pattern of Liver qi stagnation. Following a year of regular acupuncture, which was aimed at regulating the flow of Liver qi, the tongue had lost its tension, and the indentation along the edges had almost disappeared (Fig. 12.3b). In addition, the tongue body increased in volume, indicating improved circulation of blood and body fluids. This improvement was consistent with the patient's more relaxed and joyful attitude toward life, and the lack of vaginal discharge.

12.2 Changes in the Tongue Coating

The tongue coating reflects the depth (interior/exterior) of an illness; whether it is deficient or excessive in nature; the presence of heat or cold; the strength of the Stomach qi and Kidney yin; and the state of the fluids.

Analysis of the coating is extremely important in cases of acute illness as it reflects the nature, strength, and depth of penetration of an externally-contracted factor. Changes in the normal white, moist coating can occur quickly and the clinician can use the information gained from these changes to formulate a proper treatment for an acute illness.

Figs. 12.6 and 12.7 are impressive examples of this. The whitish, thick, and dry tongue coating of the patient presented in Fig. 12.6a resulted from an attack by warm-dryness. The whitish color of the coating signaled that the illness was still at a superficial stage, and its thickness reflected a condition of excess. Within four days of treatment, the patient's cough had disappeared and the tongue coating had become normal (Fig. 12.6b). The coating resumed its normal moist state in the expected time, reflecting the successful elimination of the pathogenic factor. In Fig. 12.7a, the black, slippery tongue coating reflected the penetration of a strong, externally-contracted cold pathogenic factor to the lower abdomen. This pathogenic factor had penetrated more deeply than in the preceding case, and it could therefore be expected that its elimination would take much longer. Fig. 12.7b shows the tongue of that patient after two weeks of treatment. The diminishment of the black coating correlated well with the improvement in the condition of the patient.

Figs. 12.4, 12.5, and 12.8 are examples of cases in which changes to the tongue coating were caused by interior patterns of disease. The coatings presented in Figs. 12.5 and 12.8 resulted from conditions of excess, while in Fig. 12.4 it resulted from deficiency. The patient discussed in Fig. 12.5 suffered from ulcerative colitis. Generally speaking, an important aspect in the development of this disease is the retention of damp-heat in the Large Intestine. In this case, the disease was accompanied by a thick yellow coating on the posterior third of the tongue (Fig. 12.5a). The color, texture, and thickness of the coating all pointed toward a pattern of dampness and heat, which was responsible for the patient's acute symptoms. Here the constraint of Liver qi was the primary disease factor. Fig. 12.5b shows the tongue after taking Chinese herbs for ten weeks. The yellow, greasy coating has disappeared, which correlated with the patient's feeling of well-being. The tongue edges were still curled-up, reflecting the underlying constraint of Liver qi and underlining the need for further treatment.

The tongue coating of the patient presented in Fig. 12.8a was brown, and was developing a black hue in the center. This color reflected the intensity of the heat that was developing. In this case, the color and texture of the coating were regarded as more important in terms of the treatment strategy than the color and shape of the tongue body, even though the latter suggested severe Spleen qi deficiency and accumulation of dampness. While the accumulation of dampness was understood to play a role in the disease process, it was not deemed to be responsible for the patient's painful, persistent gum infection. The treatment therefore focused on eliminating the heat toxin by purging it through the bowels. This allowed the heat to be eliminated from the yang brightness channels. After five days of Chinese herbal treatment, the heat toxin began to be eliminated, and as a result, the color and thickness of the tongue coating began to change as well (Fig. 12.8b). After eight more days of treatment, the pain began to decline as more heat toxin was eliminated. At this stage, the tongue coating was whitish, thick, and slightly dry (Fig. 12.8c), reflecting the successful elimination of heat and phlegm-heat.

The tongue coating presented in Fig. 12.4 shows a condition of deficiency. The coating in Fig. 12.4a, where the patient's major complaint involved long-standing heartburn, was without root and showed a peeled area in the center, denoting the presence of Stomach yin deficiency. In addition, the remaining coating was old and dry, signaling that the formation of new tongue coating was not occurring. As we have previously seen in other cases in this book, for example, Figs. 2.6.2 and 7.1.2.5, a tongue coating that reflects a condition of deficiency should be further evaluated in conjunction with the tongue body, and especially its color. In Fig. 12.4a, the red tongue body suggested the presence of Kidney yin deficiency. As a result, while administering herbs to regulate the qi mechanism of the middle burner, the patient was also given herbs that nourished the Stomach yin; both strategies would assist in the formation of a new tongue coating. After four weeks of treatment, the old, tofu-like coating had disappeared and the new coating was both thinner and more moist (Fig. 12.4b). The peeled area was smaller, albeit still visible, and did not seem as dry. The change in the coating occurred fairly quickly, which signifies a strong constitution.

Tongue description	**Chinese diagnosis**
Reddish	Developing heat
Reddish edges	Heat in the Liver
Tense tongue body with slight indentation along the edges	Liver qi stagnation
Thin midline crack	Slight Stomach yin deficiency
Reddish areas	Developing heat
Peeled coating	Onset of Stomach yin deficiency

Symptoms

Severe nausea
Heartburn
Feeling of epigastric fullness
Flatulence
Thirst
Tiredness

Western diagnosis

Morning sickness

Background to disease

Suppressed emotions
Overconsumption of dairy products and raw foods

Fig. 12.1
Female
40 years old

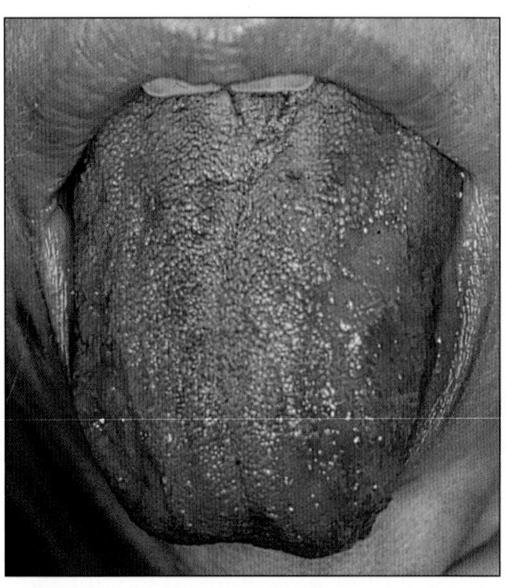

12.1a

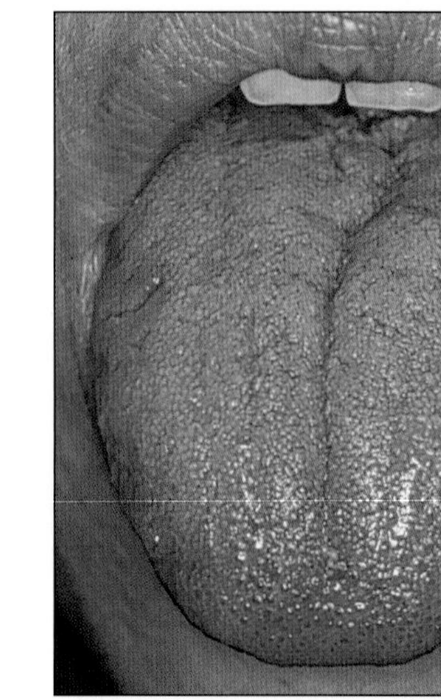

12.1b

CASE HISTORY The patient was unhappy about her third unwanted pregnancy. She came for treatment in her tenth week as she suffered from constant nausea and heartburn. She had similar symptoms in her preceding pregnancies; each time, the nausea had lasted until the fifth month. Both the nausea and heartburn improved after eating and became worse when she went without food for a long period of time. The heartburn was severe and caused a burning, hot sensation in her esophagus. Flatulence and a feeling of epigastric fullness accompanied the nausea. She was a vegetarian and mainly ate fruit, cheese, and yogurt. From the outset of this pregnancy, she had been very thirsty. Her pulse was thin and tense.

Analysis. The patient's negative feelings about the pregnancy have contributed to constraining the Liver qi. Together with the energetic changes that occur during every pregnancy, this has resulted in heat developing fairly rapidly. The red edges of the tongue clearly show this process. The pattern of Liver qi stagnation is reflected in the slight indentation along the edges of the tongue (Fig. 12.1a).

The mother's Kidney essence and blood nourish the fetus; thus, a temporary deficiency of essence and blood is engendered in the mother. Blood deficiency especially affects the Liver, the organ that stores the blood. Among its other functions, the Liver must nourish and anchor the Liver qi. If the blood is strong, it prevents the development of symptoms marked by heat and stops the qi from floating upward; that is, blood pacifies and softens the Liver and contributes to the free flow of its qi. The patient's emotional state, plus her blood deficiency, are responsible for the ensuing Liver qi stagnation, which plays an important role in morning sickness, especially during the first three months of pregnancy.[1] The Liver blood depends on nourishment from the Kidneys, which is now supplying the fetus instead. If the Kidneys are overburdened, the Liver will be undernourished, resulting in its becoming "impetuous or temperamental."[2]

The constrained Liver qi prevents the Stomach qi from descending, which results in nausea, vomiting, and choking fits. The constrained and rebellious Stomach qi is also responsible for a feeling of epigastric fullness. The constraint of qi in the Stomach also engenders heat, which ascends and causes heartburn. The development of heat in the Stomach is confirmed by the severe thirst, which was present since the beginning of the pregnancy.

As a rule, eating tends to aggravate digestive problems, especially when they are caused by a blockage of the qi mechanism of the middle burner. It is interesting that, in this case, eating eases the symptoms. This anomaly suggests the existence of deficiency. Apart from the patterns of Liver qi stagnation and constrained and rebellious Stomach qi, the patient also suffers from Spleen qi deficiency, which can be traced to her vegetarian diet as well as the overconsumption of dairy products and raw foods. In addition, the Liver qi transversely attacks the Spleen qi, which is already weakened by the pregnancy. The Spleen qi deficiency, in turn, contributes to the blood deficiency, which is reflected in the thin pulse.

The tongue coating is whitish and slightly greasy in the central part of the tongue, which signals the retention of cold and dampness in the middle burner that results from the dietary habits of the patient. The white tongue coating is not evenly distributed over the tongue body; instead, it begins to take on a peeled appearance, especially at the sides of the tongue. This could be the result of the obstruction of qi in the middle burner that gave rise to the heat. The ensuing slight injury to the fluids has contributed to the peeled coating.

Apart from these patterns, a disturbance of the Penetrating vessel is usually implicated in cases of morning sickness. During pregnancy the Penetrating vessel often develops a relative deficiency of blood and Kidney essence, especially when a woman has suffered from blood

Pathomechanism

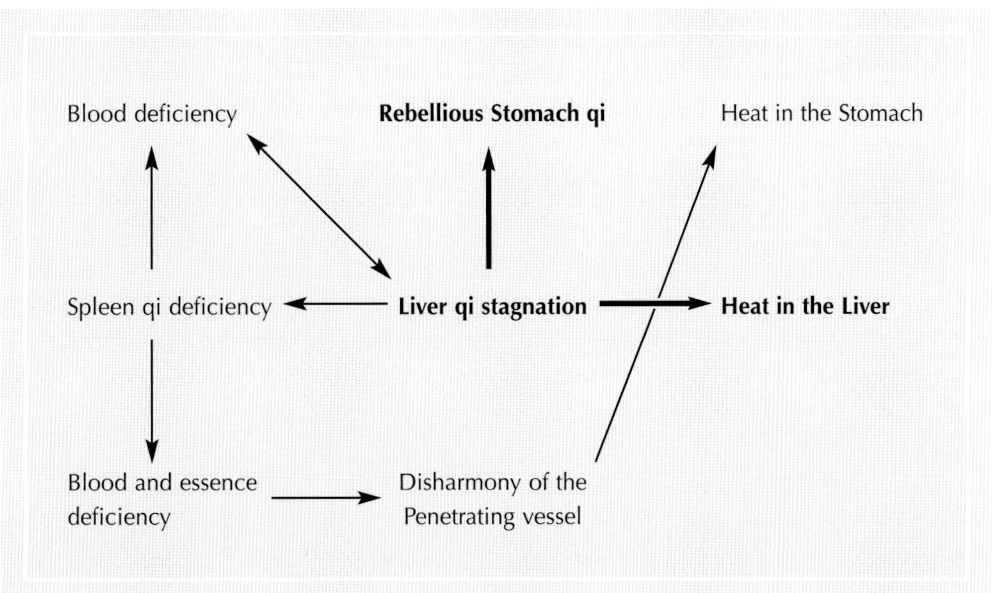

and essence deficiency prior to conception. During the first three months of pregnancy, the fetus develops rapidly, which leads to an overtaxation of the energies of the Kidneys and causes severe tiredness in most women. Because of the relative emptiness of the Penetrating vessel, especially in its lower part, rebellious qi is engendered, which eventually ascends. In addition, a disharmony in the Penetrating vessel may attack the Stomach, particularly because the Penetrating vessel is linked to the yang brightness Stomach channel at ST-30 *(qì chōng)*.

The thin midline crack in the tongue points toward Stomach yin deficiency. This sign suggests a disease pattern that began prior to this pregnancy. Generally speaking, the formation of cracks appears after a serious acute illness or a long, chronic pattern of disharmony. However, the patient had not experienced digestive problems prior to the pregnancy. Thus, this sign was not included in the final pathomechanism or treatment strategy.

Treatment strategy. Regulate the Liver qi, strengthen the Spleen qi, harmonize the Stomach qi, clear the Stomach heat, and ease the nausea.

For seven days the patient was prescribed a decoction based on Frigid Extremities Powder *(sì nì săn)* and Tangerine Peel and Bamboo Shavings Decoction *(jú pí zhú rú tāng)*. This was modified by the addition of Perillae Folium *(zǐ sū yè)* and Atractylodis macrocephalae Rhizoma *(bái zhú)*. Perillae Folium *(zǐ sū yè)* was added because of its ability to ease morning sickness, and Atractylodis macrocephalae Rhizoma *(bái zhú)* because of its action in strengthening the Spleen qi and its calming effect on the fetus. One week later, the patient felt much better. She still suffered from nausea and heartburn, but the symptoms were less intense. As a result, the above herbs were discontinued and in their place she was given Left Metal Pill *(zuǒ jīn wán)* plus Sepiae Endoconcha *(hǎi piāo xiāo)* to regulate the disharmony between the Liver and Stomach. Left Metal Pill *(zuǒ jīn wán)* consists of the two herbs Coptidis Rhizoma *(huáng lián),* to eliminate heat from the Stomach and Liver, and Evodiae Fructus *(wú zhū yú),* to regulate the Liver qi, aid the sinking of Stomach qi, and warm the Spleen qi. At the same time, the patient was prescribed Jade Fluid Decoction *(yù yè tāng),* which was modified by removing Astragali Radix *(huáng qí),* Puerariae Radix *(gé gēn),* and Schisandrae Fructus *(wǔ wèi zǐ)*. Thereafter, the patient felt much better in that she no longer suffered from heartburn, her thirst was normal, and she only experienced slight nausea. However, she then felt very tired. The above prescription was therefore repeated, but with the addition of 20 grams of Astragali Radix *(huáng qí)*. Again, the patient improved, and the nausea disappeared by the 18th week of pregnancy.

Changes in the tongue. The tongue changed considerably over the course of treatment. The tongue body is now only slightly pale and slightly swollen (Fig. 12.1b). This change signals that the heat, which was evident in the red tongue body and edges, has been cleared from the Stomach. The pale tongue body highlights the underlying pattern of the disease, Spleen qi deficiency and accumulation of dampness. Its slightly swollen quality has lost its tense appearance, showing that the flow of Liver qi has been regulated. Finally, the coating has thinned considerably and seems slightly slippery, and there are no more peeled areas. This change reflects the regeneration of Stomach yin and fluids, which could only have come about by clearing the heat.

Tongue description

Red
Bluish
Deep cracks at the sides of the tongue
Red spots at the tip of the tongue
Yellow, greasy coating with peeled areas

Chinese diagnosis

Kidney yin deficiency
Blood stasis
Spleen qi deficiency, onset of Spleen yin deficiency
Heat in the Heart
Retention of damp-heat with the onset of Stomach yin deficiency

Symptoms

Numbness of the right thigh
Pain in the bones
Dryness of the mouth
Premature ejaculation
Restlessness

Western diagnosis

Prolapsed disc

Background to disease

Injured from motorbike accidents, several operations on the lumbar spine, knees, and lower leg. Physically and mentally overworked

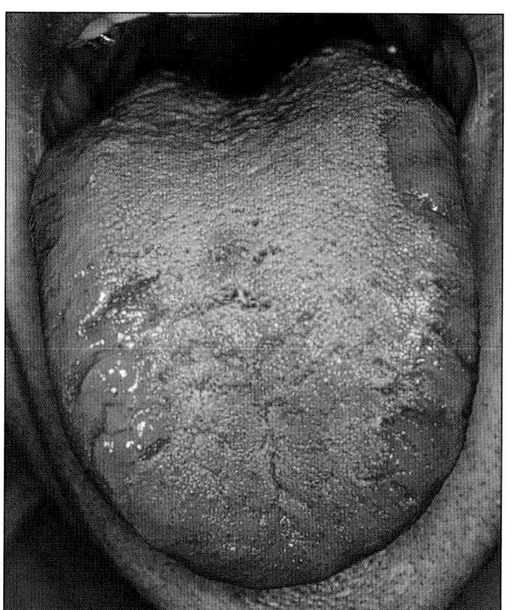

12.2a

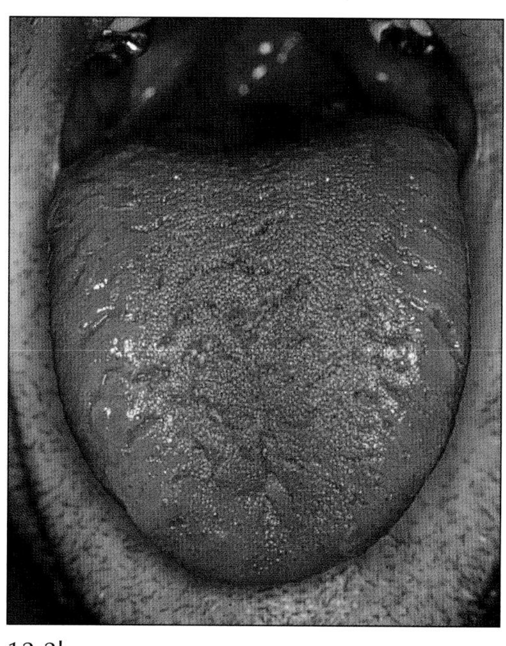

12.2b

Fig. 12.2
Male
47 years old

CASE HISTORY This patient had been a motorcycle enthusiast in his youth. He stopped riding motorcycles after several serious accidents that resulted in a number of bone fractures and contusions. Over a period of ten years, he had five operations on his lumbar spine and lower legs. He suffered from recurring pains in his knees and lower legs. The pains, which were always localized and very severe, would last for days. He felt that the bones "deep inside" caused the pain. Occasionally, the pains were so severe that his mobility was limited. His legs often felt weak. There was no recognizable pattern to the pain. A prolapsed disc between the fourth and fifth lumbar vertebrae irritated the root of the sciatic nerve, which occasionally led to numbness in the lateral aspect of his right thigh.

The patient worked with mentally ill youth, which he found to be exhausting. Shift work, especially night shifts, led to sleep deprivation. Night sweats occasionally impaired the quality of his sleep. His sexual prowess was diminished, and he frequently suffered from premature ejaculation. His appetite and thirst were normal. He ate irregularly and preferred fried and spicy foods. His pulse was deficient and floating.

Analysis. This case is an example of an obstruction syndrome caused by blood stasis in the channels, collaterals, and bones. The contusions and fractures caused qi and blood stasis in the muscles and bones, respectively, impairing the circulation of blood and thereby resulting in severe, localized pains. In this case, the channels and collaterals of the legs were affected, especially the right lower leg, since two complicated fractures had required difficult surgery and had left a large amount of scar tissue.

The bluish discoloration of the tongue body, which reflects the severe obstruction of qi and blood, was judged to be an important indication of both the chronic and intense nature of the stasis in the channels and bones. The pain did not react to changes in the climate, nor did it improve or worsen with hot or cold applications. This suggests an external pathogenic factor could be excluded as the basis for the pain.

Apart from this condition of excess—qi and blood stasis in the channels—the body of the tongue indicates a pattern of deficiency. Important signs include the deep cracks at the sides of the tongue and the peeled areas on the tongue coating, which together indicate a long-standing weakness of Stomach and Spleen yin. The depth and width of the cracks suggest a possible constitutional weakness. A long-term disease process can lead to deficiency of Spleen yin. The patient's dry mouth and obvious red lips are a reflection of this deficiency. Spleen yin deficiency impairs the transformation and transportation of food essence, which will adversely affect the Spleen as well as the rest of the body,[3] principally the muscles. This will result in a feeling of weakness in the legs. In addition, one branch of the Spleen sinew channel adheres to the spine.[4] It unites with the Governing vessel at GV-11 *(shén dào)* and thus contributes to the spine's stability.

Apart from the pain in his legs, the patient suffered from a prolapsed disc and irritation of the sciatic nerve, resulting in numbness of the lateral aspect of the right thigh. From the perspective of Chinese medicine, numbness and one-sided symptoms can be used to confirm a diagnosis of blood stasis in the channels, especially of the lesser yang Gallbladder channel.

Underlying Kidney yin deficiency is responsible for the patient's premature ejaculation. Since the Kidney energy is too weak, it cannot contain the sperm. In addition, the yin deficiency results in the flaring of fire from deficiency, which also contributes to the premature ejaculation. The red tongue body, the peeled tongue coating, and the deficient, floating pulse confirm this

Pathomechanism

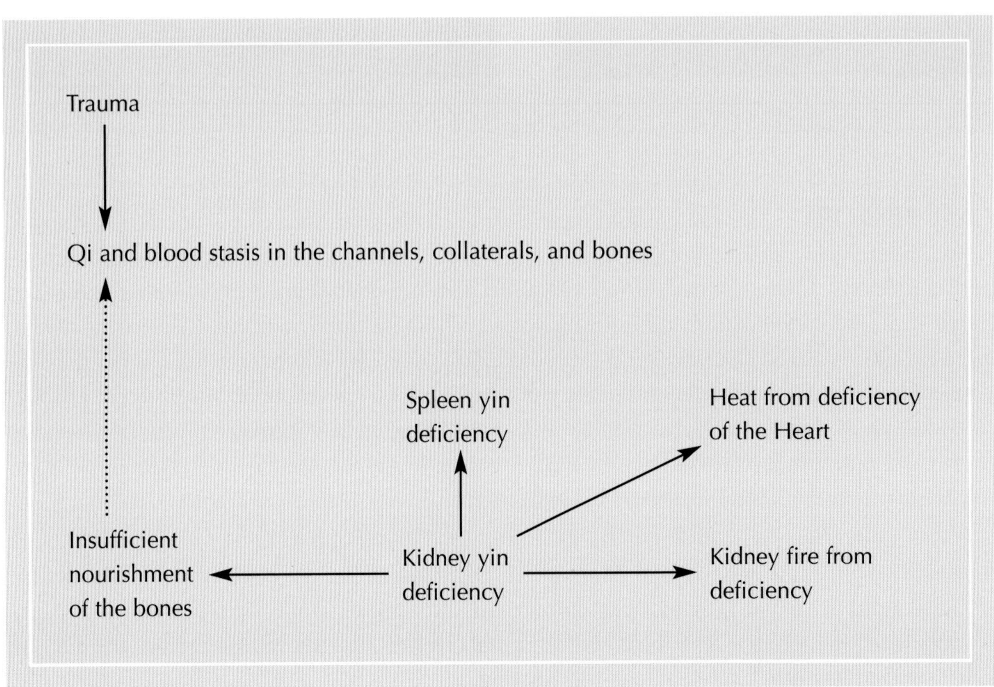

diagnosis. The pattern is probably aggravated by the Spleen yin deficiency and his continual lack of sleep. The Kidney yin deficiency contributes to the patient's dryness of the mouth and the occasional night sweats.

As previously noted, the lifestyle of this patient exacerbates the Kidney yin deficiency and allows for the development of heat from deficiency, as reflected in the red spots at the tip of the tongue. The Kidney yin deficiency can lead to heat from deficiency of the Heart, which agitates the spirit; this is reflected in the restlessness of the patient. Finally, the underlying Kidney yin deficiency also contributes to insufficient nourishment of the bones, since the Kidneys govern the bones; this has contributed to the weakness of the spine and the slow healing process.

A yellow, greasy tongue coating is a result of the patient's improper diet of mainly fried, fatty foods. Since he did not have symptoms suggesting retention of damp-heat, this pattern was largely ignored in evaluating the overall pathomechanism and treatment strategy.

Treatment strategy. Invigorate the qi and blood in the channels and strengthen and nourish the Spleen, Stomach, and Kidney yin.

The patient was treated over a period of 12 weeks with acupuncture and Chinese herbs. Initially, the emphasis was on reducing the stasis of qi and blood in the channels and collaterals. After 12 acupuncture treatments the pain had diminished and the numbness in the left thigh had disappeared. Xi-cleft points were frequently used because of their ability to move qi and blood in the channels and to ease pain. A draining needle technique was frequently used at LR-6 *(zhōng dū)*, GB-36 *(wài qiū)*, and BL-63 *(jīn mén)*. Other frequently used points included BL-11 *(dà zhù)*, BL-17 *(gé shū)*, BL-23 *(shèn shū)*, BL-60 *(kūn lún)*, KI-3 *(tài xī)*, SP-3 *(tài bái)*, and HT-6 *(yīn xī)*. At the onset of treatment, the patient also received a modified version of Trauma Pill *(diē dǎ wán)*.

After the fifth week of treatment, when the pain became less intense, the patient was given Anemarrhena, Phellodendron, and Rehmannia Pill *(zhī bái dì huáng wán)* in tablet form. After four weeks of taking these tablets, he felt better. The night sweats had not recurred. After another eight weeks of taking the tablets, his sexual strength had increased.

Changes in the tongue. The tongue body color and coating reflect the improvement in the condition of the patient. The tongue body color is less red, and the coating shows no peeled areas (Fig. 12.2b). These changes signal a strengthening of the Kidney yin and a reduction in the heat from deficiency. The bluish discoloration of the tongue body is no longer visible. This corresponds to the reduction in the level of pain. The patient occasionally suffers from lower leg pain, which is successfully eased with acupuncture.

Tongue description	Chinese diagnosis
Reddish	Developing heat
Reddish, curled-up edges	Liver qi stagnation with heat in the Liver
Reddish tip	Heat in the Heart
Yellow, dry coating	Retention of damp-heat
Yellow, thick coating with red points in the posterior third of the tongue	Retention of damp-heat in the lower burner

Symptoms

Irritability, anger, dissatisfaction
Restlessness
Smelly, yellowish, itchy vaginal discharge
Tiredness

Western diagnosis

Vaginal candidiaisis

Background to disease

Disappointed relationships
Dissatisfaction with her job

Fig. 12.3
Female
36 years old

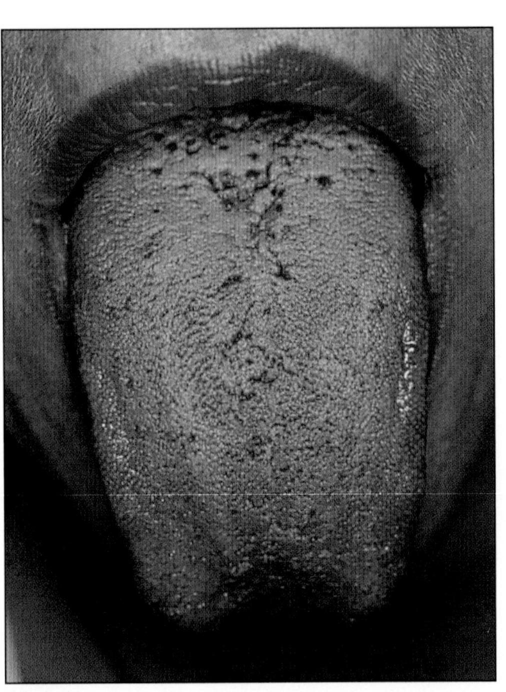
12.3a

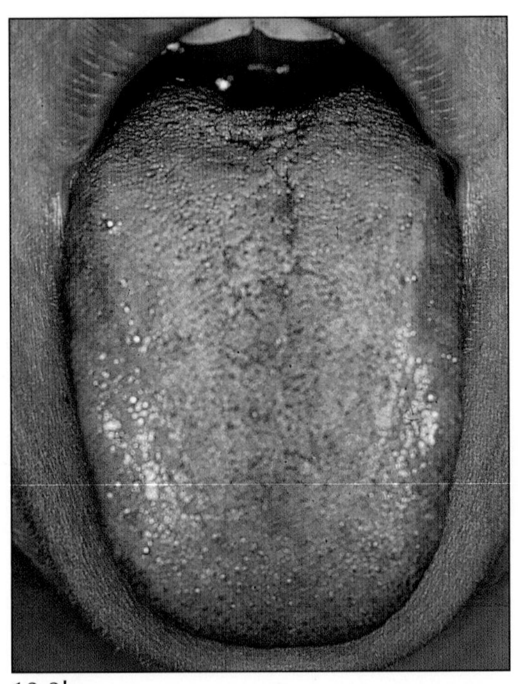
12.3b

CASE HISTORY Despite years of psychotherapy, the patient could not rid herself of a constant feeling of dissatisfaction, as she experienced life as exhausting and joyless. The slightest thing annoyed her, and she was always irritable. In addition, she had no life vision and was unable to develop plans.

She had a yellowish, smelly, itchy vaginal discharge from a *Candida albicans* infection that had lasted for several days. Her only other complaint was that she often felt tired. Her pulse was slightly rapid and wiry.

Analysis. The patient's constitution was obvious from both her symptoms and the shape of the tongue body. The thin, curled-up edges of the tongue reflect a long-standing disharmony of the wood phase (Fig. 12.3a). An indentation that seems to separate the tongue edges from the body of the tongue is noteworthy; often this sign shows a deep and chronic pattern of Liver qi constraint. The wiry pulse confirms the presence of this pattern.

The patient could not remember ever feeling content or being carefree. Long-standing Liver qi stagnation causes the development of heat in the Liver, as reflected in the tongue's red edges and the slightly rapid and wiry pulse. The Liver stores the blood, and because of the Liver's close relationship to blood, heat in the Liver can readily impair the anchoring and housing of the spirit and ethereal soul. Liver blood has the function of nourishing and rooting the ethereal soul. In this case, because the ethereal soul is inadequately nourished and anchored, the patient's ability to develop plans and form a vision of the future is diminished.[5] Lastly, since the Heart controls the blood, heat in the blood will always affect the spirit. The red tip of the tongue reflects heat in the Heart.

The constraint of Liver qi and its transformation into heat are readily discernible in the patient's behavior. She appears tense, and is very critical and skeptical. The constraint of Liver qi manifests as irritability and a readiness to react with anger. These symptoms, and the nature of the tongue edges, are important indications of the intensity of the constraint.

The Liver qi controls the movement of fluids as well as the free flow of qi. Long-standing constraint of the Liver qi may lead to an accumulation of fluids, which eventually transforms into dampness. Dampness can join with heat and sink to the lower burner where they can block the flow of qi in the Liver channel that traverses the genitals. The yellow, itchy vaginal discharge here is a manifestation of the damp-heat in the Liver and Gallbladder channels.[6]

A frequent pathomechanism involved in the formation of damp-heat is underlying Spleen qi deficiency. However, the body of this patient's tongue is not swollen or pale, so this pattern can be discounted. The tiredness of the patient is the only symptom suggesting Spleen qi deficiency. But here, the tiredness is interpreted to arise from the improper flow and constraint of qi.

Treatment strategy. Eliminate the dampness and clear the heat from the Liver and Gallbladder, resolve the constraint of Liver qi, and calm the spirit.

First, the acute vaginal infection needed to be addressed. The first treatments consisted of eliminating dampness and clearing heat from the Liver and Gallbladder channels and relieving the itching. Over the long term, it was deemed necessary to resolve the constraint of Liver qi and calm the spirit.

The patient was treated over a period of one year with acupuncture. She sometimes felt well and contented. She found a new job, and to her surprise, she had no arguments with her colleagues. The vaginal discharge disappeared. The following points were frequently used: GB-41 *(zú lín qì)*, GB-34 *(yáng líng quán)*, LR-2 *(xíng jiān)*, LR-3 *(tài chōng)*, LR-8 *(qū quán)*, SP-9 *(yīn líng quán)*, CV-2 *(qū gǔ)*, CV-3 *(zhōng jí)*, PC-6 *(nèi guān)*, and HT-5 *(tōng lǐ)*.

Changes in the tongue. The resolution of the Liver qi constraint changed the attitude of the patient as well as the shape of her tongue body. The indentation of the edges disappeared (Fig. 12.3b) and the tongue body took on a normal shape and color. The red points at the tip of the tongue were no longer visible; heat was cleared from the Heart, which made the patient feel much calmer. The yellow, thick coating on the posterior third of the tongue thinned out, and the color of the red points became less intense. This change in the tongue coating correlated with the absence of vaginal discharge.

Pathomechanism

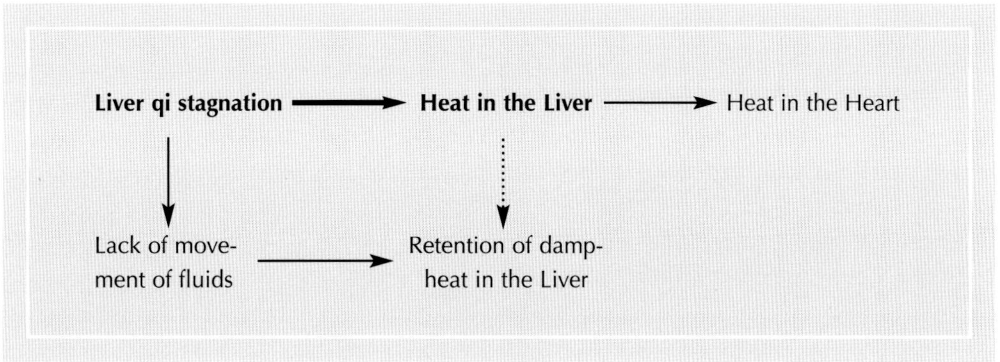

Tongue description	**Chinese diagnosis**
Red	Kidney yin deficiency
Peeled coating in the center	Stomach yin deficiency
Light yellow, tofu-like[7] coating	Retention of damp-heat
Yellow, thick coating with red points on the posterior third of the tongue	Food stagnation with developing heat

Symptoms

Heartburn
Stomach pain, feeling of pressure in the epigastric region
Urge to heave, vomit of white, blood-tinged sputum
Thirsty at night, dryness of the mouth
Dry, hard stools
Exhaustion

Western diagnosis

Chronic reflux esophagitis

Background to disease

Symptoms for the last 30 years
Condition after a fundoplication[8] two years before

Fig. 12.4
Female
75 years old

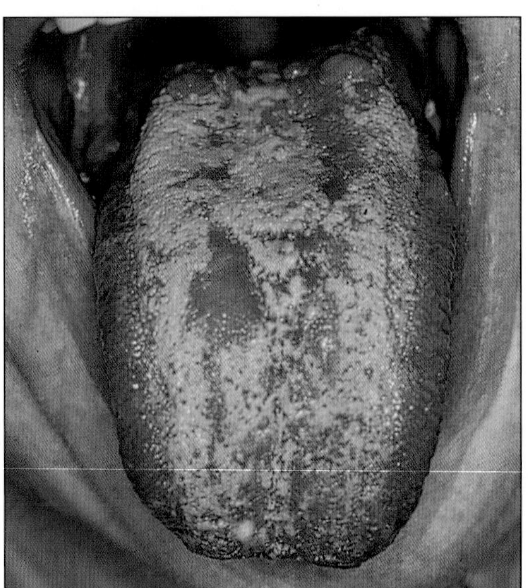

12.4a

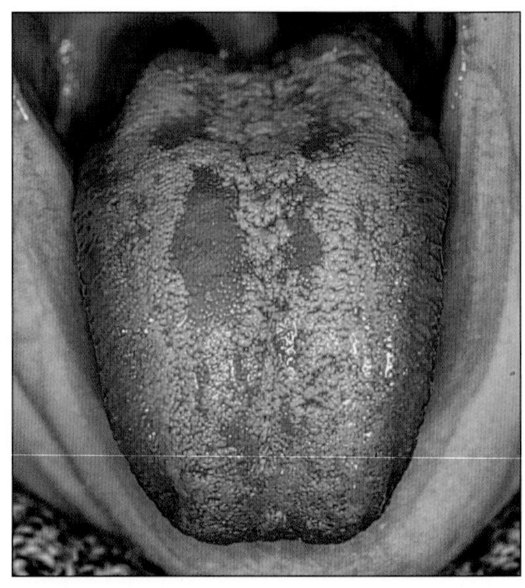

12.4b

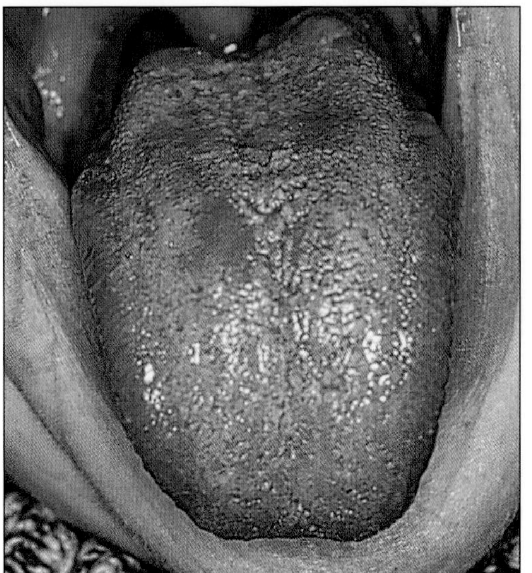

12.4c

CASE HISTORY For 30 years the patient suffered from chronic reflux esophagitis. The condition did not improve after an operation two years earlier during which she lost a large amount of blood. Since the operation, she was exhausted and felt that her health had declined. Prior to the operation, she had always been strong and fit.

When treatment began, she was troubled by vomiting that generally started in the early evening and that contained white, blood-tinged mucus. She slept poorly because lying down caused severe stomach pain and a feeling of pressure in the stomach area. At night, she was very thirsty and suffered from dryness of the mouth. Since the operation, she suffered from rhagades—fissures in the skin—at the corner of her mouth. Her stools were also dry and hard. Her appetite was good, but she ate very little for fear of triggering the stomach pain. Heartburn and stomach pain were brought on by the consumption of fatty foods, spices, alcohol, and meat. She also felt that fluids would "gather" in her stomach.

The patient had been married for 50 years; her husband suffered from depression, which forced her to deny her own needs. Her pulse was floating, deficient, and rapid. The left distal position was noticeably wiry.

Analysis. For many years the patient suppressed her own needs. Thus the origin of her chronic symptoms may be found in constraint of Liver qi, as reflected in the wiry pulse. The tongue, however, does not show any corresponding signs. A discrepancy between the tongue and pulse is not uncommon, especially in cases of Liver qi constraint. For example, in Fig. 12.8, the tongue does not present any specific signs, such as curled-up edges, but the pulse is wiry.

The acute condition of the patient was dominated by a disharmony of the Stomach. The color of the tongue body is red and the coating is peeled in the center (Fig. 12.4a), reflecting a deficiency of Stomach and Kidney yin. This deficiency is perhaps expected in a 75-year-old individual, but it is probably intensified by the blood loss she experienced two years earlier during her operation. The operation is also responsible for a weakening of her source qi and Kidney essence, resulting in exhaustion and decline in health. The yin deficiency and the resulting lack of body fluids results in the dryness of the mouth and the excessive thirst at night, both of which are characteristic of this deficiency. Because these symptoms appeared only after the operation, it is clear that the operation adversely affected the strength of the Kidney yin. Prior to the surgery, she apparently did not have symptoms of Kidney yin deficiency, and despite her stomach pain and other symptoms, she still lives an active life.

The shape of the tongue body underscores the strong constitution of the patient. The form and texture of the tongue body are normal, while the color and coating reflect the acute pathology. The floating, deficient, rapid pulse correlates well with the findings on the tongue, that is, Kidney yin deficiency with developing heat.

The tongue's dry consistency and tofu-like coating plus its slightly dirty yellowish hue point toward a pattern of food stagnation and heat in the Stomach. This has caused rebellious Stomach qi, resulting in heartburn and the urge to vomit. Repeated vomiting has injured the Stomach qi, which eventually impaired the Stomach functions. Protracted vomiting has also contributed to a deficiency of Stomach yin, which manifests in the peeled coating in the center

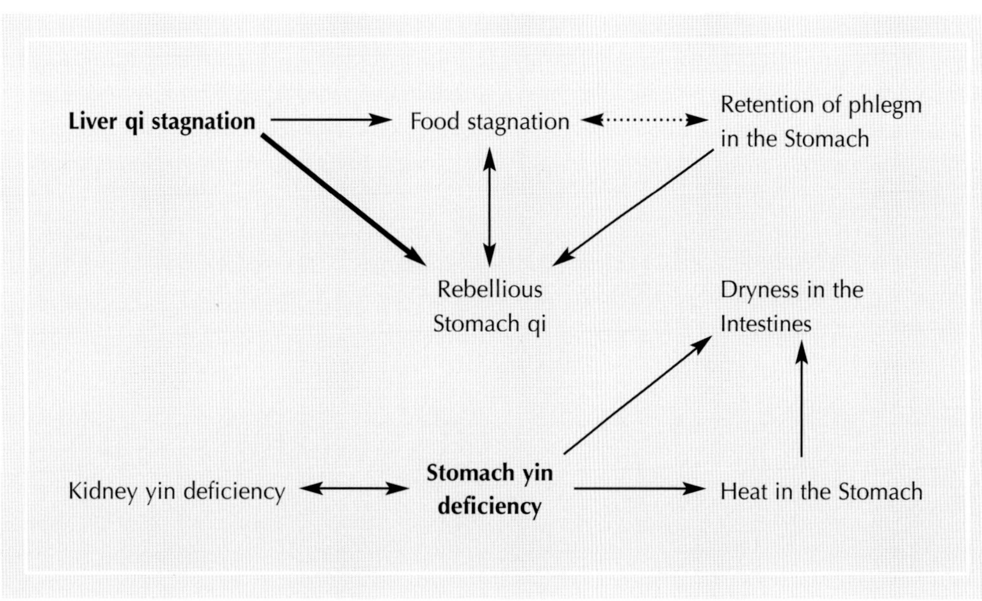

Pathomechanism

of the tongue. The Stomach yin deficiency led to the development of heat in the Stomach, which has subsequently injured the fluids. The Stomach is the source of fluids. Without sufficient fluids and Stomach yin, new coating cannot form, which is evident here in the peeled, dry coating.

The heat in the Stomach has also prevented the sinking of the Stomach qi, causing a blockage of the qi mechanism in the middle burner and making the digestion sluggish. In this case, the resulting food stagnation has manifested in stomach pain that is aggravated when food is consumed. The fact that the stomach pain increases when the patient lies down indicates that the obstruction of the qi mechanism in the middle burner is a condition of excess. In the recumbent position, the phlegm gathers, aggravating the obstruction of qi. The heat in the Stomach is also responsible for the appearance of the rhagades at the corner of the mouth and the traces of blood in the vomit. Finally, the heat in the Stomach and deficiency of fluids and yin has led to dryness of the Intestines, evident here in the dry and hard feces.

The patient tried to ease her pain by eating large amounts of yogurt and curd. Overconsumption of these foods leads to an accumulation of dampness in the Stomach. The presence of heat in the Stomach will transform the dampness into phlegm, which is responsible for the consistency of the patient's vomit, and which has further aggravated the rebellion (counterflow) of Stomach qi.

Chronic Stomach yin deficiency will eventually result in Kidney yin deficiency because a dry Stomach, which is 'the sea of fluids,' will inevitably injure the root of all yin the Kidneys. As previously noted, the combination of Stomach and Kidney yin deficiency engenders the formation of heat in the body, which in turn injures the fluids. Here, the strength of this pathomechanism is reflected in the red discoloration of the tongue body and the peeled coating.

Treatment strategy. Direct the rebellious Stomach qi downward, stop the vomiting, harmonize the Stomach and clear the heat, and nourish the Stomach and Kidney yin.

For a period of four weeks, the patient was prescribed a modified version of Tangerine Peel and Bamboo Shavings Decoction (*jú pí zhú rú tāng*), with the addition of Glehniae/Adenophorae Radix (*[běi/nán] shā shēn*), Polygonati odorati Rhizoma *(yù zhú)*, and Sepiae Endoconcha *(hǎi piāo xiāo)*.

Changes in the tongue. After only two weeks of treatment, the patient's vomiting disappeared. The changes in the tongue correlated with the improvement in her condition. The tongue body was less red, and the tongue coating was thinner and more moist (Fig. 12.4b). The coating still showed peeled areas, however, and its color was still dirty yellow.

After two more weeks of treatment, the patient was free of pain. For the first time in 20 years, she ate a Christmas goose without any problems. However, her thirst and dry mouth persisted. Again the tongue reflected the improvement in the patient's condition. A new coating had formed, a sign of regeneration of the Stomach yin (Fig. 12.4c). Only a small area of peeled coating was visible in the center of the tongue. The patient then chose to discontinue treatment because she felt so much better.

Tongue description	**Chinese diagnosis**
Pale red	Normal
Curled-up edges	Liver qi stagnation
Red in the anterior third	Heat in the Heart
Vertical midline crack with light yellow, greasy coating	Retention of phlegm-heat in the Stomach
Yellow, thick coating with red points at the root of the tongue	Retention of damp-heat in the Large Intestine

Symptoms

Severe abdominal pain
Urge to defecate
Frequent bowel movements that contained blood and mucus
Flatulence
Night sweats
Insomnia
Restlessness and irritability
Depressive moods

Western diagnosis

Ulcerative colitis

Background to disease

Sexual abuse in her youth
Long-standing emotional problems

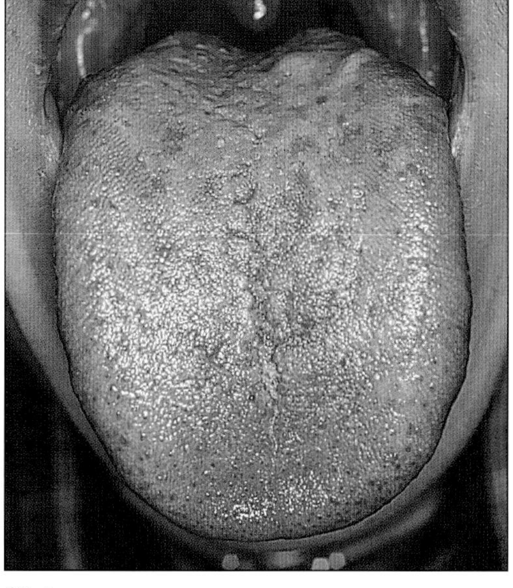

12.5a

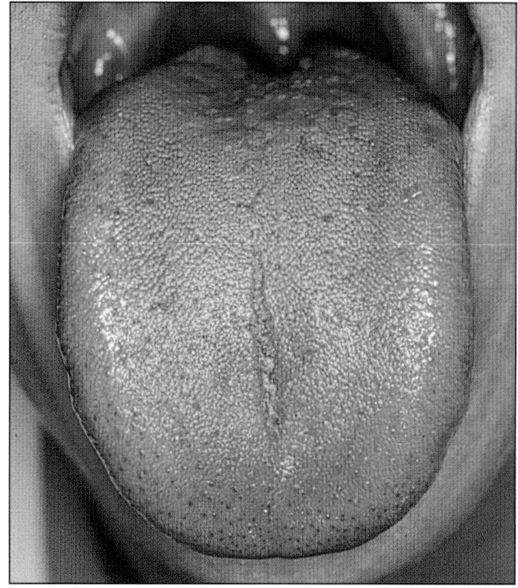

12.5b

Fig. 12.5
Female
32 years old

CASE HISTORY The patient was restless, discontented, irritable, and very frightened about her illness. She started experiencing the symptoms associated with ulcerative colitis twelve months earlier. The illness began during a stay in a clinic specializing in the treatment of psychosomatic illnesses. Constant abdominal pain troubled her. The urge to defecate was strong and nearly uncontrollable. She emptied her bowels about three times a day, which improved the pain. The feces were soft and contained blood, mucus, and pus. She also suffered from smelly flatulence. She felt thirsty but had almost no appetite. She was constantly exhausted. Her sleep was disturbed, and she often woke during the night. She occasionally had night sweats. She refused medical drugs as she believed a healing process could take place with the aid of psychotherapy. Her pulse was slightly rapid and wiry.

Analysis. This case is an example of a pattern where Liver qi stagnation is the primary cause of a dysfunction in the Large Intestine. A combination of long-standing constraint of Liver qi and retention of damp-heat in the Large Intestine is responsible for the prevailing disease mechanism. The stagnation of Liver qi is responsible for the heat that inhibits the proper flow of qi in the middle burner and disturbs the qi mechanism of the Spleen and Stomach. The impairment in the Spleen's functions of transformation and transportation leads to an accumulation of dampness. Since dampness is heavy, it sinks down to the Intestines where it gathers and transforms into heat.

Constraint of Liver qi is reflected in the curled-up edges. Yet there are important differences. The distribution of the coating is irregular and much thinner in the middle portion of the tongue than at the root. This gives the coating a peeled appearance, suggesting a pattern of deficiency. However, the thickness and yellow hue of the coating reflects a condition of excess caused by heat and dampness. The intensity of heat and dampness, reflected in the almost uncontrollable urge to defecate and in the frequent bowel movements, equally determine this disease process, as the amount of excreted blood, pus, and mucus are of the same proportion. The secretion of pus is a sign of the generation and accumulation of heat toxin from the damp-heat in the Large Intestine. The presence of mucus in the stools is indicative of the accumulation of dampness and its transformation in the lower burner. The presence of blood in the stool is the result of the intense heat in the lower burner that has injured the blood vessels. The retained damp-heat in the lower burner has led to the constraint of qi and stagnation of blood, resulting in abdominal pain; the damp-heat is also responsible for the smelly flatulence and stools.

The emotional state of the patient has led to constraint of Liver qi, as reflected in the wiry pulse and the curled-up edges of the tongue. Sexual abuse in her youth changed the patient and led to feelings of frustration, bitterness, and irritability. These emotions agitated the spirit and manifest now in restlessness and sleeping problems. The reddish tip and red anterior third of the tongue reflect heat in the upper burner, specifically the Heart. The slightly rapid pulse is a reflection of this developing heat.

Pathomechanism

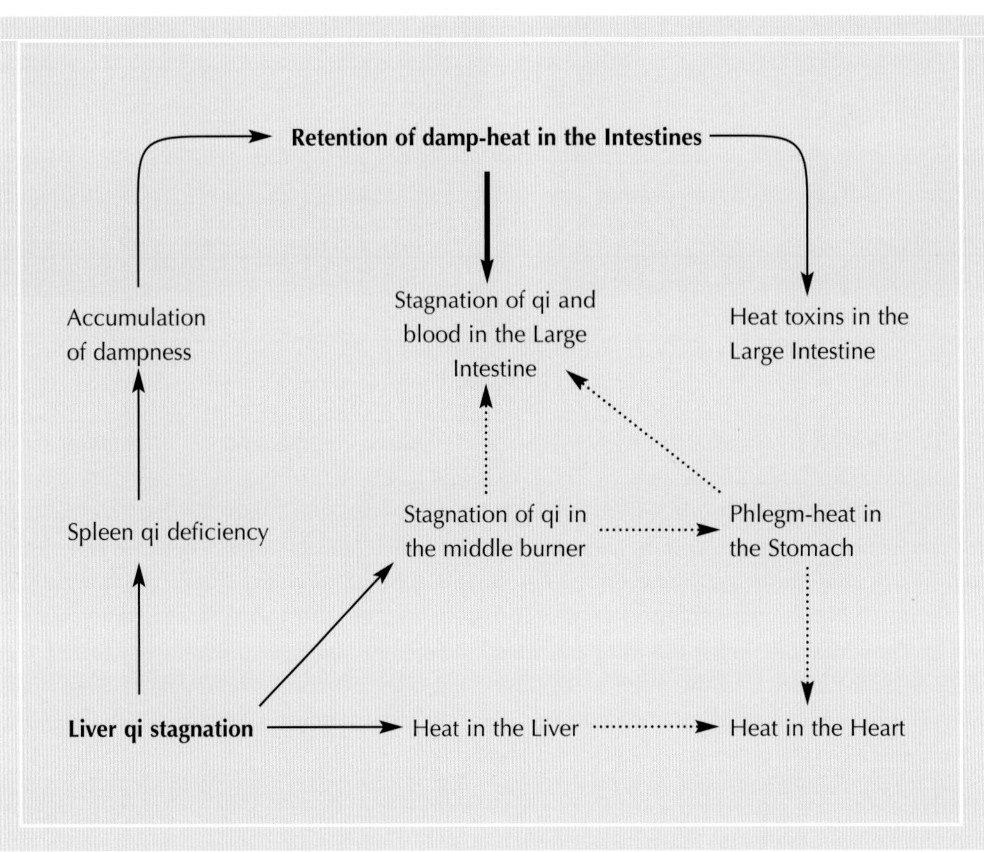

The vertical midline crack covered with a yellow, greasy coating signals phlegm-heat in the Stomach. This disease pattern agitates her spirit and is responsible for the patient's mental imbalance and sleeping problems. The occasional feeling of thirst suggests a flaring of Heart fire.

Treatment strategy. Eliminate the dampness, clear the heat and eliminate heat toxin from the Large Intestine, regulate the Liver qi, ease the abdominal pain, and calm the spirit.

Over a period of two weeks, a modified version of Peony Decoction *(sháo yào tāng)* was prescribed, with the addition of Rehmanniae Radix *(shēng dì huáng),* Lophateri Herba *(dàn zhú yè),* Picrorhizae Rhizoma *(hú huáng lián),* and Sophorae Flos *(huái huā).* The urge to defecate and her abdominal pain thereupon declined, and the stools were free of pus and blood. However, she still had the feeling that stress could trigger a recurrence of the symptoms. The prescription was then modified and she received Frigid Extremities Powder *(sì nì săn),* with the addition of Coptidis Rhizoma *(huáng lián),* Scutellariae Radix *(huáng qín),* Salviae miltiorrhizae Radix *(dān shēn),* and Atractylodis macrocephalae Rhizoma *(bái zhú).*

Changes in the tongue. After three months of treatment the patient was free of symptoms, although she still seemed to be emotionally unstable. Her depressive mood swings persisted without causing symptoms on a physical level. The tongue reflected the improvement in the patient's condition (Fig. 12.5b). The reddish tip and the yellow coating had disappeared. However, the curled-up edges did not change, reflecting the unresolved constraint of Liver qi.

CASE HISTORY During the spring the patient had been in charge of a workshop in Italy. The weather was sunny but still cool. She wore light clothing as she taught in overheated rooms. After three days, she developed a temperature of 102.2°F (39°C). She felt ill and exhausted. A loud, barking cough developed that caused pain in her chest. She expelled sparse but thick yellow mucus. In addition, it was difficult for her to exhale, and she experienced tightness in the chest. She consulted her physician and had an x-ray taken of her lungs so that pneumonia could be ruled out.

She came for treatment on her third day of being sick. Her fever had dropped to 100°F (37.8°C). The cough still troubled her, especially because it disturbed her sleep. She had no appetite, but did have a strong thirst. Her bowels were normal. She seldom caught colds. In general, she was healthy and fit. A year before, she had been successfully treated with acupuncture for insomnia. Her pulse was rapid and floating.

Analysis. The patient's exterior had not been sufficiently protected because of inappropriate clothing. In addition, her protective qi did not adjust adequately to the change from cool,

Pathomechanism

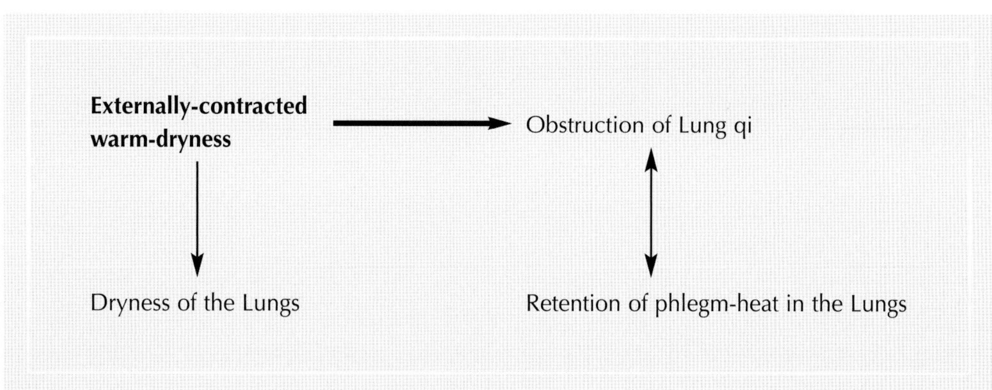

Tongue description	**Chinese diagnosis**
Pale red	Normal
Slightly slack, soft tongue body	Spleen qi deficiency
Whitish, thick, dry coating in the middle portion of the tongue	Externally-contracted warm-dryness

Symptoms

Coughing fits, loud, barking cough
Cough with sparse yellow mucus
Tightness of the chest
Difficulty exhaling
Slight fever
Thirst
Feeling of malaise

Western diagnosis

Acute bronchitis

Background to disease

Inappropriate clothing in cool climate
Overworked

Fig. 12.6
Female
38 years old

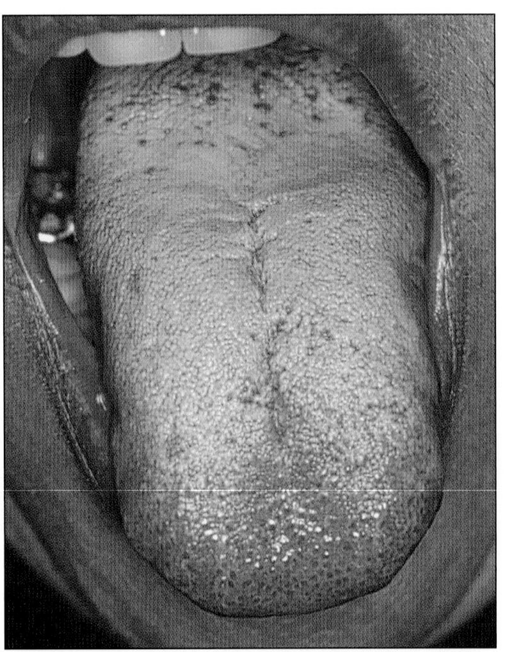

12.6a

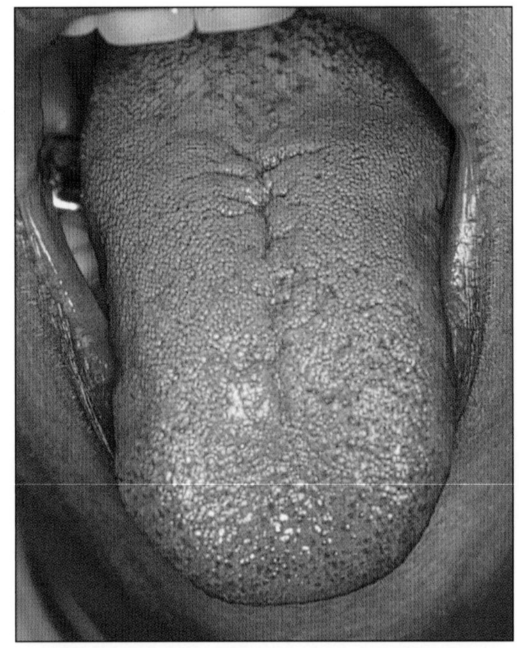

12.6b

dry weather to a warm, dry 'climate,' that of the overheated rooms; this allowed the external pathogenic factors to readily invade her body. Because of her overall good health, the externally-contracted warm-dryness had affected the Lung qi at a relatively superficial level. The whitish color of the tongue coating showed that the pathogenic factors had not deeply penetrated the interior.

The dryness of the coating indicates that external dryness is the dominant pathogenic factor. The warm and dry external pathogenic factors have caused a constraint of heat in the Lungs and have injured the fluids. The mucus is yellow, indicating the development of heat in the Lungs. The pathogenic factors have produced a condition of excess, which is reflected in the thickness of the tongue coating. The floating, rapid pulse reflects the development of heat at a relatively superficial level, plus the presence of external pathogens.

The pathogenic factors are hindering the descent of Lung qi, which accounts for the loud cough. Tightness in the chest and difficulty exhaling are characteristic of the obstruction of Lung qi. Together with the heat in the Lungs, this helped produce the thick but sparse mucus that she found difficult to expectorate. Heat and dryness are also responsible for the patient's thirst. The fever fell at the onset of treatment; its presence is a reflection of the struggle between the protective qi and the externally-contracted pathogens.

Treatment strategy. Disperse and eliminate the warm-dryness and stop the coughing.

A modified version of Mulberry Leaf and Apricot Kernel Decoction *(sāng xìng tāng)* was prescribed. To ease the cough, the following herbs were added: Platycodi Radix *(jié gěng)*, Peucedani Radix *(qián hú)*, Asteris Radix *(zǐ wǎn)*, and Stemonae Radix *(bǎi bù)*. To eliminate heat and phlegm from the Lungs, the following herbs were added: Benincasae Semen *(dōng guā zǐ)*, and Mori Cortex *(sāng bái pí)*. After taking this decoction for four days, the patient was much better and only a slight cough remained. Her chest felt free and her breathing was again harmonious.

Changes in the tongue. Four days later the tongue coating reflected the improvement in the patient's condition (Fig. 12.6b). The tongue was now moist and the coating had normalized. As expected, the soft tongue body had not changed. This indicates Spleen qi deficiency that causes tiredness from time to time. The patient did not take enough time off to rest.

Tongue description	**Chinese diagnosis**
Pale	Spleen qi deficiency → blood deficiency
Teeth marks	Spleen qi deficiency
Black, slippery coating	Penetration of externally-contracted cold

Symptoms

Irregular menstrual bleeding
Protracted flow of blood with large clots
Feeling of cold in the lower abdomen
Backache with radiating pain toward the thigh
Exhaustion, lack of drive
Mood swings, lack of concentration

Western diagnosis

Uterine fibroid, uterine polyp
Acute sciatica

Background to disease

Condition followed laparoscopy
Long-standing emotional problems

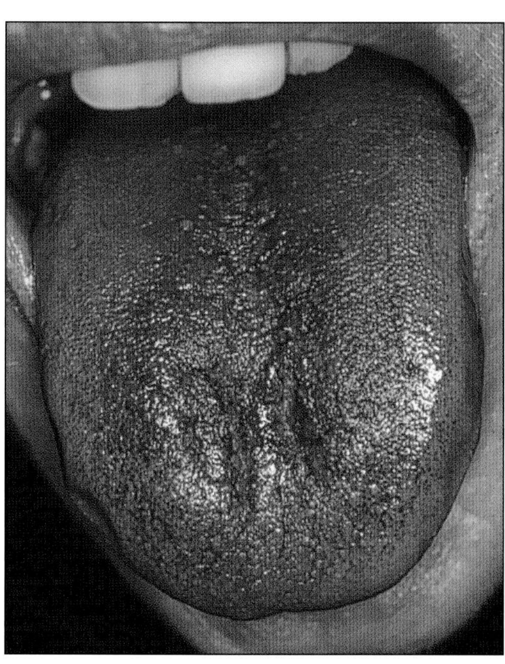

12.7a

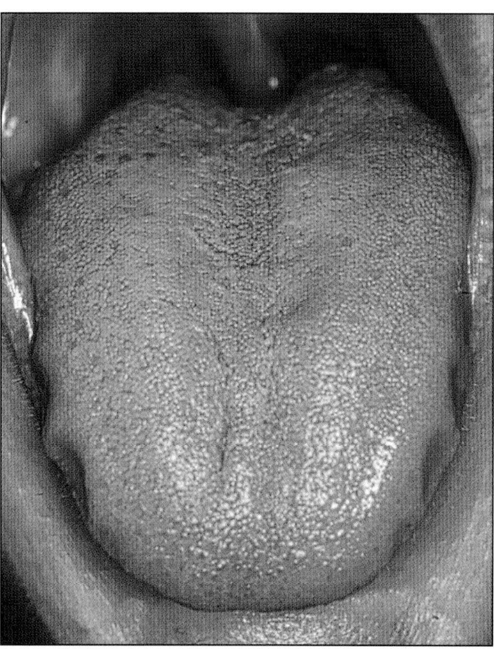

12.7b

Fig. 12.7
Female
49 years old

CASE HISTORY At the onset of menopause the patient suffered from irregular menstrual bleeding. Gynecological examinations revealed a small uterine fibroid and polyp. The regularity of her menstrual cycle fluctuated. Often, the strong bleeding occurred after 45 to 60 days, and the menstrual blood was red, consisting of large (2cm) clots. The bleeding could last up to 20 days. After the first seven days of bleeding, it became lighter. Nevertheless, the patient lost large amounts of blood. In addition, she often experienced a drawing sensation in the lower abdomen, and her abdomen felt cold. Since the protracted bleeding weakened her considerably, surgery was recommended to remove the uterine polyp.

Fig. 12.7a was taken three days after the operation, which included the introduction of cold carbon dioxide into the abdominal cavity. Following the anesthesia, she woke with a distinct feeling of cold in her lower abdomen. This feeling persisted for three days after the operation when she also experienced acute sciatica. Her left leg felt slightly numb and was painful. There was still some slight menstrual bleeding.

The patient was often depressed and dejected, and sometimes aggressive and irritable. She felt that her life was stagnating and could not imagine any improvement. Her memory and concentration were poor. Her sleep was good although she had occasional night sweats. Her pulse was sinking, frail, and noticeably wiry at the Liver position.

Analysis. The black coating covers the entire tongue body and signals the penetration of externally-contracted cold. Although the remaining white coating is no longer visible, the diagnosis of externally-contracted cold can be confirmed by the slippery texture of the coating. If a black coating arises from injury to the fluids due to intense heat, the coating would be dry or yellow in color.

The feeling of cold following the operation is localized in the lower abdomen and is accompanied by a drawing sensation and a sense of malaise. A uterine polyp was removed during a laparoscopy, which included introducing cold carbon dioxide into the abdominal cavity. This process can be seen as a direct invasion of external cold into the abdomen where it caused acute local stasis of qi and blood, manifested as a cold sensation and drawing pain

Pathomechanism

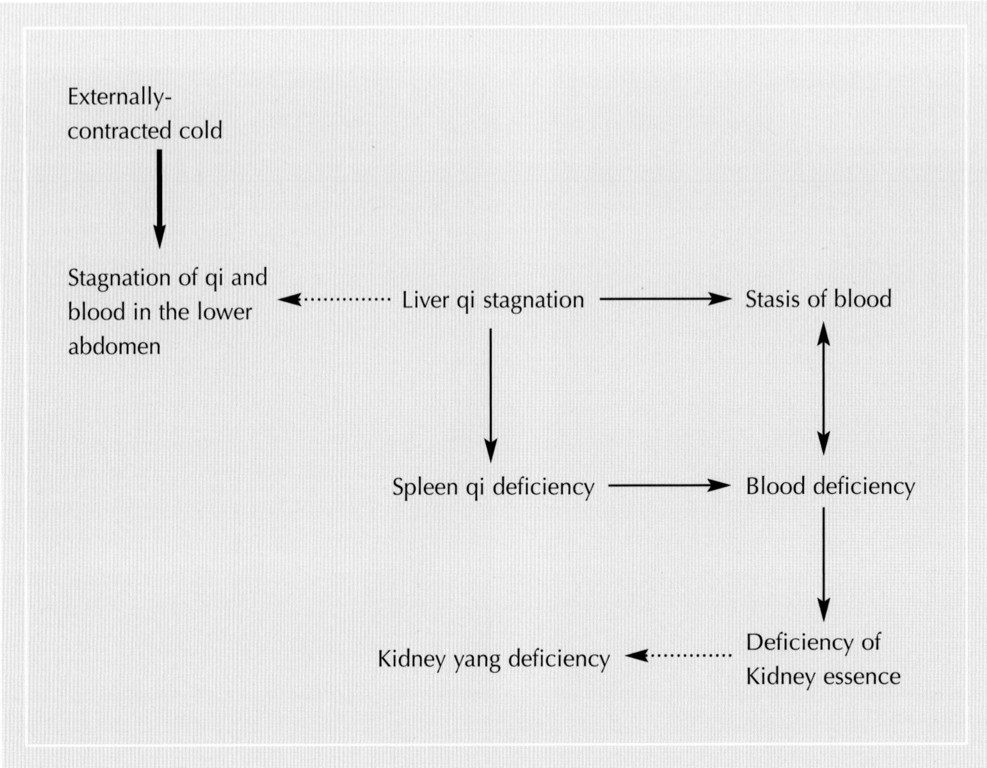

in the abdomen. The black coating reflects the intensity of the cold. The acute stasis that has developed blocks the transportation and transformation of fluids, causing the discoloration and slippery texture of the coating.

The patient's source qi has been weakened by the cold in the abdomen and the operation, and this has deprived the lower back of nourishment, resulting in acute sciatica. It is possible that the pathogenic cold blocked the flow of qi and blood in the leg greater yang Bladder channel, contributing to the pain and numbness in the thigh.

The underlying energetic disharmony of the patient is a result of pronounced constraint of Liver qi, which is confirmed by the wiry pulse. This pattern arose because of her long-standing unresolved emotional problems and unsatisfactory personal relationships. The constraint of Liver qi has led to insufficient movement of blood in the lower burner, which has contributed to the formation of the fibroid and polyp in the uterus. In addition, the constrained Liver qi has attacked the Spleen qi and impaired its function of holding the blood. While the Liver qi constraint is deemed responsible for the formation of the blood stasis, the tongue, nevertheless, does not present any specific signs of this pattern, such as curled-up edges. In this case, the pulse is more accurate than the tongue, and the patient's mood swings are also characteristic of constrained Liver qi. Finally, because of the blood deficiency, the Liver is not softened and pacified, which accounts for her aggressive and irritable behavior, nor is the ethereal soul sufficiently nourished, which impairs her ability to make plans and develop a vision for herself.

In all, there are three mechanisms responsible for the protracted menstrual bleeding, which was the patient's main complaint:

- Blood stasis in the Penetrating vessel and uterus prevented a regular flow of blood. In addition, the newly-formed blood could not be held in the uterus because of the preexisting blood stasis, resulting in an uncontrollable flow. The big clots are an indication of a pattern of blood stasis in the Womb.
- The Spleen qi was too weak to hold the blood, as is evident from the protracted bleeding that lasts up to 20 days.
- Because of the patient's age, the menstrual bleeding, which occurs at irregular and long intervals, could signify the onset of menopause. Kidney essence contributes to the regularity of the menstrual cycle. According to traditional Chinese medicine, from the 49th year, the Kidney energy loses its strength, which manifests, depending on the woman's constitution, as signs and symptoms characteristic of yin or yang deficiency. In this case, the Kidneys lost their astringing function, which contributes to the blood loss.

The weakened Kidney essence is also not strong enough to adequately nourish the brain, resulting in poor memory and lack of concentration. Finally, the source qi and Kidney yang have weakened, as reflected in the lower backache, tiredness, lack of drive, and the frail, sinking pulse.

The teeth marks and paleness of the tongue body signal Spleen qi deficiency. Together with the protracted loss of blood, this is responsible for the pattern of blood deficiency. This deficiency, in turn, contributes to a weakening of the Kidney essence. Because the Kidney essence and Kidney yin have a close affinity, the lack of one may cause a weakness in the other. The slight Kidney yin and blood deficiency engender heat from deficiency, resulting in occasional night sweats. Nevertheless, the tongue body has a good shape and texture, and it does not show any marked signs of Kidney yin or yang deficiency. It is therefore assumed that regulating the qi and blood in this patient will result in a speedy recovery.

Treatment strategy. Expel the cold from the Womb, nourish the Kidneys, regulate the Liver qi, and invigorate the blood.

A modified version of Warm the Menses Decoction *(wēn jīng tāng)* was prescribed. The sensation of cold in the lower abdomen disappeared after seven days of treatment and the patient recovered quickly after the operation. Rambling Powder *(xiāo yáo sǎn)* was then prescribed to treat her underlying constitution. She took the patent formula for a period of four months, but even so, her menstrual cycle remained irregular. To further the healing process, the patient undertook an intensive energetic exercise program. Two years later, she is very well and enjoys her life again.

Changes in the tongue. The photograph in Fig. 12.7b was taken two weeks after the surgery. The black coating has disappeared, reflecting the successful expulsion of cold from the lower abdomen and Womb. However, the pale tongue body reflects the persistence of the underlying Spleen and blood deficiency.

Tongue description	Chinese diagnosis
Pale	Spleen qi deficiency → blood deficiency
Very swollen with teeth marks	Spleen qi deficiency with accumulation of dampness and phlegm
Slight indentation of the tip	Heart blood deficiency
Slightly reddish tip	Heat from deficiency of the Heart
Yellow coating at the sides, brownish black coating in the central area	Heat accumulation in the Stomach and Large Intestine, transforming to heat toxin

Symptoms

Severe pain in the upper jaw
Bad breath
Constipation
Tiredness

Western diagnosis

Early stage of necrosis of the gingiva

Background to disease

Alcohol abuse

Fig. 12.8
Female
31 years old

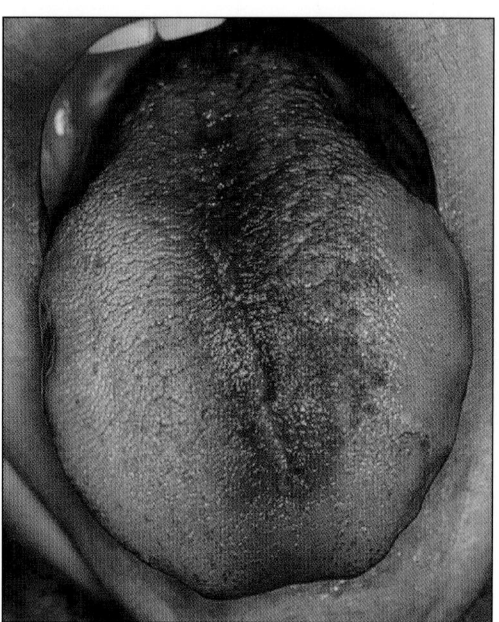

12.8a

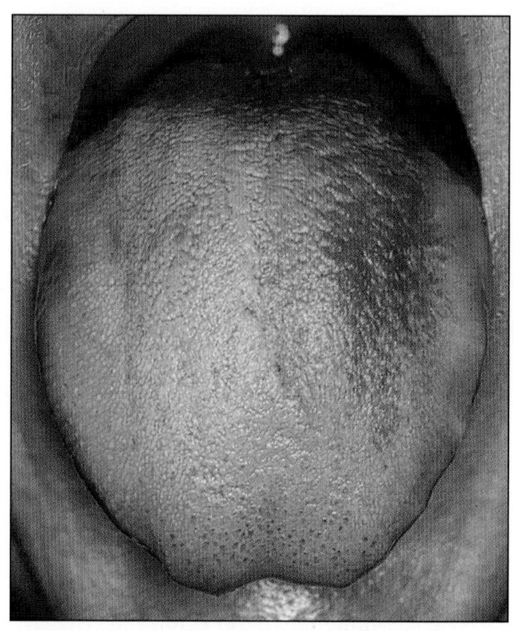

12.8b

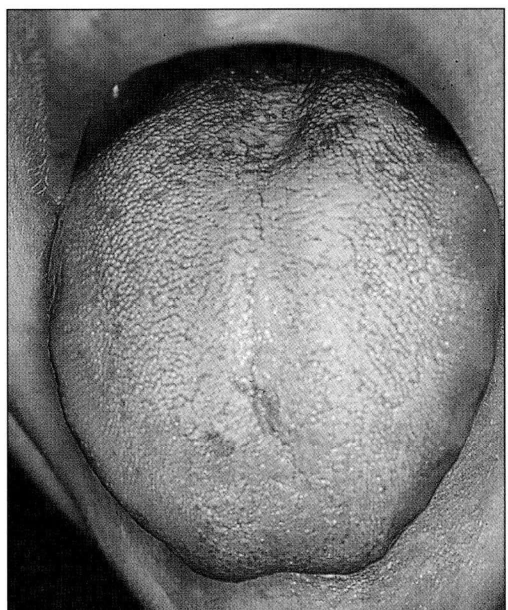

12.8c

CASE HISTORY The patient suffered from severe and constant pain in her jaw after the extraction of three teeth in the upper left quadrant. The extractions were necessary because granulomas had formed as the result of the chronic inflammation of the jawbone.[9] The tissue around the areas of the extracted teeth unfortunately did not heal. The dentist diagnosed necrotic changes in the tissue that showed blackish areas. He treated the infected region daily with antiseptic medicines and simultaneously prescribed antibiotics, which brought no improvement. The patient was incapable of chewing, and wearing a dental prosthesis was impossible because of the intense pain. She suffered from noticeably bad breath and was very thirsty. The pain made her depressed and irritable and she felt very unwell.

The patient had phases of alcohol abuse triggered, as a rule, by depressive moods. During these periods, which lasted for about three weeks, she would consume about a pint-and-a-half of whiskey a day. She would then avoid alcohol altogether for about two to three months. The patient looked bloated and puffy and was about 44 pounds overweight. Her stools were hard, and she had a bowel movement only once every two or three days. Her pulse was slippery and full.

Analysis. This is an example of a wound—the result of the extraction of three teeth—being damaged by the accumulation of heat toxin. The tongue coating clearly illustrates the intensity of the heat and of the heat toxin. The change from a yellow, dry coating at the sides of the tongue to a brownish black coating in the central area signals the penetration of the heat and heat toxin from the exterior toward the interior, the growing intensity of the heat and heat toxin, and the destructive effect of the heat on the fluids.

The symptoms are characteristic of an accumulation of fire toxin and phlegm-fire. An accumulation of toxin causes necrotic lesions as well as a feeling of malaise. The granulomas located at the roots of the teeth are manifestations of phlegm-fire, which contributed to the inflammation of the upper jaw. Because of the intensity of the pathogens, the heat simmered and caused the qi and blood to stagnate in the area between the skin and flesh. The yang brightness Stomach and Large Intestine channels and collaterals, which supply this area with qi and blood, are particularly vulnerable to heat from excess. Thus, the intense heat caused the clumping of qi and blood in these channels, resulting in inflammation and necrotic lesions in the upper jaw. The stagnation of qi and blood is so pronounced that the ensuing pain is severe. The intense heat in the yang brightness Stomach and Large Intestine channels and organs is also responsible for the bad breath, thirst, constipation, and irritability.

The accumulation of heat toxin has at least one of the following causes:

- Externally-contracted heat if present in large amounts can transform into heat toxin.
- Epidemic heat can penetrate the body and produce heat toxin.
- A traumatic injury, like the extraction of the teeth in this case, can transfer toxic qi into the body. The combination of toxic qi and underlying retention of damp-heat or accumulation of phlegm-heat can block the movement of qi, blood, and fluids so severely that heat toxin is formed. The ensuing clumping often results in sores, skin erosions, or inflammation.

Pathomechanism

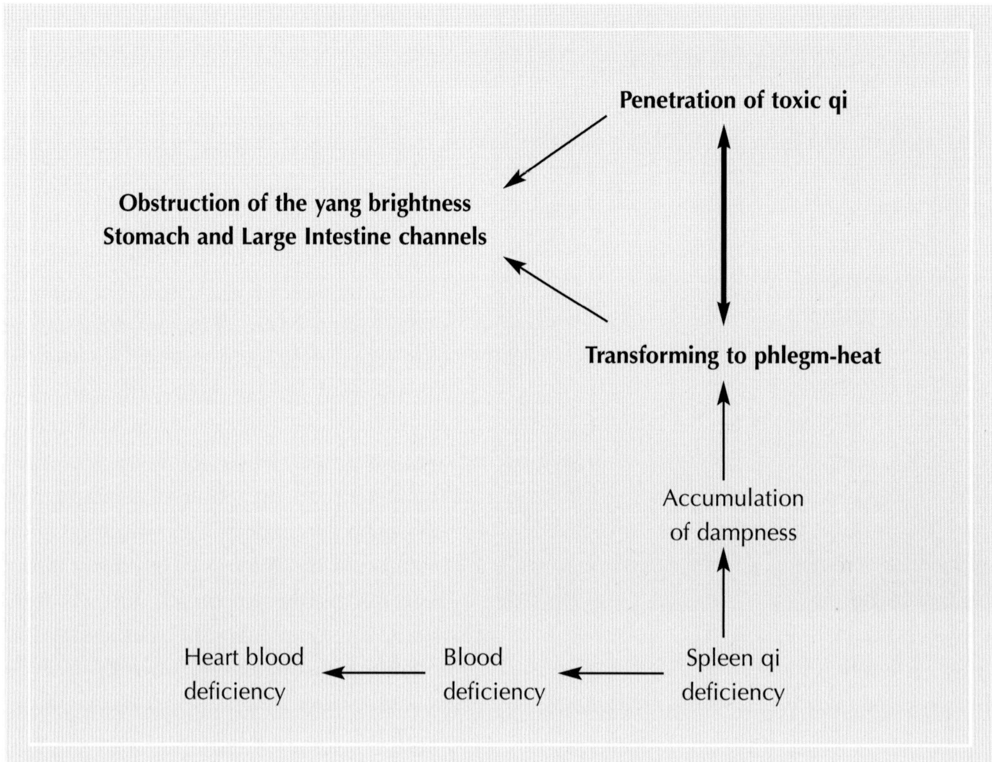

In this case, the accumulation of heat toxin has its origin in the underlying accumulation of phlegm-heat as well as the presence of toxic qi in the body.

The extremely swollen tongue body denotes an accumulation of dampness. Together with the pale color of the tongue body, this would suggest that an underlying pattern of Spleen qi deficiency is responsible for the accumulation of dampness. Because of her irregular, but excessive, abuse of alcohol, the dampness has transformed into phlegm-heat. Whiskey has a yang quality. It is sweet and slightly acrid. Taken in small amounts, it supports the circulation of qi and blood and opens the channels and collaterals. But consumed in large amounts, it engenders heat that affects the Stomach and Liver. Its sweet, rich taste may also contribute to the formation of dampness and phlegm. In this case, the pathogens joined with the heat and formed phlegm-heat, which is reflected in the full and slippery pulse. The accumulated phlegm manifests, as it does with many alcoholics, in a puffy face and weight gain.

Based on the above evidence, the treatment strategy should be two-fold. First, the acute condition must be addressed. Once this has been resolved, the patterns revealed in the tongue color and shape of the tongue body should be addressed; in other words, it is important to treat the underlying constitution and/or root of the disease. The tongue body here is very pale, implying that the Spleen qi is too weak to provide sufficient essence for the production of blood. As a result, the Heart is not adequately supplied with blood, which means that the spirit is undernourished. The tip of the tongue shows a slight indentation, suggesting deficiency of Heart blood. This is the basis for her depressive moods, which trigger the uncontrollable need for alcohol. The slight reddening at the tip of the tongue signals the development of heat in the Heart, exacerbating the emotional instability of the patient.

Treatment strategy. Eliminate the fire toxin, clear the heat, transform the phlegm, and drain the heat from the Stomach and Large Intestine.

The first prescription consisted of Sublime Formula for Sustaining Life (*xiān fāng huó mìng yǐn*), with the addition of Coptidis Rhizoma *(huáng lián)* and Rhei Radix et Rhizoma *(dà huáng)*. The daily dosage amounted to 120 grams, and the prescription was administered for a period of five days. By this time the bowel movements occurred daily, but the stools were still very hard. Her thirst was also considerably reduced. The intensity of the pain in the jaw, however, had not been affected.

Changes in the tongue. By this point the tongue coating had changed (Fig. 12.8b). It was lighter in color and less thick. This initial change in the coating probably indicates a clearing of the heat via the stool. The accumulation of heat toxin was still evident on the tongue, and the obstruction of qi and blood as evidenced by the intensity of the pain was obviously still present. The prescription was therefore modified to reflect the changes in the patient's condition. Coptis Decoction to Resolve Toxicity (*huáng lián jiě dú tāng*) was prescribed, with the following additions: Forsythiae Fructus *(lián qiào)*, Lonicerae Flos *(jīn yín huā)*, Taraxaci Herba *(pú gōng yīng)*, Violae Herba (*zǐ huā dì dīng*), and Cimicifugae Rhizoma *(shēng má)*. Again, the daily dosage amounted to about 120 grams.

After taking the modified decoction for five days, the patient felt much better. The pain had noticeably declined and the dentist found an improvement in the affected tissue. The prescription was repeated for another seven days. Following this period, the patient was free of pain and resumed further dental treatment. The tongue coating was still dry (Fig. 12.8c), reflecting the past injury to the fluids. Its color was whitish yellow, a sure sign that the heat and heat toxin had been successfully cleared. However, the consistency of the coating was greasy, denoting the continued presence of phlegm, but the redness at the tip of the tongue had disappeared. Three months later, the patient was able to wear a dental prosthesis without any pain.

Endnotes

1 Fu Qing-Zhu. *Fu Qing-Zhu's Gynecology,* translated by Yang S-Z and Liu D-W. Boulder, CO: Blue Poppy Press, 1992: 61-62.

2 Ibid.

3 Clavey S. Spleen and stomach yin deficiency. *The Journal of Chinese Medicine* 1995: 47:23-29.

4 Maciocia G. *The Foundations of Chinese Medicine.* Edinburgh: Churchill Livingstone, 1989: 393.

5 Anonymous. *Su wen* [Basic Questions], edited by He W-B et al. Beijing: China Medicine Science and Technology Press, 1996: 8:49.

6 Clavey S. *Fluid Physiology and Pathology in Traditional Chinese Medicine.* Edinburgh: Churchill Livingstone, 1995: 247.

7 Song T-B. *Atlas of the Tongue and Coatings in Chinese Medicine.* Beijing: Joint publication of People's Medical Publishing House and Editions Sinomedic, 1995: Figs. 225 and 226.

8 This involves mobilization of the lower end of the esophagus and wrapping of the fundus of the stomach around it. The procedure is also called a Nissen operation.

9 Granulomas can be initiated by various infectious and noninfectious agents.

BIBLIOGRAPHY

Chinese Language Publications

Anonymous. *Huang di nei jing ling shu yi shi* [Translation and Explanation of the Yellow Emperor's Inner Classic: Divine Pivot], edit. by Nanjing College of Traditional Chinese Medicine, Traditional Chinese Medicine Department. Shanghai: Shanghai Science and Technology Press, 1997.

Anonymous. *Su wen* [Basic Questions], edit. by He Wen-Bin et al. Beijing: China Medicine Science and Technology Press, 1996.

Chen Meng-Lei et al. *Gu jin tu shu ji cheng, yi bu quan lu* [Collection of Writings Past and Present: Complete Medical Section], vol. 5. Peoples Medical Publishing House: Beijing, 1995.

Li Nai-Min. *Zhong guo she zhen da quan* [Compendium of Chinese Tongue Diagnosis]. Beijing: Xueyuan Press, 1994.

Wei Yi-Lin. *Shi yi de xiao fang.* In *Gu jin tu shu ji cheng* [Collection of Writings Past and Present]. Shanghai: China Press, 1934.

Zhu Zhen-Heng. *Ge zhi yu lun* [Extra Treatises Based on Investigation and Inquiry]. In *Zhong guo xue shu ming zhu* (rev. ed.) Taibei: World Press, 1962.

English Language Publications

Anonymous. *Essential Subtleties on the Silver Sea, Yin hai jing wei,* trans. by Jurgen Kovacs and Paul Unschuld. Berkeley: University of California Press, 1998.

Anonymous. *Nan-Ching, The Classic of Difficult Issues,* trans. by Paul Unschuld. Berkeley: University of California Press, 1986.

Beaven, Donald and Ward, Brooks. *Color Atlas of the Tongue in Clinical Diagnosis.* London: Wolfe Medical Publications, 1988.

Bensky, Dan and Barolet, Randall. *Chinese Herbal Medicine: Formulas & Strategies.* Seattle: Eastland Press, 1990.

Chace, Charles. *A Qin Bo Wei Anthology.* Brookline, MA: Paradigm Publications, 1997.

Chen Zelin and Chen Mei-Fang. *The Essence and Scientific Background of Tongue Diagnosis.* Long Beach, CA: Oriental Healing Arts Institute, 1989.

Clavey, Steven. *Fluid Physiology and Pathology in Traditional Chinese Medicine.* Edinburgh: Churchill Livingstone, 1995.

Clavey, Steven. Spleen and stomach yin deficiency. *The Journal of Chinese Medicine* 1995; 47:23-29.

Deadman, Peter, Al-Kafaji, Mazin, and Baker, Kevin. *A Manual of Acupuncture.* London: Chinese Medicine Publications, 1998.

Fu Qing-Zhu. *Fu Qing-Zhu's Gynecology,* trans. by Yang Shou-Zhong and Liu Da-Wei. Boulder, CO: Blue Poppy Press, 1992.

Hsu Ta-Chun. *Forgotten Traditions of Ancient Chinese Medicine, I-Hsueh Yuan Liu Lun,* trans. by Paul Unschuld. Brookline, MA: Paradigm Publications, 1990.

Huang Fu-Mi. *The Systematic Classic of Acupuncture and Moxibustion (Zhen jiu jia yi jing),* trans. by Charles Chace and Yang Shou-Zhong. Boulder, CO: Blue Poppy Press, 1995.

Kirschbaum, Barbara. *Atlas of Chinese Tongue Diagnosis,* vol. 1. Seattle: Eastland Press, 2000.

Kirschbaum, Barbara. *Atlas of Chinese Tongue Diagnosis,* vol. 2. Seattle: Eastland Press, 2003.

Li Dong-Yuan. *Treatise on the Spleen and Stomach,* trans. by Yang Shou-Zhong and Li Jian-Yong. Boulder, CO: Blue Poppy Press, 1993.

Maciocia, Giovanni. *The Foundations of Chinese Medicine.* Edinburgh: Churchill Livingstone, 1989.

Maciocia, Giovanni. *Obstetrics and Gynecology in Chinese Medicine.* London: Churchill Livingstone, 1998.

Maciocia, Giovanni. *The Practice of Chinese Medicine.* Edinburgh: Churchill Livingstone, 1994.

Maciocia, Giovanni. *Tongue Diagnosis in Chinese Medicine,* rev. ed. Seattle: Eastland Press, 1995.

Scheid, Volker. Mume pill (*wū méi wán*): a clinical history. *Orientation,* November, 1999.

Shen De-Hui, Wu Xiu-Fen, and Nissi Wang. *Manual of Dermatology in Chinese Medicine.* Seattle: Eastland Press, 1995.

Song Tian-Bin. *Atlas of the Tongue and Lingual Coatings in Chinese Medicine.* Beijing: People's Medical Publishing House and Editions Sinomedic, 1995.

Wang Shu-He. *The Pulse Classic: A Translation of the Mai Jing,* trans. by Yang Shou-Zhong. Boulder, CO: Blue Poppy Press, 1997.

Zhong Bo Li. "Diagnosis of sublingual veins in Chinese medicine." Lecture presented at the 31st Congress for Traditional Chinese Medicine, Rothenburg, Germany, 2001.

Zhu Dan-Xi. *Extra Treatises Based on Investigation and Inquiry: A Translation of Zhu Dan-Xi's Ge Zhi Yu Lun,* trans. by Yang Shou-Zhong and Duan Wu-Jin. Boulder, CO: Blue Poppy Press, 1994.

Zhu Dan-Xi. *The Heart and Essence of Dan Xi's Methods of Treatmeny,* trans. by Yang Shou-Zhong. Boulder, CO: Blue Poppy Press, 1993.

German Language Publications

Darga, Matina. *Das Alchemistische Buch von Innerem Wesen und Lebensenergie (Xing min gui zhi).* Munich: Hugendubel, 1999.

Liu Lin and Wang Jin-Hong. Überblick über chinesische arzneimittel, die tumorzellen gegen über radioaktiver bestrahlung sensibilisieren. *Zeitschrift für Traditionelle Chinesische Medizin* 2000;1:47-50.

INDEX

C

D

E

F

G

H

I

J

K

L

M

N

O

P

Q

R

T